POCKETBOOK OF
EMERGENCY CARE

Commissioning Editor: **Robert Edwards**
Development Editor: **Nicola Lally**
Project Manager: **Janaki Srinivasan Kumar**
Designer/Design Direction: **Charles Gray**
Illustration Manager: **Gillian Richards**

POCKETBOOK OF
EMERGENCY CARE
A Quick Reference Guide for Paramedics

Ian Greaves QHS, FRCP, FCEM, FRCSEd(Hon.), FIMC, RCS(Ed), DTM&H, DMCC, DipMedEd, L/RAMC
Visiting Professor of Emergency Medicine, University of Teesside and Consultant in Emergency Medicine, British Army, UK

Chris Wright FCEM, DipIMC RCS(Ed), RAMC
Specialist Registrar in Emergency Medicine and Prehospital Care, Academic Department of Military Emergency Medicine, HEMS Doctor, British Army, UK

Keith Porter FRCS(Eng), FRCS(Ed), FIMC, RCS(Ed), FSEM, FCEM
Consultant Trauma Surgeon, Selly Queen Elizabeth Hospital, Birmingham, UK and Professor of Clinical Traumatology, University of Birmingham, Birmingham, UK

Timothy J Hodgetts CBE, OStJ, MMEd, MBA, CMgr, FRCP, FRCSEd, FCEM, FIMCRCSEd, FIHM, FCMI, L/RAMC
Emeritus Defence Professor of Emergency Medicine, College of Emergency Medicine, Chief Medical Adviser Allied Rapid Reaction Corps, Birmingham, UK

Malcolm Woollard PA02584, MPH, MBA, MA(Ed), Dip IMC (RCSEd), PGCE, RN, FCPara, NFESC, FASI, FHEA, FACAP
Professor in Pre-hospital and Emergency Care and Director, Pre-hospital, Emergency and Cardiovascular Care Applied Research Group, Coventry University, Past Chair, College of Paramedics

Foreword by
Fionna Moore
Medical Director
London Ambulance Service

SAUNDERS
ELSEVIER

Edinburgh London New York Oxford Philadelphia St Louis Sydney Toronto 2012

SAUNDERS
ELSEVIER

ISBN 978-0-7020-2891-5

British Library Cataloguing in Publication Data
A catalogue record for this book is available from the British Library

Library of Congress Cataloging in Publication Data
A catalog record for this book is available from the Library of Congress

Notices
Knowledge and best practice in this field are constantly changing. As new research and experience broaden our understanding, changes in research methods, professional practices, or medical treatment may become necessary.

Practitioners and researchers must always rely on their own experience and knowledge in evaluating and using any information, methods, compounds, or experiments described herein. In using such information or methods they should be mindful of their own safety and the safety of others, including parties for whom they have a professional responsibility.

With respect to any drug or pharmaceutical products identified, readers are advised to check the most current information provided (i) on procedures featured or (ii) by the manufacturer of each product to be administered, to verify the recommended dose or formula, the method and duration of administration, and contraindications. It is the responsibility of practitioners, relying on their own experience and knowledge of their patients, to make diagnoses, to determine dosages and the best treatment for each individual patient, and to take all appropriate safety precautions.

To the fullest extent of the law, neither the Publisher nor the authors, contributors, or editors, assume any liability for any injury and/or damage to persons or property as a matter of products liability, negligence or otherwise, or from any use or operation of any methods, products, instructions, or ideas contained in the material herein.

ELSEVIER your source for books, journals and multimedia in the health sciences
www.elsevierhealth.com

Working together to grow libraries in developing countries
www.elsevier.com | www.bookaid.org | www.sabre.org
ELSEVIER BOOK AID International Sabre Foundation

The Publisher's policy is to use paper manufactured from sustainable forests

Printed in China

Contents

Contents

Foreword

Being a paramedic is an immensely challenging professional role and one that is constantly changing and developing. It is more than a decade since the two senior editors of this pocketbook launched *Emergency Care: A Textbook for Paramedics*, which is now established as a core textbook for pre-hospital clinicians in the UK. They have now been joined by a member of the growing younger generation of pre-hospital specialists in producing a pocket-sized distillation of the second edition of *Emergency Care*, which is intended as a practical guide on the streets rather than a detailed reference text. Reflecting the structure of *Emergency Care*, the pocketbook contains the essentials of every aspect of clinical practice in an easily accessible and convenient form. This pocketbook is intended to be a pocket companion in clinical practice, for instant reference and individual customisation. I have no doubt that it will be successful, just as *Emergency Care* has proved so successful in establishing a core reference for consultation in less stressful times.

Professors Greaves and Porter remain immensely active in pre-hospital care and their commitment to assisting practitioners, as well as shaping the future of the speciality, based on their own extensive experience is undimmed. I share their hope that this little book will help paramedics and other pre-hospital practitioners with the day-to-day problems of their professional lives and I am confident that it will be become an essential item in every practitioner's pocket or in every ambulance.

Fionna Moore
Medical Director
London Ambulance Service.

Preface

When *Emergency Care: A Textbook for Paramedics* was first published in 1997, we hoped that it would be a significant step forward in making sound, evidence-based practical advice available to pre-hospital care practitioners in an attractive and easy to use format. We believed that it was particularly important that *Emergency Care* was a textbook of British practice and chose our contributors accordingly. The response to the first edition and to the second in 2004 confirmed that we were on the right lines although it would be extraordinarily foolish ever to assume that a book of this kind was the definitive word on the subject. Indeed, in response to changes in clinical practice and the structure of the National Health Service, we hope that work will soon commence on the third edition.

As part of our aim with *Emergency Care*, we also wished to produce a pocket-sized volume which might be useful to the pre-hospital practitioner "on the ground" rather than as a reference text. This pocketbook is the result, based section by section on its larger companion text. We hope that this little book contains everything the practitioner is likely to want to know in a hurry when faced with a challenging patient or difficult situation. Inevitably, therefore, we have had to make choices regarding what is included or left out. Equally inevitably, our selection will not please everybody. Thus, whilst we believe that the pocketbook is a significant step forward, it is undoubtedly "work in progress" which we hope will be refined as clinical practices change and in the light of comments from readers which we would encourage and which are always most welcome.

We hope that as users of the pocketbook become more familiar with it, they will add their own notes and stick in their own additions to make it very much a personalised companion in their clinical practice.

Built as it is on *Emergency Care*, this pocketbook would not have been possible without the work of the contributors to both first and second editions. We are grateful to all of them, to the team at Elsevier and as ever to our families for their assistance and forbearance in bringing this project to completion.

Birmingham, January 2011

Ian Greaves
Chris Wright
Keith Porter
Timothy J. Hodgetts
Malcolm Woollard

Acknowledgements

The core of this book is based on the contents of *Emergency Care: A Textbook for Paramedics*, with material extracted and re-edited to suit the format of this book. Although some chapters and topics have of necessity been cut or substantially edited, authors of all chapters drawn upon have been acknowledged here in recognition of their contribution to the parent textbook.

Bruce Armstrong RGN, RMN
Consultant Nurse, Basingstoke Hospital
Formerly Consultant Anaesthetist, Frenchay Hospital, Bristol

James Briscoe MRCPsych
Honorary Clinical Lecturer, Department of Psychiatry, University of Birmingham, Birmingham

Christopher Carney DipIMC.RCS(Ed)
Chief Executive, East Anglia Ambulance Service Trust, Norwich

Timothy Coats FRCS
Professor of Accident & Emergency Medicine,
Leicester Royal Infirmary

Peter Driscoll MD, FRCS, FCEM
Consultant and Senior Lecturer, Department of Emergency Medicine, Hope Hospital, Salford

Peter Dyer FRCS(Ed), FFD.RCSI
Consultant in Maxillofacial Surgery, Royal Lancaster Infirmary

Judith Fisher FRCGP
Formerly Consultant in Primary Care, Royal London Hospital, London

Ian Greaves QHS, FRCP, FCEM, FRCSEd(Hon.) FIMC, RCS(Ed), DTM&H, DMCC, DipMedEd, L/RAMC
Visiting Professor of Emergency Medicine, University of Teesside, Consultant in Emergency Medicine British Army

Carl Gwinnutt FRCA
Consultant Anaesthetist, Hope Hospital, Salford

Jacqueline Hanson FRCS, FCEM
Consultant in Accident & Emergency Medicine,
Preston Royal Infirmary, Preston

Timothy Hodgetts CBE, OStJ, MMEd, MBA, CMgr, FRCP, FRCSEd, FCEM, FIMCRCSEd, FIHM, FCMI, L/RAMC
Emeritus Defence Professor of Emergency Medicine, College of Emergency Medicine, Chief Medical Adviser Allied Rapid Reaction Corps, Birmingham

Graham Johnson FRCS, FCEM
Consultant in Emergency Medicine, St James University Hospital, Leeds

Jason Kendall MRCP(UK), FCEM, DipIMC.RCS(Ed), MD
Consultant in Accident & Emergency Medicine, Frenchay Hospital, Bristol

Alastair Main MD, FRCP
Consultant in Geriatric Medicine, Queen Elizabeth Hospital, Birmingham

David Morgan-Jones
General Practitioner, Royal Army Medical Corps

Gordon JA Morris MRCGP, AFOM, DRCOG
Senior Medical Officer, Occupational Health Care Services, Glasgow

Julie Nancarrow MB, ChB, DipIMC, FRCSEd, MRCGP, FCEM
Consultant in Emergency Medicine, Warwick University

Jerry Nolan FRCA
Department of Anaesthesia, Royal United Hospital, Bath

Mike Parr FRCA
Intensive Care Unit, Royal North Shore Hospital, Sydney, Australia

Gavin Perkins MRCP
Consultant in Respiratory Medicine, Heartlands Hospital, Birmingham

Keith Porter FRCS(Eng), FRCS(Ed), FIMC, RCS(Ed), FSEM, FCEM
Consultant Trauma Surgeon, Queen Elizabeth Hospital, Birmingham, Professor of Clinical Traumatology, University of Birmingham, Birmingham

James Ryan MCh, FRCS
Formerly Leonard Cheshire Professor of Post Conflict Recovery, University College London

John Scott DipIMC.RCS(Ed), DA
Senior Lecturer, University of Aberdeen

Jason Smith MRCP(UK), FCEM, RN
Consultant in Emergency Medicine, Royal Navy

Andrew Thurgood MSc, RGN, DIMC RSC Ed, Dip HS, SRPara
Immediate Care Practitioner & Nurse Consultant, Birmingham

Ian Todd LLB(Hons), DipIMC.RCS(Ed), SRPara
Formerly Paramedic Officer, Warwickshire Ambulance Service NHS Trust; Visiting Research Fellow, University of Warwick

Lee Wallis MRCP(UK)
Professor of Emergency Medicine, Johannesburg, South Africa

Malcolm Woollard PA02584, MPH, MBA, MA(Ed), Dip IMC (RCSEd), PGCE, RN, FCPara, NFESC, FASI, FHEA, FACAP
Professor, Pre-hospital and Emergency Care and Director, Pre-hospital, Emergency and Cardiovascular Care Applied Research Group, Coventry University, Past Chair, College of Paramedics

Chris Wright FCEM, DipIMC, RCS(Ed), RAMC
Specialist Registrar in Emergency Medicine and Prehospital Care, Academic Department of Military Emergency Medicine, HEMS Doctor, British Army

CHAPTER 1

Approaching the scene

Heading to the scene

- The Road Traffic Act allows certain exemptions to drivers of emergency vehicles who may:
  - Exceed the statutory speed limit by 20 mph
  - Treat red traffic lights as give-way indicators
  - Pass on the off-side of a keep left sign
  - Turn right where this is not normally permitted
  - Use a bus lane
  - Stop and park on clear ways
  - Stop and park on a pedestrian crossing and its controlled area
  - Park on double yellow lines
- Drivers of emergency vehicles are specifically NOT ALLOWED to:
  - Park dangerously
  - Drive without reasonable care and attention for other road users
  - Ignore one-way signs
  - Ignore stop signs
  - Go the wrong way round a roundabout
  - Cross double white lines
  - Fail to stop after an accident
  - Fail to provide information after being involved in an accident
  - Ignore directions from police officers
- The public road user may react in a variety of ways to an approaching ambulance:
  - Sudden braking
  - Sudden changing of lane
  - Failure to give-way

- There should be a 2 second gap between your vehicle and the vehicle in front
- Lights and sirens provide no legal protection in the event of an accident.

Accidents while driving

- Ambulance personnel have the same duties as the general public under the Road Traffic Act if involved in an accident, regardless of whether they are responding to an emergency call or not
- This Act requires that the driver stops and provides to persons having reasonable grounds for requesting it, the following information:
  1. Name and address
  2. Name and address of the owner of the vehicle
  3. Registration number of the vehicle
  4. Insurance certificate
- If this information cannot be provided, then the accident must be reported to a police officer as soon as possible and within 24 hours
- An NHS Traffic Accident Report form should be completed
- DO NOT accept liability for an accident; the circumstances will be established by investigation.

Parking at the scene

- Double-parking may be unavoidable, which may obstruct the flow of traffic – hazard lights or beacons are then used at the driver's discretion
- When an ambulance is the first or only emergency vehicle to arrive at the scene of a road traffic accident, the vehicle is parked in the fend-off or in-line position to protect the incident
- If the ambulance is left unattended it should be locked.

Immediate-care doctors

A green beacon identifies a registered medical practitioner – sirens can only be used by doctors with the approval of the county's Chief Police Officer after the completion of appropriate training.

Priorities at the scene

The priorities at the scene can be remembered as CONTROL then ACT. Overall scene control and traffic management is the responsibility of the police. The police are also responsible for establishing and controlling the outer cordon.

Control

- Beacons should be left switched on
- Members of the public should be cleared from obstructing the road
- The engine of the vehicle involved in the accident should be turned off.

Protecting oneself

Individual emergency service personnel must be responsible for their own safety. Suitable protective clothing includes:

- A high-visibility jacket marked with the level of training: a class 3 jacket is required for any incident on a road with traffic speeds above 30 mph (the classification of a jacket is clearly marked inside and is based on the amount of fluorescent and reflective material)
- A helmet with integral visor fitted with a secure chin strap (ideally marked with skill level and rank)
- Debris gloves must be worn in the presence of glass and cut metal
- Goggles should always be worn when working near fire service hydraulic lines and if there is a risk of splashing from body fluids
- Ear protection must also be worn when working in noisy environments (e.g. Fire service cutting equipment)
- Latex free gloves to protect from body fluids – wearing two layers is wise where glass fragments or cut metal are present
- Long sleeves must always be worn in the presence of body fluids, cut metal and glass fragments.

Always think of your own safety first, then the safety of other rescuers and bystanders and finally, the safety of the casualties. This is the 1-2-3 of safety. All patients should be assumed to be infectious in terms of communicable diseases such as hepatitis B and C or human immunodeficiency virus (HIV).

Ambulance officer's personal protective equipment

- Hard hat with chin strap
- Eye protection (goggles, glasses or visor)
- Ear protection
- High-visibility jacket, with identifying markings
- Heavy-duty gloves
- Patient treatment gloves
- Robust footwear.

Protecting casualties

- The safety of the casualties is ensured by protecting the scene with the emergency service vehicles and a cordon
- It is the responsibility of the fire service to rescue casualties from a hazardous environment
- A snatch rescue may be appropriate when the patient's life is in immediate danger, e.g. from fire or toxic chemicals. Every reasonable attempt should be made to extricate the patient safely, but spinal immobilisation in particular may have to be compromised in order to save life.

ACT

A – Assess

C – Communicate

T – Triage, treat and transport.

Assess the scene

After taking control of an incident the next priority is to assess the scene. There are three important elements to the scene assessment:

1. Assessment of hazards, both present and potential
2. Reading the scene
3. Rapid assessment of the number and severity of casualties.

An assessment of hazards will include:

- Actual hazards (fire, chemical spillage)
- Potential hazards (fire due to ignition of petrol on the road)
- Specific hazards (e.g. the electricity supply through overhead or broken cables).

Reading the scene:

- Observe the nature of deformation of a vehicle and its position
- At a medical incident there may be vital clues to the nature of a medical illness (bottles of pills, Medic-Alert bracelets, etc.).

Number and severity of casualties:

- Do not miss casualties hidden under vehicles or in undergrowth.

> Read the scene for clues to injuries following trauma or to the reason for medical illness.

Communicate

- There are several levels of communication to consider:
  - with the patient
  - between ambulance crew members
  - with ambulance control
  - with other emergency services at the scene
  - with the hospital
- When assistance is required at an incident scene, it is useful to remember the mnemonic METHANE when communicating with ambulance control:
  - M – My call sign (Major Incident standby or declared if appropriate)
  - E – Exact location
  - T – Type of incident
  - H – Hazards, present and potential

- A – Access
- N – Number, severity and type of casualties
- E – Emergency services, present and required.

The essential information the hospital will require in order to be able to assemble the appropriate staff and prepare equipment is:

- Age of the patient (the age of a child allows the hospital to prepare equipment such as endotracheal tubes and to calculate drug doses)
- Sex
- History
- Injuries/illness
- Condition of patient (vital signs and level of consciousness; Glasgow coma scale, GCS)
- Expected time of arrival (ETA).

> Good communication is central to effective emergency service teamwork.

Triage, treat and transport

- Triage requires a rapid assessment and prioritisation of each patient
- Transfer to hospital must not be delayed by unnecessary treatment
- The golden hour is the time from injury to the time that definitive treatment is given (such as surgery for a trauma patient).

> The golden hour does not start when the ambulance arrives on the scene but when the incident occurs.

- In prehospital care, it is more appropriate to think in terms of the platinum 10 minutes to stabilise the patient before moving to hospital.

For further information, see Ch. 1 in *Emergency Care: A Textbook for Paramedics*.

CHAPTER 2

Approach to the patient

The approach to the patient follows scene safety and scene assessment. In trauma cases you will already have information about the patient's likely injuries after 'reading the wreckage' or understanding the nature of the accident. In medical cases, important clues will be gained on approach such as looking at the patient's medications on the bedside table. While examining a patient, any Medic-Alert bracelet or card should be identified.

- Wherever possible, relevant medical history, current medication and allergies should be established. Use the mnemonic SAMPLE:
  - S – Signs and symptoms
  - A – Allergies
  - M – Medication
  - P – Past history
  - L – Last meal
  - E – Event (i.e. current problem).

Life-threatening associations

- Patient falling from a height greater than 5 metres
- Road traffic collision with an extrication time greater than 20 minutes
- Patient ejected from a vehicle
- Loss of life in the same vehicle
- Child (less than 12 years old), pedestrian or cyclist struck by a vehicle
- Pedestrian struck by a vehicle and thrown
- Vehicle intrusion greater than 30 cm.

Primary and secondary surveys

The patients seen by ambulance personnel may be divided broadly into two groups:
1. Medical patients
2. Trauma patients.

The initial approach to these two groups is similar. The components of the systematic approach are:
- Primary survey
- Resuscitation
- Secondary survey
- Definitive care.

The role of the primary survey is to identify any life-threatening problems or injuries. Whenever possible, treatment of any life-threatening problem is carried out as soon as that problem is identified and before moving on to the next stage of the assessment.

> - Primary survey and resuscitation take place simultaneously
> - The primary survey identifies life-threatening problems
> - The secondary survey identifies non-life-threatening problems.

The primary survey

The primary survey follows the simple system of <C>ABCDE.
   Although this system was originally designed for use in trauma, it is equally relevant to the management of life-threatening medical conditions.

<C> – Identify and manage catastrophic external haemorrhage

- Rapid bleeding from a main vessel requires immediate management with direct pressure and elevation
- Rarely it may be necessary to apply pressure over a pressure point or to use a designated tourniquet (never use improvised tourniquets)
- Remember that blood may be hidden under the patient or within thick clothing
- Can be skipped if external haemorrhage is clearly not an issue.

A – Airway with cervical spine control

- Assess the airway
- Anticipate the development of problems. In burns patients, for example, it is important to check for evidence of soot in the nose and on the lips or evidence of oedema of the upper airway
- Establish and maintain a patent airway

- In-line cervical immobilisation should be maintained during all airway manoeuvres in trauma patients.

> Of unconscious trauma patients, 5% have a cervical spine injury.

- Patients with injury above the clavicle should be assumed to have a cervical spine injury until proved otherwise
- Medical patients with rheumatoid arthritis are at higher risk of having cervical spine injury.

> The airway takes priority over the cervical spine.

B – Breathing with adequate ventilation/oxygenation

- Look, listen and feel for 10 seconds to ascertain whether the patient is breathing
- Assess rate and effort.

> The normal respiratory rate in adults is between 12 and 18 breaths/minute.

- All patients with a reduced (<12) or increased (>18) respiratory rate should receive oxygen and if the rate is below 10 or above 29, assisted ventilation may be required
- A raised respiratory rate is a sign of both hypoxia and hypovolaemia
- In trauma patients, a structured approach to the assessment of the respiratory system can help to identify time-critical life-threatening problems (e.g. 'TWELVE FLAPS' acronym):

- **T**rachea – is it central?
- **W**ounds in the neck – must be sealed to prevent air embolus and to control haemorrhage
- **E**mphysema – is surgical emphysema present (potentially indicating tension pneumothorax)?
- **L**aryngeal crepitus present (indicating fracture)?
- **V**eins – is there distension of the neck veins (indicating tension pneumothorax or cardiac tamponade)
- **E**xpose the thorax
- **F**eel the chest for symmetrical expansion, crepitus, rib fractures, flail segments
- **L**ook at the chest for bruising, wounds (seal sucking wounds immediately), patterning from clothes or seatbelts, asymmetrical or see-sawing movement
- **A**uscultate – equality of breath sounds, added sounds
- **P**ercuss – dullness, hyper-resonance, symmetry
- **S**ides – check under the sides of the chest and the shoulders for bleeding and deformity.

C – Circulation with control of external haemorrhage

- It is first essential to determine if the patient has a cardiac output and to start basic life support (BLS) if this is absent
- Think 'blood on the floor and four more' (chest, abdomen, pelvis, long bones)
    Check the entire surface of the patient for bleeding
    Chest (already assessed)
    Abdomen
    Femurs
- Assess rate and strength of radial pulses bilaterally (if absent check a central pulse), a radial pulse in the supine adult trauma patient implies a systolic blood pressure of ≥ 90 mmHg
- Assess colour and temperature of skin and measure the blood pressure in all patients
- Obtain intravenous access (this should not delay transfer to hospital)
- 250 mL boluses of (warm) intravenous crystalloid may be required to bring the systolic blood pressure to 90 mmHg or to achieve a radial pulse.

D – Disability and neurological examination

- Pupils (PEARL, **P**upils **E**qual **A**nd **R**eactive to **L**ight)
- AVPU
    A – alert
    V – responds to verbal stimuli
    P – responds to painful stimuli
    U – unresponsive
- Posture.

E – Evaluation and environment

- Is this a time-critical patient?
- Are they protected from the elements (trauma patients who are allowed to become cold have significantly higher rates of mortality and morbidity).

If the patient's condition deteriorates, always revert to the ABCs and repeat the primary survey.

Handover

A clear handover of the patient in hospital is essential. Take 45 seconds to hand-over the patient, during which all members of the receiving medical team listen, unless there is a problem with the airway or cardiopulmonary resuscitation is in progress. Only key information needs to be given at this stage. This can be remembered by the acronym MIST:

- M – Mechanism of injury
- I – Injuries – apparent and suspected
- S – Signs – abnormal vital signs
- T – Treatment given.

Secondary survey

In trauma cases, a secondary survey may be performed in order to identify non-life-threatening injuries. In medical emergencies, a similar approach to the patient may uncover vital clues to the patient's condition – injection marks, bruises, rashes or scars.

If the patient's injuries are non-critical, then a secondary survey may be undertaken. Depending on circumstances, this may best be done in the shelter and protection of the ambulance. The secondary survey should begin with reassessing the airway.

> The secondary survey must never delay transfer to definitive care.

Head

Assess:

- Pupil size and reaction
- For evidence of bruising, lacerations, tenderness and other signs of fractures
- The nose and ears for blood and cerebrospinal fluid leakage.

Neck

Assess:

- For signs of trauma, although in-line stabilisation must be maintained
- Larynx and trachea for evidence of injury and for tracheal deviation
- Neck veins (distended in tension pneumothorax and cardiac tamponade)
- Carotid pulse.

Chest

The chest is inspected for:

- Open wounds
- Contusion (bruising)
- Seatbelt markings
- Flail segment
- Respiratory rate and effort.

Palpation may reveal:

- Local tenderness indicative of rib fractures
- Chest wall instability with a flail segment
- Surgical emphysema following a pneumothorax.

Auscultation may demonstrate:

- Reduced air entry
- Added sounds (e.g. wheeze).

Percussion may be used to identify a haemothorax (dull, like a full barrel) or pneumothorax (resonant, like an empty barrel).

Abdomen

The abdomen is inspected or palpated for:

- Open wounds
- Seatbelt markings and contusion
- Tenderness in all four quadrants.

Pelvis

Examination of the pelvis may precipitate deterioration in its patient's condition. Splintage should be undertaken on the basis of risk of injury determined by the mechanism of injury.

Upper and lower limbs

Major injuries which might be associated with life-threatening haemorrhage should be identified in the primary survey.

The limbs are inspected for swelling, deformity and wounds. They are palpated for fractures (a step in the cortex) or crepitus (broken ends grating together – very painful).

The limb examination should include assessment of:

- Motor response – test for active movements
- Sensation – response to touch
- Circulation – pulse and skin temperature.

Limb injuries are treated as necessary, with dressings and splintage. Analgesia should be a high priority with suspected long-bone fractures. The choice may include:

- Reassurance
- Splintage (possibly with traction splint)
- Nitrous oxide inhalation (Entonox, Nitronox)
- Morphine.

Be aware that unnecessary delay at the scene may well jeopardise patient outcome.

For further information, see Ch. 2 in *Emergency Care: A Textbook for Paramedics*.

CHAPTER 3

An introduction to clinical examination

Examination will be described in the order used in the standard approach which is a common theme throughout this book – the <C>ABCDE system.

No examination is performed without clues from the history and attention should be paid to other information such as mechanism of injury, patterns of vehicle damage and damage to protective clothing or helmets.

Often an assessment of A–D is made by a simple question: 'Are you OK?' If this elicits a response such as 'Yes, but my ankle hurts', this means the airway is clear, the patient is breathing enough to speak clearly, the brain is adequately perfused and the Glasgow Coma Score is either 14 or 15.

<C> is applied in cases of catastrophic haemorrhage where control of bleeding takes priority over the rest of the primary survey.

Airway

Possible abnormal noises originating in the upper airway include the following:

Gurgling

Gurgling suggests the presence of fluid in the airway, possibly blood, saliva or stomach contents that have been regurgitated. This will require suction.

Snoring

This is usually caused by the soft tissues of the nasopharynx and oropharynx flopping back against the posterior wall of the throat, partially obstructing the flow of air.

Stridor

Stridor is caused by partial blockage of the upper airway by swelling (due to burns, infection or anaphylaxis) or a foreign body.

Hoarseness

Hoarseness has many causes, all relating to pathology around the larynx and vocal cords.

A more formal visual inspection is then carried out to assess for swelling, the presence of a foreign body, trauma or bleeding that may compromise the airway. An assessment of the airway goes hand in hand with an assessment of breathing and if there is no evidence of breathing, airway opening manoeuvres should be performed to ascertain if there is respiratory effort.

Other features which should be sought when examining the neck are summarised in Box 3.1.

Box 3.1 **Findings on neck examination**

- Tracheal deviation
- Swelling
- Surgical emphysema
- Wounds
- Distended neck veins.

Breathing

The assessment of breathing (and the respiratory system) should involve a four-stage process.

- Look
- Feel
- Auscultate
- Percuss.

Looking for visual clues

A great deal of important information can be gained from careful inspection of the chest:

- How hard is the patient working to breathe?
- Are there any external signs of injury such as pattern bruising or abrasions?
- What is the respiratory rate (normally 12–18/minutes)?
- Are there signs of respiratory distress?

- What is the position of the patient (the patient sitting forward using the arms to support the chest is in respiratory distress)?

If there is unequal movement of the chest, this suggests a problem on one side such as a pneumothorax, haemothorax or collapse of one lung.

General hyperinflation of the chest may suggest chronic obstructive pulmonary disease (COPD) or may occur in severe asthma.

> Always count and record the respiratory rate.
>
> DO NOT FORGET TO ADMINISTER OXYGEN.

Feel

Once visual inspection is complete, the chest should be palpated for equal expansion and, in trauma, for any evidence of tenderness over the ribs or sternum.

Auscultation

Problems include:

- Stridor – a harsh noise produced on inspiration, e.g. due to inhalation of foreign body, swelling due to airway burn, croup or epiglottitis
- Wheeze – a higher pitched noise on expiration due to obstruction lower down in the lungs in the smaller air passages
- Bronchial breathing – the noise that is transmitted from the larger airways through solid lung, the result of infection or collapse
- Crepitations – crackling sounds that are typically heard in the lung bases in the presence of pulmonary oedema.

During auscultation, the stethoscope should be placed on the front of the chest on both sides, in the axillae and at the bases.

Table 3.1 Added sounds on auscultation

Added sound	Clinical meaning	Clinical example
Wheeze	Lower airway obstruction	Asthma
Stridor	Upper airway obstruction	Airway burn
Bronchial breathing	Solid lung	Pneumonia
Crepitations	Air spaces popping open	Pulmonary oedema

Table 3.2 Clinical findings in lung pathology

Condition	Chest expansion	Trachea	Percussion	Breath sounds
Pneumothorax	Decreased	Unchanged	Resonant	Reduced
Tension pneumothorax	Hyperexpanded	Deviated away from tension	Hyper-resonant	Absent on affected side
Haemothorax	Possibly reduced	Undeviated	Dullness	Reduced or absent
Collapse/consolidation	Reduced	May deviate towards the collapse	May be dull	Reduced or bronchial breathing
Pleural effusion	Possibly reduced	Undeviated	Dullness	Reduced or absent

Pulse oximetry should be considered routine in the examination of the sick or injured patient.

Percussion

Percussion is performed by tapping the end of the middle finger of one hand onto the middle phalanx of the same finger of the other hand, which should rest flat on the surface being examined. Use the tip of the finger and not the pad of the finger, and only one finger should be used as the 'hammer'.

A more hollow (resonant) sound than normal suggests an air-filled cavity beneath; a dull sound suggests a solid organ (e.g. liver) and fluid is revealed by 'stony' dullness.

Circulation

After establishing the presence of a pulse, the next thing to do is establish its rate. This should be done by counting how many beats occur in a given time, usually 15 seconds, and multiplying by four to give a heart rate per minute.

The normal heart rate for an adult is 60–100 beats per minute (bpm). A pulse faster than 100 bpm is by definition a tachycardia.

A weak and thready pulse suggests a low blood pressure and a compromised cardiovascular state, whereas a strong and bounding pulse may indicate a hyperdynamic circulation and is found in conditions such as chronic lung disease and carbon monoxide poisoning.

Non-invasive blood pressure measurement and a three-lead electrocardiogram trace are also essential parts of the assessment of the circulation.

Disability

Disability assessment should include examination of the conscious level, pupils and gross motor function. The conscious level can be assessed quickly using an AVPU score or more thoroughly using the Glasgow Coma Score.

The AVPU score

The AVPU score is a quick and easy assessment of conscious level.

- A – alert
- V – responds to voice
- P – responds to a painful stimulus
- U – unresponsive.

The painful stimulus should be applied above the clavicles, e.g. by applying pressure on the forehead. Pressure on a finger nail bed should not be used as no response would be elicited in a patient with a spinal injury.

The Glasgow Coma Score

The Glasgow Coma Score (GCS) is used to make a more formal assessment of conscious level during the secondary survey. It involves three components: the eye opening (E), verbal (V) and motor (M) responses, as outlined in Box 3.2.

Box 3.2 **The Glasgow Coma Scale (*Note*: the BEST response is scored)**

Eye opening response

Spontaneous	=	4
To verbal stimuli	=	3
To painful stimuli	=	2
No response	=	1

Best verbal response

Orientated	=	5
Confused	=	4
Inappropriate words	=	3
Incomprehensible sounds	=	2
No response	=	1

Best motor response

Obeys commands	=	6
Localises pain	=	5
Withdraws from pain	=	4
Abnormal flexion	=	3
Abnormal extension	=	2
No movement	=	1

When handing over information about a GCS, it should always be broken down into its three components (e.g. 'a GCS of 8 with E2 V3 M3').

Pupil response

After an assessment of conscious level, the pupils should be examined with a bright light source.

- The size, symmetry and reaction to light should be assessed
- The pupils should constrict equally to a light stimulus
- A unilateral dilated unreactive pupil may be a sign of III cranial nerve damage due to intracranial swelling or haematoma on that side (a late sign)
- Bilateral pinpoint pupils may suggest administration of opiates and dilated pupils can be the result of drugs or activation of the sympathetic nervous system.

The signs of rising intracranial pressure are:

- Bradycardia
- Hypertension (blood pressure falls as a pre-terminal event)
- Alteration in conscious level
- Unilateral then bilateral pupillary dilation
- Irregular ventilatory pattern
- Dysrhythmias (preterminal).

Table 3.3 Pupillary responses

Pupils	Common causes
Bilaterally constricted	Opiate overdose
Bilaterally dilated	Drugs, e.g. tricyclics Sympathetic response Dead
Unilaterally dilated	Raised ICP (see below) III cranial nerve palsy Traumatic mydriasis

Finally, a gross assessment of peripheral motor and sensory function can be made by asking the patient to clench the fists and wiggle the toes and whether she/he can feel you touching his/her hands and feet. In this way, a map of normal sensation over the body can be made and should be documented.

In the case of stroke, one side of the body may be paralysed, or in the case of spinal injury, there will be loss of sensory and motor function below the level of injury.

Examination of the limbs

Each limb should be examined in turn, using the following method:

- Look for bruising, swelling or deformity
- Actively move (patient moves each joint)
- Passively move (practitioner moves each of the joints in the affected limb)
- Feel for swelling, crepitus, bruising and tenderness.

For further information, see Ch. 3 in *Emergency Care: A Textbook for Paramedics.*

The emergency services

Box 4.1 **The emergency services**

- Ambulance services
- Police services
- Fire services
- HM Coastguard (part of the Maritime and Coastguard Agency)
- Air Sea Rescue
- Mountain Rescue
- Voluntary Aid Societies (St John and St Andrew Ambulance Associations, British Red Cross)
- Volunteer organisations (e.g. British Association for Immediate Care, Women's Royal Voluntary Service).

The fire and rescue service

Functions of the Fire service:

- Rescue of casualties from fire incidents
- Neutralisation of hazardous materials – chemicals, radiation
- Release of entrapped casualty (transport and industrial accidents)
- Extrication of patients from inaccessible areas (e.g. steep slope rescue)
- Assistance at major incidents (lighting, shelter, personnel for stretcher carry).

Command structure

The Fire service has a formal system of command. When attending an incident involving the Fire service, it is important to identify and speak to the senior officer in order to ensure a coordinated response.

Junior ranks wear yellow helmets, while officers wear white helmets.

The helmets of anyone above the grade of Fire-fighter will also be marked with black bands of varying number and thickness. The greater the number and width of the bands, the greater the seniority.

The rank markings of the Fire service are shown in Figure 4.1.

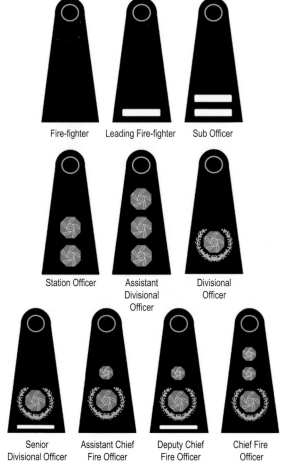

Figure 4.1 Fire service rank markings.

Entrapments

The successful and orderly management of an entrapment can be divided into six phases commonly used by Senior Fire Officers:

- Assessment and making the scene safe
- Stabilisation and initial access
- Glass management
- Space creation
- Access
- Extrication.

An initial assessment of the scene is made on arrival to ensure safety for the patient and any personnel involved in the rescue. On arriving at the scene of an accident, the paramedic should contact the Senior Fire Officer in order to determine whether it is safe to approach the patient.

Incidents involving chemical or radioactive contamination

It is important for ambulance service staff to establish early liaison with the Senior Fire Officer to determine the nature of the hazard and the involvement of any casualties.

It is a responsibility of the ambulance service to provide adequate decontamination facilities for patients.

Although the Fire service has been issued with equipment for mass-decontamination, this is aimed at uninjured survivors.

Major incidents

The primary objectives of the Fire and rescue service at a major incident are shown in Box 4.2. The emergency services will generally adopt a rigid command structure at a major incident. The Gold Commander is usually located away from the incident and maintains a strategic oversight of the incident. The Silver Commander is on-site and delegates specific tasks to the Bronze (or sector) Commanders who are each responsible for a defined area of the incident.

Box 4.2 **Objectives of the fire and rescue service at a major incident**

- Saving life
- Prevention of escalation of the incident (control fires, contain chemicals)
- Protection of rescuers and casualties
- Extrication of casualties, including first aid where necessary, and assistance with movement of the injured to the casualty clearing station
- Control of access and egress from the inner cordon where hazards are existent
- Assistance in investigating the cause of the incident.

The Police service

The primary duty of the police is to uphold the law and to bring to the justice system those who break it. The police will be involved jointly with the Ambulance service in incidents where a crime has been committed such as an assault, a road traffic accident and a major incident (see below).

Command structure

Specialised areas of policing include traffic, firearms teams and air support. Police service rank markings are shown in Figures 4.2 and 4.3.

The crime scene

At a crime scene, the police will be primarily concerned with the preservation of evidence where an offence may have been committed.

The treatment and evacuation of patients from the scene of an incident will inevitably risk disturbing forensic evidence but the preservation of life is the first priority.

Ambulance service staff should therefore be aware of the police requirements to preserve evidence and avoid unnecessary contamination of a crime scene.

Ambulance service staff may subsequently be asked to provide a witness statement as a professional witness.

The police role at major incidents

Police roles at a major incident are given in Box 4.3.

HM coastguard

HM Coastguard (part of the Maritime and Coastguard Agency) is accessible through the 999 operator and is the fourth emergency service. In incidents in coastal waters, they have primacy over other services and will take the traditional coordinator role that the police assume on land. Large multi-agency incidents will commonly be coordinated from the regional coastguard headquarters. Primacy is handed back to the police when on land.

Box 4.3 **Responsibilities of the police at a major incident**

- Preservation of life
- Emergency services coordination
- Preservation of evidence
- Control of access to the scene
- Identification of the victims
- Removal of bodies of fatalities to mortuary facilities
- Collection of evidence.

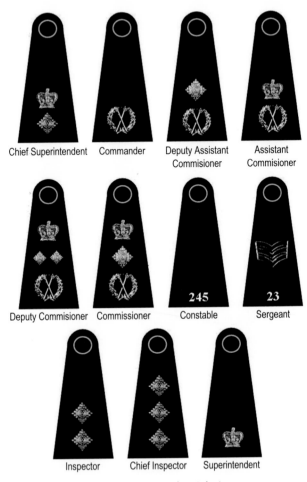

Chief Superintendent   Commander   Deputy Assistant Commisioner   Assistant Commisioner

Deputy Commisioner   Commissioner   Constable   Sergeant

Inspector   Chief Inspector   Superintendent

Figure 4.2 Police service rank markings (Metropolitan Police).

Voluntary aid societies

The Voluntary Aid Societies (VAS) (British Red Cross, St John and St Andrew Ambulance Associations) commonly provide care at mass gathering events. Their principal capability is to provide first-aid but the societies will also deploy

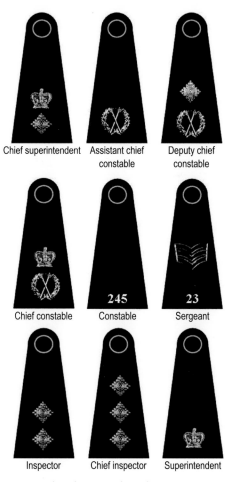

Figure 4.3 Police service rank markings (outside London).

volunteer nurses, doctors and off-duty ambulance personnel to augment the statutory emergency services.

In the context of a major incident, all voluntary aid society members will be responsible to the Ambulance Commander from the statutory ambulance service, who will determine how VAS staff and VAS ambulances are utilised.

BASICS

The British Association for Immediate Care (BASICS) consists of volunteer doctors functioning independently or in organised schemes to support their local ambulance service. There is no statutory role for this organisation, although some ambulance services rely on these volunteers to assist in the management of difficult cases at the roadside or in the home.

For further information, see Ch. 4 in *Emergency Care: A Textbook for Paramedics*.

CHAPTER 5

Basic life support

The Resuscitation Council (UK) algorithms for basic, advanced, paediatric and neonatal resuscitation can be accessed via their website at: www.resus.org.uk, and are based on European and International consensus of the research evidence.

A patient's best chance of survival occurs when the collapse is witnessed and basic life support (BLS) techniques are started immediately.

The main sign of cardiac arrest is the absence of normal breathing in a non-responsive patient.

The sequence of BLS for laypersons

1. Safety check: to ensure that rescuer, bystanders and patient are not in danger
2. Evaluation of the patient: to identify whether the patient is unresponsive and not breathing normally
3. Airway control: to obtain and maintain a patent airway
4. Circulatory support: to establish an artificial circulation by external cardiac compression
5. Ventilatory support: to establish artificial ventilation using exhaled air.

The algorithm recognises the importance of starting chest compressions as soon as cardiac arrest is suspected; for this reason circulatory support is placed before ventilatory support.

The SAFE approach

S – Shout for help

A – Approach with care

F – Free from danger

E – Evaluate the patient.

- On discovering or being asked to attend to a collapsed patient, the first response must be to shout for help
- BLS techniques are more effective if performed by two rescuers
- Rescuers should approach a collapsed person with care, never putting themselves or others at risk
- If there are risks either to the victim or rescuer, then the patient must be moved to a place of greater safety which is free from danger before starting resuscitation. This decision will inevitably result in a delay to instituting BLS
- Finally, the rescuer must evaluate the patient's airway, breathing and circulation. Not all collapsed patients will need artificial ventilation and external cardiac compressions.

Patient evaluation

Check the patient for a response: place one hand on the patient's forehead and shake the shoulder gently with the other hand. At the same time, ask loudly, 'Are you all right?'

The patient responds by either talking or moving:

- If it is safe to do so, leave the patient in the position in which he or she was found and summon medical assistance or prepare for transfer. Regular reassessment is mandatory
- The head is held stable during the evaluation to guard against the possibility of aggravating an injury to the cervical spine and where there is obvious trauma, the cervical spine must then be immobilised by manual in-line stabilisation
- The patient may be deaf, therefore ensure he or she can see your lips moving when assessing responsiveness.

There is no response to voice or touch:

- If no assistance has arrived, shout for help again and then turn the patient onto their back in a controlled manner. BLS cannot be performed on a patient who is prone or lying awkwardly
- Evaluate the state of the patient's airway, breathing and circulation.

Open the airway

- In most unconscious patients, the reduced tone in the muscles of the tongue, jaw and neck allow the tongue to fall against the posterior pharyngeal wall
- If a foreign body in the airway is suspected, then the procedure for the choking patient should be followed
- The following manoeuvres are designed to achieve a clear airway.

Head tilt plus chin lift

- This manoeuvre is not recommended if there is any possibility that the patient has a cervical spine injury
- The rescuer's hand nearest the head is placed on the forehead, gently tilting (extending) the head backwards as though the patient is sniffing
- The chin is then lifted using the index and middle finger of the rescuer's other hand. If this causes the mouth to close, the lower lip should be retracted downwards by the thumb
- This is the 'triple airway manoeuvre' – head tilt, chin lift, mouth open.

Jaw thrust

- If there is a suspicion that the cervical spine may have been injured, then the jaw thrust alone is used
- The patient's jaw is thrust upwards (forwards) by applying pressure behind the angles of the mandible
- The rescuer uses the fingers, with the base of the thumbs resting on the patient's cheeks
- When performed correctly, this manoeuvre is uncomfortable for the patient and is generally not tolerated if the patient is conscious.

Patients with suspected cervical spine injury

- Great care should be taken with airway alignment in patients with suspected cervical spine injury. Flexion and rotation of the neck are the most dangerous movements. At all times manual in-line stabilisation should be applied by an assistant
- The safest way to achieve airway patency in patients with suspected cervical spine injury is by jaw thrust
- Extension of the head on the neck should be minimised to that just necessary to establish an airway. It is important to remember, however, that airway obstruction is immediately lethal and airway management takes precedence.

Assess breathing

Keep the airway patent while now assessing breathing for no longer than 10 seconds:

- Look down the line of the chest to see if it is rising and falling
- Listen at the mouth and nose for breath sounds, gurgling or snoring sounds

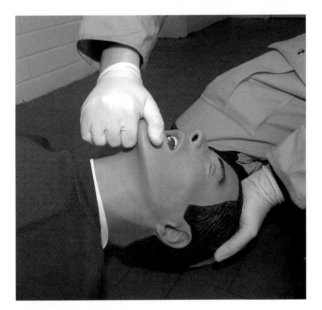

Figure 5.1 Head tilt, chin lift.

- Feel for breathing at the patient's mouth and nose with the side of your cheek.

The professional medical responder may check the carotid pulse at the same time. Agonal gasps are present in 40% of cardiac arrest patients and must not be misdiagnosed as normal breathing.

The patient is breathing

- Place the patient in the recovery position unless it is unsafe to do so because of other injuries
- Check regularly for breathing
- The majority of these patients will require urgent hospital transfer. It is essential at this point that either someone is sent to summon such help or, if you are alone, you must leave the patient and go for help.

The patient is not breathing

- Help must be sought immediately, either by sending someone else or going yourself, even if this means temporarily leaving the patient
- On return, begin chest compressions

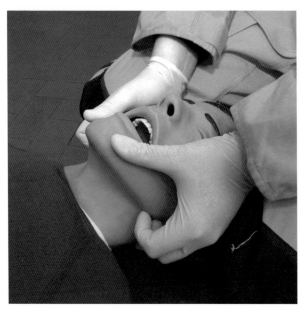

Figure 5.2 Jaw thrust.

- Exhaled air ventilation (rescue breaths) are started once the first set of 30 chest compressions have been performed.

> 30 chest compressions to 2 ventilations.

The only exceptions to this sequence of events are cases of drowning or infants and children, when a single rescuer may give five rescue breaths and perform resuscitation for 1 minute before going for help. In these situations, hypoxia is more likely to be the underlying cause of the arrest and so attempts to correct this are made immediately.

Cardiopulmonary resuscitation

- A patient who is unresponsive and is not breathing or has agonal breathing should be placed in the supine position on a firm surface and cardiopulmonary resuscitation (CPR) started

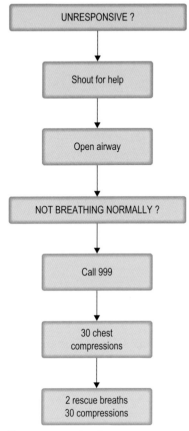

Figure 5.3 The basic life support (BLS) algorithm.

- The patient is in a safe place, the airway is open, help has been sought and cardiac arrest identified
- The first action at this point is to administer 30 chest compressions
- Once the first set of chest compressions has been given, then the rescuer can administer two exhaled air ventilations
  1. The ratio is 30 compressions:2 breaths
  2. Should be performed with as few interruptions as possible
  3. Assign tasks: e.g. one person for ventilations and a second for compressions

4. The person performing compressions should be changed every 1–2 minutes
5. If the patient shows signs of spontaneous ventilation or movement, then re-evaluate from the beginning of the BLS algorithm (unfortunately very rare).

External cardiac (closed chest) compression

- At best, chest compressions only achieve a maximum blood flow of 20% of normal
- Emphasis is on beginning chest compressions rather than the exact position of the hands:
  1. Kneel by the side of the patient
  2. Place the heel of one hand in the centre of the patient's chest (which is the lower half of the victim's sternum breastbone)
  3. Place the heel of the other hand on top of the first hand
  4. Interlock the fingers of your hands and ensure that pressure is not applied over the victim's ribs. Do not apply any pressure over the upper abdomen or the bottom end of the bony sternum
  5. Position yourself vertically above the victim's chest and, with your arms straight, press down on the sternum 5–6 cm
  6. After each compression, release all the pressure on the chest without losing contact between your hands and the sternum. Repeat at a rate of about 100–120 times/minute. Compression and release should take an equal amount of time
  7. External cardiac compressions are best performed with the rescuer leaning well forward over the patient, with straight arms.

Techniques of exhaled air ventilation

To successfully ventilate a patient with exhaled air, there must be a clear path, with no leaks, between the rescuer's lungs and the patient's lungs.

Mouth-to-mouth ventilation

1. The patient's airway is kept patent by the rescuer using the palm of the uppermost hand to perform a head tilt, leaving the index finger and thumb free to pinch the patient's nose to prevent leaks. The fingers of the lower hand are then used to perform a chin lift and if necessary, the thumb is used to open the mouth
2. The rescuer takes a deep breath in and makes a seal with his or her lips around the patient's mouth. Well-fitting dentures should be left in place
3. The rescuer blows into the patient's mouth for 1 second, at the same time listening for leaks and looking down the patient's chest to ensure that it rises

---

Box 5.1 **Common causes of ineffective external chest compressions**

1. Wrong hand position
   - Too high: the heart is not compressed
   - Too low: the stomach is compressed and the risk of aspiration increased
   - Too far laterally: will injure underlying organs
2. Over-enthusiastic effort
   - Causes cardiac damage
   - Fractures ribs, causing damage to underlying organs, particularly lungs and liver
3. Inadequate effort
   - The rescuer is not high enough above the patient to use his or her body weight
   - Fatigue during prolonged resuscitation or poor technique
4. Failure to release between compressions
   - Prevents venous return and filling of the heart
5. Inadequate or excessive rate.

---

4. While maintaining the head tilt and chin lift, the rescuer moves away from the patient's mouth to allow passive exhalation, watching to make sure the chest falls.

Mouth-to-nose ventilation

Mouth-to-nose ventilation is used where mouth-to-mouth ventilation is unsuccessful, e.g. if an obstruction in the mouth cannot be relieved or when the rescuer is a child (a child's mouth would not completely cover an adult's mouth). The airway is maintained as already described but the mouth is closed with the fingers of the lower hand. The seal is made with the rescuer's lips around the base of the patient's nose. Inflation is as above, checking to ensure that the chest rises. The mouth is opened to assist expiration, with the rescuer watching to ensure that the chest falls.

Box 5.2 **Common causes of inadequate ventilation**

- Obstruction – failing to maintain head tilt or chin lift
- Leaks – inadequate seal around the mouth or failure to occlude the patient's nose
- Inflating too hard – trying to overcome an obstructed airway, resulting in gastric distension and regurgitation
- Foreign body – unrecognised in the patient's airway.

Transmission of disease during resuscitation

The safety of both the rescuer and victim are paramount during a resuscitation attempt. There have been few incidents of rescuers suffering adverse effects from undertaking CPR, with only isolated reports of infections such as tuberculosis (TB) and severe acute respiratory distress syndrome (SARS). Transmission of HIV during CPR has never been reported. If the rescuer is unwilling, or unable, to perform exhaled air ventilation, then chest compression only CPR can be performed, although the efficacy of the resuscitation attempt declines after about 5 minutes.

Paramedic basic life support

As there will generally be more than one trained person present, it will be possible for a paramedic crew to undertake actions simultaneously.

1. Having established that the victim is unresponsive, one person should check for breathing, at the same time assessing for signs of a circulation and feeling for a carotid pulse
2. The second person should rapidly collect the appropriate resuscitation equipment, including a defibrillator
3. Having confirmed the diagnosis of cardiac arrest, the defibrillator electrodes should be applied as quickly as possible
4. At the same time, ventilation should commence using a bag-valve-mask with supplemental oxygen rather than exhaled air ventilation
5. If indicated, a shock must be administered, either manually or via an automated external defibrillator (AED)
6. If there is any delay or a shock is not indicated, chest compressions and ventilations in a ratio of 30:2 should commence.

> Attempts at defibrillation must not be delayed while basic life support is performed.

The recovery position

In the unconscious patient who is breathing and has a pulse, the airway is best maintained and the risk of aspiration of gastric contents minimised by placing the patient in the recovery position.

1. Remove the patient's glasses if present
2. Place the patient supine, with legs extended, and ensure the airway is open (head tilt, chin lift)
3. Kneeling against the patient's chest, move the patient's closest arm away from the body so that it lies at 90°, and then flex the elbow to 90° so that the palm lies facing upwards

4. Bring the patient's far arm to lie across the chest, so that the back of the hand lies against the cheek
5. Flex the far leg at the hip and knee, keeping the foot on the ground. Grasp the far shoulder
6. Roll the patient by pulling the shoulders towards you, while using the bent leg as a lever – this is achieved by gently pulling the flexed knee towards you and pressing down
7. Adjust the upper leg so that both the hip and the knee are flexed to 90°. Adjust the hand under the cheek to help maintain the head tilt
8. Finally, the airway, breathing and pulse are checked regularly.

In the recovery position, gravity helps keep the tongue away from the posterior pharyngeal wall; the airway takes precedence over possible cervical spine injuries.

After 30 minutes, the patient should be placed in the recovery position on their other side in order to minimise the chance of developing pressure sores.

Management of choking (foreign body airway obstruction)

- In adults, the obstruction is usually food. In these circumstances, adults show signs of acute airway obstruction, with extreme distress and activity to try to dislodge an obstruction
- If the obstruction is incomplete, there may be severe coughing and inspiratory stridor
- If the patient is still conscious and unable to cough, then back blows should be used initially.

Back blows

- Standing to one side of the patient, the rescuer should encourage the patient to lean forwards
- While supporting the chest with one hand, five firm blows are delivered between the scapulae. If the obstruction is relieved quickly, all five blows need not be delivered
- If this fails then proceed rapidly to the abdominal thrusts.

Abdominal thrusts

- These can be performed with the patient standing, sitting or kneeling down. The aim is to produce a rapid rise in the intrathoracic pressure (by forcing the diaphragm into the chest), which will expel the foreign body
- If the patient is standing, the rescuer should move behind the patient and pass both arms around the body at the level of the upper abdomen
- The rescuer makes one hand into a fist and places it firmly in the patient's epigastrium
- The rescuer's other hand is then placed over the fist and both together forced vigorously upwards and backwards into the epigastrium; this should be repeated up to five times

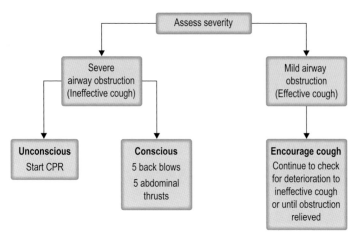

Figure 5.4 Management of foreign body airway obstruction algorithm in adults (Resuscitation Council, UK). The authors are aware of impending changes in resuscitation guidelines (late 2010). Refer to www.resus.org.uk for up-to-date information.

- This manoeuvre is not without danger of causing visceral injury to the stomach, spleen and liver and it is not recommended for infants and small children
- With luck, this will force the object into a position where the patient can remove it by coughing or it can be hooked out with a finger
- If this fails to dislodge the foreign body, the sequence of five back blows and five abdominal thrusts should be repeated until the patient recovers or becomes unconscious.

Continued deterioration

- When the patient is unconscious, he or she should be placed supine. Tilt the head back and remove any visible obstruction. Perform a chin lift and check for breathing; if absent, then begin chest compressions and follow the algorithm for cardiac arrest
- As soon as ALS equipment is available, perform a laryngoscopy and visualise the object. If it is possible to do so without risk of worsening the obstruction, remove the object using Magill's forceps. If this proves impossible, a cricothyroidotomy should be performed without further delay and the patient transferred urgently to hospital.

For further information, see Ch. 5 in *Emergency Care: A Textbook for Paramedics*.

Basic management of the airway and ventilation

- Airway management is the cornerstone of emergency care
- Airway obstruction producing hypoxia will lead to circulatory arrest and irreversible central nervous system damage within 3–4 minutes
- Often the application of basic skills is all that is required.

Simple airway management

Upper airway patency can generally be re-established by correctly positioning the head and by use of the head tilt, the chin lift or if the cervical spine may be damaged, the jaw thrust. Simple adjuncts may further improve the situation.

Foreign body airway obstruction

- The algorithm for the management of choking in the adult is on p. 37. In patients who are (or become) unconscious due to airway destruction, tilt the head back and remove any visible foreign object. Perform a chin lift and check for breathing: if this is absent, begin CPR with chest compressions and continue until ALS equipment (laryngoscope, Magill's forceps, and cricothyroidotomy kit) is available. Ideally the suction end should be manipulated under direct vision using a laryngoscope
- A flexible catheter can be used to clear the lumen of an airway adjunct, such as a nasopharyngeal airway, tracheal tube or laryngeal mask.

Table 6.1 Causes of airway obstruction

Cause:	Leads to:
Coma Mandible trauma	Tongue displacement
Anaphylaxis	Tongue oedema
Foreign body Maxillary trauma	Oropharynx obstruction
Irritants	Laryngeal spasm
Foreign body	Laryngeal obstruction
Laryngeal trauma	Laryngeal oedema/obstruction
Infection Anaphylaxis	Laryngeal oedema
Foreign body	Tracheal or bronchial obstruction
Irritants Anaphylaxis Infection Near-drowning Neurogenic shock Cardiac failure	Pulmonary oedema

Liquid in the airway

- The best way of removing liquid from the oropharynx is by direct suction using a wide-bore or Yankauer suction catheter
- Suction should only be performed under direct vision. 'Blind' suctioning may lead to airway injuries or oedema
- Adult suction devices must not be used on neonates. Specialist suction devices (soft tipped, dual chamber) should be used.

Respiratory control

Central control

The brainstem controls respiration. Sleep, sedatives, alcohol, many analgesic drugs and injury to the respiratory centres result in hypoventilation. This reduction in ventilation may result from a fall in respiratory rate or tidal volume or both. Ventilation is stimulated by a rise in arterial carbon dioxide or a fall in arterial oxygen and is also stimulated by a fall in blood pH which may occur, e.g. in a hyperglycaemic diabetic coma.

Chronic obstructive pulmonary disease

Patients with chronic obstructive pulmonary disease tend to have high levels of carbon dioxide in their blood. Some of these patients will have adapted to these high levels and their stimulus to breathing will be provided only by low oxygen levels rather than by increases in carbon dioxide.

Thus, if high inspired concentrations of oxygen are given to these patients they may lose their respiratory drive leading to carbon dioxide retention and decreasing consciousness. It is important to remember that a high carbon dioxide content kills slowly, but a low oxygen content kills quickly. Thus the need to provide immediate adequate oxygenation takes precedence. Hence cyanotic patients should always be treated with high oxygen concentrations.

Peripheral control

- Adequate ventilation also requires an intact chest wall and intrapulmonary mechanics
- Peripheral causes of impaired ventilation include obstruction of the upper airway, most commonly due to the tongue
- The phrenic nerves originate from cervical spinal roots C3–5; therefore diaphragmatic function will be maintained with cord lesions below this level.

Airway and ventilation assessment

- Establish the circumstances of the immediate event and any pre-existing conditions of relevance, such as asthma
- Airway and ventilation problems may be delayed in onset. The effects of smoke or chemical inhalation may not develop until hours after the event
- Physical assessment of the airway and ventilation involves looking, listening and feeling for chest movement and air flow
- Check the respiratory rate, the presence of cyanosis and/or agitation and the use of the accessory muscles of respiration and abnormal movement of the abdominal muscles
- Noisy breathing during inspiration generally indicates obstruction above the level of the larynx, whereas an expiratory wheeze usually indicates that the problem lies at or below the larynx
- Auscultation will give added information about air flow into the lungs.

Simple airway adjuncts

The use of these devices makes the task of keeping an airway open considerably easier.

Table 6.2 Assessment of the airway and ventilation

	Airway	**Ventilation**
Check for:	Unconsciousness	Unconsciousness
Look for:	Cyanosis Pallor Blood Excessive salivation Stomach contents Foreign body Maxillofacial injury Neck trauma Broken dentures	Penetrating injury Cyanosis Pallor Respiratory rate Chest movements (adequate/flail/equal) Use of accessory muscles Use of abdominal muscles Chest wall bruising
Listen for:	Voice quality Air entry Wheeze inspiratory/expiratory Abnormal sounds (stridor)	Voice quality Air entry Wheeze inspiratory/expiratory Abnormal sounds (crackles)
Feel for:	Airflow on your cheek Subcutaneous emphysema (neck)	Chest movement Subcutaneous emphysema (chest)

Oropharyngeal airway

- The oropharyngeal airway stops the tongue falling backwards and may reduce the need for a jaw thrust
- The airway is introduced through the mouth in an inverted position and rotated through 180° as it passes the edge of the palate
- The distal end locates in the oropharynx
- The airway may also be introduced directly using a tongue spatula or laryngoscope. This method is recommended in infants and small children
- The oropharyngeal airway comes in a range of six sizes suitable for an infant (size 000) to a large adult (size 4)
- The correct size for any individual equates to the distance from the mid-point of the incisors to the angle of the mandible
- The airway must be removed if it induces vomiting or coughing in the patient.

Nasopharyngeal airway

- The nasopharyngeal airway consists of a bevelled tube with a flange at the proximal end
- The airway is introduced, well lubricated, into either nostril (generally the right is attempted first because of the direction of the distal bevel)

- It should be directed backwards (not upwards) along the roof of the palate so that the tip lies in the hypopharynx, just above the larynx
- If resistance to the passage of the airway is encountered, it should be withdrawn and an attempt made through the other nostril
- Suction should be on hand to control any bleeding
- The correct size of airway equates approximately with the diameter of the patient's nostril – an airway of 6.0 or 6.5 mm internal diameter will be suitable for the majority of adults
- The nasopharyngeal airway is particularly valuable in patients with maxillofacial injuries or a clenched jaw. Once in place, it is better tolerated than an oropharyngeal airway
- If a basal skull fracture is suspected then extra care should be taken when inserting the device.

Simple ventilation aids

The simple foil

- Foil devices provide a barrier between patient and rescuer during expired air ventilation
- A plastic film with a central orifice and a textile filter or one-way valve which is aligned with the patient's mouth is applied to the oronasal region
- Expired air ventilation is applied in the usual way with the patient's nostrils occluded with the fingers of one hand, while the other hand applies chin lift and seals the foil to the face.

The face mask device

- A moulded face mask, made from transparent material, is fitted with an inflation port incorporating a one-way valve which directs the patient's exhaled air away from the rescuer and traps macroscopic particles
- Some models incorporate an additional port for supplemental oxygen. The oxygen flow rate should be set at the maximum available
- The mask is applied over the mouth and nose with both hands, applying jaw thrust and head tilt to draw the face into the mask and sealed to the face with the index fingers and thumb of each hand.

The self-inflating bag valve device

- Use of a self-inflating bag with valve allows the rescuer to ventilate the patient by hand instead of using expired air
- Inflation of the lungs is provided through a valve which directs the air/oxygen to the patient and vents exhaled air to the atmosphere

- Oxygen enrichment (only achieving an inspired concentration of up to 50% – FiO2 0.5) can be provided through a port adjacent to the unidirectional air inlet valve
- Much better inspired concentrations can be achieved (FiO2 0.9, an inspired oxygen concentration of 90%) when an oxygen reservoir bag is attached to the air inlet valve and the flow rate adjusted to 10–15 L/min
- The aim is to adjust the flow rate to ensure that the reservoir bag remains at least partially inflated at all times. If this is achievable with a flow rate of 10 L/min then oxygen can be conserved
- The self-inflating bag may be used with a face mask or may be attached to a tracheal tube or laryngeal mask airway
- A two-person technique is advocated, one person using two hands to hold the mask with the airway aligned and the other inflating the patient's lungs by squeezing the bag
- A modified patient valve can permit positive end-expiratory pressure (PEEP) to be applied when the bag is used with a tracheal tube
- The use of PEEP may be particularly valuable in patients with pulmonary oedema by reversing the leakage of fluid into the alveoli
- A filter can be fitted on the intake valve to permit operation in contaminated atmospheres.

Ventilation volumes

Inflation volumes of 10 mL/kg (600–900 mL in an adult) should be used if ventilating on air. If supplemental oxygen is available, the volume of each inflation should be limited to 400–600 mL (7 mL/kg). Overinflation will lead to gastric inflation and increased risk of regurgitation, as well as the possibility of barotrauma (lung damage).

Cricoid pressure

The unconscious patient with an insecure airway is continually at risk of regurgitation of gastric contents and pulmonary aspiration. True security of the airway can only be provided by placing a cuffed tube within the trachea but cricoid pressure (Sellick's manoeuvre) during artificial ventilation in the patient with the unsecured airway substantially reduces the risk of gastric regurgitation. The technique should always be used when endotracheal intubation is to be attempted. Cricoid pressure is applied to either side of the cricoid cartilage using the thumb and forefinger of one hand at a pressure of 30 Newtons (which feels equivalent to the weight of three 1 kg bags of sugar).

Oxygen therapy in the spontaneously breathing patient

Patients with airway or ventilatory compromise, major trauma or chest disease should be given oxygen. High inspired concentrations can only be achieved with an oxygen mask that incorporates a reservoir bag. The oxygen flow rate should be set at 10–15 L/min, to ensure the reservoir bag remains inflated.

If a pulse-oximeter is available then patient saturations should be kept above 94%. However, in patients with COPD, oxygen should be administered at a concentration of 24–28% using a Venturi mask. Lower saturations of 88–92% are acceptable.

Some COPD patients may be on long-term home oxygen, which means high flow oxygen can be used safely as they will not have developed a hypoxic ventilation drive.

For further information, see Ch. 6 in *Emergency Care: A Textbook for Paramedics*.

CHAPTER 7

Advanced management of the airway and ventilation

The gold standard for airway control in prehospital care is endotracheal intubation using a cuffed tracheal tube, however basic airway management must be mastered before learning advanced techniques.

Accidental and unrecognised oesophageal intubation is likely to be fatal. Excessive movement of the head and neck during laryngoscopy and intubation may aggravate a cervical spine injury.

Tracheal intubation

The trachea can be intubated via the oropharynx or via the nasopharynx. Oropharyngeal endotracheal intubation requires a laryngoscope for successful placement.

Indications

- Airway obstruction or potential airway obstruction in the profoundly unconscious patient with no gag reflex
- Patient at risk of aspiration of foreign material (e.g. gastric contents, blood from maxillofacial trauma)
- Patient requiring positive pressure ventilation, e.g. in cardiorespiratory arrest
- To gain access to the lower respiratory tract to aspirate secretions or foreign material.

Contraindications

Box 7.1 **Contraindications to tracheal intubation**

- Insufficient operator skill or experience
- Conscious or semiconscious patient
- Immobility of the head and neck (relative)
- Distorted anatomy (relative)
- In children:
  - Croup
  - Epiglottitis
- Gag reflex present.

> On NO ACCOUNT should attempts be made to intubate children with croup or infections such as acute epiglottitis.

However, if the child loses their airway anyway, then cautious intubation or surgical airway may be life-saving.

Equipment for conventional endotracheal intubation

The following equipment is required:

- Appropriate sized laryngoscope in working order, different size blades
- Appropriate range of tubes cut to correct length with connections (15 mm) to fit the bag valve device
- Suction apparatus
- Lubricant on a gauze swab (only occasionally required in the prehospital setting)
- 20 mL syringe for cuff inflation
- Flexible bougie and stylet
- Magill's forceps
- Tape or tie to secure tube in place
- Apparatus to inflate the lungs (bag valve device or ventilator)
- Pulse oximeter to monitor patient during and after intubation attempt
- End-tidal CO_2 apparatus to detect correct tube placement
- Rescue equipment including laryngeal mask airway and surgical airway.

Size of endotracheal tube

ET tubes of size 7–9 mm will fit most adults. ET tubes are made longer than is generally needed and should be cut to a length of 21–25 cm in order to reduce dead space. The length required in any individual will be twice the distance from the corner of the mouth to the angle of the jaw.

For children, the correct size can be calculated using the following formulae:

Correct internal diameter (mm) = (age of child in years/4) + 4

Correct length (cm) = (age of child in years/2) + 12

Once the correct diameter has been calculated, have the next biggest and the next smallest tube available to ensure a good fit.

In children it is important that the full range of ET tube sizes (including half sizes) are available. ET tubes <6.5 mm are not supplied with an inflatable cuff, in order to avoid pressure damage to the trachea.

Technique for endotracheal intubation using laryngoscopy

1. Ensure that all equipment functions correctly and that tubes and bougies are well lubricated if necessary
2. The patient should be supine with the head and neck aligned in the clear airway position (preferably with the head on a small pillow or rolled-up blanket). Apply cricoid pressure if possible
3. Holding the laryngoscope in the left hand, insert the curved blade into the right-hand corner of the patient's mouth, ensuring that the lip is not caught between the blade and lower teeth
4. Advance the blade, aiming for the larynx in the midline, and displacing the tongue towards the left-hand side of the mouth to leave a clear view
5. When the tip of the blade reaches laryngeal level, lift the handle forwards and upwards. Slide the tip of the blade into the recess between the epiglottis and the base of the tongue
6. Maintain the backwards tilt of the head by pressing on the occiput with your other hand and against the tip of the blade to get the best view of the glottic opening. Cricoid pressure will generally improve the view and should be used in all patients in the field
7. Pass the tracheal tube from the right-hand side of the mouth through the glottic opening, rotating it 90° counter-clockwise if necessary, to ease entry between the vocal cords
8. If a full view of the glottis is not possible a bougie may be passed under direct vision through the cords and the tube introduced over the bougie into the trachea. The bougie is then withdrawn. Alternatively, a malleable stylet may be placed inside the lumen of the tube and bent to a curve suitable for introduction of the tube through the glottis
9. Once the tube has passed between the vocal cords it should be advanced so that the cuff lies below the larynx
10. The cuff should be inflated with air (or sterile water if the patient is to be transported at altitude or in a decompression chamber). Sufficient air should be introduced to eliminate any leak at the peak of positive pressure ventilation. Cuff inflation volumes requiring more than 15 mL should lead

to a suspicion that the tube is misplaced in the oesophagus or that the cuff itself has developed a leak

11. Check that the tube is in the trachea by observing bilateral chest movement and listening for air entry over both upper lobes. Unilateral chest movement (generally on the right) may indicate that the tube has gone down too far and has entered the main bronchus. A check should also be made that air entry is not heard in the epigastric area. However end tidal CO_2 monitoring is the gold standard

12. Secure the tube in place with a tie or tape. Remove cricoid pressure.

The entire process of intubation should be accomplished in 30 seconds or less. If the attempt is taking longer, then it should be temporarily abandoned and the patient ventilated with oxygen via a face mask for 1–2 minutes before trying again. Note that ventilation via a mask between intubation attempts is pointless if the airway remains obstructed. No more than two attempts should be made before moving to other measures.

Complications of endotracheal intubation

- Trauma to lips, teeth, tongue and structures in the pharynx and larynx (a common problem is using the teeth as a fulcrum, causing damage to crowns particularly)
- Oesophageal intubation likely to guarantee patient death
- Intubation of a single bronchus will lead to hypoxia and collapse of the opposite lung
- Aspiration of foreign material such as stomach contents or blood during the intubation attempt
- Kinking of the tracheal tube
- Overinflation of the cuff leading to pressure damage of the tracheal mucous membrane or ballooning of the cuff over the lumen of the tube
- Exacerbation of cervical spine injury
- Beginning positive pressure ventilation may convert an open pneumothorax to a tension pneumothorax in the trauma patient.

Aids to orotracheal intubation

The intubating laryngeal mask

The intubating laryngeal mask (ILM) is a variant of the conventional laryngeal mask airway which is specifically designed to facilitate blind tracheal intubation. The midline position of the bevel of this tube is designed to increase the chances of successful blind intubation by passing a conventional endotracheal tube down the lumen of the ILM. A handle is fitted at the proximal end to introduce the device and manipulate it to the correct position.

- Size 3 (child age 10–14)
- Size 4 (adult female or small male)
- Size 5 (normal to large adult male).

The device is introduced in the head and neck neutral position, which is of value in patients with suspected cervical spine injury.

Indications

The device should be used, by trained personnel, in unconscious patients with suspected cervical spine injury when an airway is required. It may also be used in patients with known or anticipated difficult intubation or if access to above the patient's head is difficult or impossible.

Technique

1. Test the cuff for leaks and lubricate the back and sides, but not the aperture, of the laryngeal mask airway (LMA) at the distal end
2. Test the tracheal tube cuff for leaks
3. Lubricate the tracheal tube and slide it in and out of the ILM until it moves easily
4. Deflate the cuff of the ILM completely
5. With the head and neck in the neutral position, grasp the handle of the ILM and position it over the patient's lower neck and upper chest
6. Introduce the top of the mask behind the upper incisors and, using a rotating movement, roll the mask along the surface of the palate and down into the hypopharynx
7. Inflate the cuff of the ILM (20 mL for size 3; 30 mL for size 4; and 35–40 mL for size 5)
8. Connect a ventilating device to the ILM and check for chest movement and leaks around the cuffs
9. Make final adjustments to the position with the handle to achieve inflation with least resistance. Usually a slight elevation of the mask will achieve the best position
10. Holding the handle firmly in this position, introduce the tracheal tube into the ILM and attempt to pass it through into the trachea. Passage without resistance will occur in the majority of cases
11. If resistance occurs, partially remove the ILM by rotation of the handle and then reintroduce it. This may dislodge a down-folded epiglottis
12. When it is thought that the tracheal tube is in position, inflate the cuff and check for bilateral lung inflation and the absence of gastric inflation
13. The ILM can now be removed. Deflate the cuff of the ILM
14. Remove the connector from the tracheal tube and, using a pusher, hold the tracheal tube in place while removing the ILM with a rotation action
15. Once removal of the ILM is nearly complete, grasp the tracheal tube in the mouth to prevent its dislocation and complete removal of the ILM, ensuring the tracheal tube pilot balloon passes easily through the ILM
16. Replace the tracheal tube connector and check again for correct tracheal tube placement.

The lighted stylet

Another intubation aid uses a malleable lighted stylet passed through the lumen of the tracheal tube so that the light at the end does not quite emerge from the distal end of the tube. Bent to a 'J' shape, the tube is introduced directly through the glottis into the trachea. Correct positioning just above the glottic opening is confirmed by maximal transillumination in the midline. Once the tube is correctly placed, the lighted stylet should be unclipped from the proximal end and withdrawn from the tube.

Alternatives to tracheal intubation

The laryngeal mask airway

The LMA consists of a wide-bore tube with a standard 15 mm connector at the proximal end. At the distal end is an elliptical cuff designed to seal the hypopharynx around the laryngeal opening.

Table 7.1 Laryngeal mask sizes

Patient	Weight (kg)	Size	Cuff volume (mL)
Neonate/infant	<6.5	1	2–4
Infant/child	6.5–15	2	10
Child	15–30	2.5	15
Small adult/child	30–50	3	20
Adult	50–75	4	30
Large adult	>75	5	40

Indications

The LMA is indicated when an airway is required in an unconscious patient and tracheal intubation is precluded by lack of available expertise or equipment or has proved difficult or impossible.

Technique

1. Test the cuff inflation for leaks and then lubricate the back and sides, but not the aperture, of the cuff and the distal part of the tube
2. Deflate the cuff completely
3. The patient should be supine with the head and neck in the clear airway position

4. The mouth should be opened by an assistant depressing the chin
5. The tube is held like a pen in the gloved hand and introduced into the mouth with the aperture facing the tongue. *As the LMA is advanced it should be applied to the roof of the palate*
6. Once the hand cannot go further inside the mouth, it should be moved to the proximal end of the tube and the mask pressed into position until resistance is felt as it locates in the hypopharynx. The coloured line on the tube should be aligned with the nasal septum
7. The cuff is inflated with the correct amount of air for the size (Table 7.1). As the cuff is inflated, the tube rises out of the mouth by approximately 1 cm
8. Confirm that a clear airway exists by listening for spontaneous breathing or check for chest movement and breath sounds during inflation with a bag attached to the tube
9. Insert the bite block or oropharyngeal airway alongside the tube and secure it in place with a tie or tape.

> Normally the operator will be positioned at the head of the patient to introduce the tube, but if access to this position is impossible the operator may stand or kneel in front of the patient and introduce the tube from below.

Detection of correct tube placement

An undetected misplaced tracheal tube is the most serious complication of airway management. A protocol to check correct placement should follow each intubation attempt.

> If there is any doubt about the correct placement of a tracheal tube – *remove it.*

Clinical methods
- Visualising the tube passing between the vocal cords during the intubation attempt
- Palpation of the tube as it passes through the larynx
- During positive pressure inflation applied to the tube – *Note*:
  - Absence of leak around the inflated cuff
  - Bilateral chest expansion
  - Breath sounds in both axillae
  - Absence of sounds in the epigastric area.

Detection of carbon dioxide emerging from the tube generally indicates that it is in the trachea:
- Simple, inexpensive and reliable colorimetric devices such as Easy Cap® can be used

- Easy Cap® will turn from purple to yellow with six breaths/ventilations if CO_2 is passing through it
- Carbon dioxide can emerge from the oesophagus if the patient has recently had a carbonated drink
- Miniaturised electronic devices are also available which provide a capnograph trace and digital readings
- End-tidal CO_2 monitoring represents the gold standard for confirming ET tube placement
- Effective BLS may produce measurable carbon dioxide levels in patients in cardiac arrest.

Airway management in suspected cervical spine injury

Special care must be taken during management of the airway in patients with suspected cervical spine injury. However, securing the airway remains the higher priority.

Flexion and rotation of the head and neck are the most dangerous movements.

Oral intubation using direct laryngoscopy can be safely accomplished by a skilled operator in the vast majority of cases.

Airway management in patients with pharyngeal or laryngeal oedema

Oedema in the pharyngeal or laryngeal region can be related to thermal injury, anaphylaxis or acute infection such as epiglottitis.

In the prehospital setting, the airway should be managed by basic positional methods and a high inspired oxygen concentration, with rapid transfer to a hospital.

Life-threatening airway obstruction should be treated by needle cricothyroidotomy and jet ventilation or surgical cricothyroidotomy.

Patients with inhalational thermal injury should be intubated early before serious oedema develops, however, there is usually time for this to be achieved following arrival in the hospital.

The surgical airway

The surgical airway is indicated in patients with life-threatening airway obstruction where basic positional methods and endotracheal intubation (or alternatives) have failed. Access to the trachea should be made through the cricothyroid membrane. In the first instance, the recommended method is needle cricothyroidotomy, however ventilation provided by this method is marginal and sufficient only to buy a few minutes' time until an alternative is available.

Needle cricothyroidotomy

1. A 14-gauge intravenous cannula directed slightly towards the feet (caudally) is introduced through the cricothyroid membrane, while aspirating continually through an attached 20 mL syringe until a free flow of air is obtained
2. The needle is withdrawn, leaving the cannula *in situ*
3. The cannula is secured, the safest way is to hold it
4. A 14-gauge cannula is of insufficient diameter to allow any significant spontaneous ventilation to occur. Positive pressure ventilation can be provided using a self-inflating bag attached to a 3 mm tracheal tube connector which will fit a Luer intravenous connection
5. Adequate insufflation *can* be provided using a high-pressure jet injector system. The cannula is connected by non-compliant tubing to an oxygen cylinder fitted with a regulator, which will produce a pressure in the region of 400 kPa. This is the pressure produced by an oxygen cylinder before a flow meter is attached and requires a special fitting. This system can not be relied upon for more than 20 minutes due to build up of carbon dioxide
6. Inflation is produced by a finger intermittently occluding a hole in the tubing or by a specially designed system with a manually operated trigger which produces inflation when depressed. Alternatively, a 'Y' connector may be used to connect the tubing to the cannula, with the stem of the 'Y' towards the patient and one of the top ends attached via the tubing to the oxygen supply. The open branch can be intermittently occluded to produce insufflation
7. Time must be left for lung deflation (1 second inflation: 4 seconds deflation). For the technique to be safe there must be a clear route through the larynx and mouth for the expired gases, otherwise lung barotrauma will occur.

Surgical cricothyroidotomy

Surgical cricothyroidotomy may occasionally be performed by a medical practitioner before the patient reaches hospital.

1. A 2–3 cm transverse stab incision is made through the cricothyroid membrane
2. The membrane is widened using forceps or by using a tracheal hook
3. The forceps may be left in the wound to maintain the track
4. A 6–7 mm lubricated tracheal tube (tracheal/tracheotomy) is inserted through the incision and directed towards the lower trachea
5. The cuff is inflated and the tube is secured with a tape and connected to the ventilating apparatus.

Blind stab techniques

Devices such as the Portex Mini-Trach® II or expandable trochar systems such as Nu-Trach® use a combination of both techniques allowing wider lumen devices to be inserted giving better ventilation. Even with these devices ventilation is unlikely to be successful for more than 1 hour.

Ventilators

- Oxygen-powered ventilators have been designed to take over from the self-inflating bag
- They are driven from a high-pressure (400 kPa) oxygen source, so are valuable in contaminated atmospheres
- Ventilators may be connected to a tracheal tube or laryngeal mask
- The inspiratory flow rates should be restricted to a maximum of 40 L/min and should incorporate a blow-off valve with automatic warning if the inflation pressure exceeds 60 cmH$_2$O in adults (this level can be altered in some models)
- Intubated patients with head injury will receive better ventilation from an automatic ventilator than can be achieved even by practised personnel with a hand bag-valve system.

Ventilator settings

Inspiratory flow rates (if available)

Generally 1.5–2 seconds (longer if there is an increased resistance to inspiration).

Expiratory flow rates (if available)

Generally, the expiratory time should be twice as long as the inspiratory time. It may need to be longer in patients with increased expiratory resistance such as asthma.

Ventilation rate

Generally, rates should be similar to natural breathing, i.e. 20 breaths/minute in an infant; 15 in a child and 12 in an adult. Shocked patients may require higher rates and rates may be adjusted in response to end-tidal capnography.

Relief/alarm pressure

This should be set to = 60 cmH$_2$O. Start at a much lower setting such as 30 cmH$_2$O so that problems with ventilation are identified immediately.

Tidal volumes

Normally 7–8 mL/kg body weight (approximately 500 mL in a 70 kg patient).

Epiglottitis

Epiglottitis is a bacterial infection of the epiglottis, seen most often in children. It leads to marked swelling of the epiglottis, with a typical 'cherry red' appearance.

The patient will often be grey, distressed, drooling at the mouth and leaning forward. There is severe continuous stridor.

> Examination of the mouth and pharynx must not be attempted in suspected epiglottitis.

Complete airway obstruction can develop within minutes. Any procedure that can cause crying or gagging, including simple examination of the throat, can precipitate laryngeal spasm and airway obstruction.

If the condition is suspected, the patient should be calmed, given high-concentration oxygen, sat forward and transported quickly to hospital. A paediatric team and senior anaesthetist should be requested to stand by. If airway obstruction occurs before arrival at hospital, intubation or needle cricothyroidotomy may be required.

For further information, see Ch. 7 in *Emergency Care: A Textbook for Paramedics*.

CHAPTER 8

Vascular access

Intravenous access allows fluids or drugs to be administered. In children, the intra-osseous (IO) route is often used. This route is increasingly being used in shocked adults in whom intravenous access may be difficult or impossible.

Technique of intravenous cannulation

The largest cannula which can *successfully* be inserted into the vein should always be chosen. As with any procedure where there is a risk of contact with body fluids, gloves should be worn by the operator, then:

1. Choose a vein capable of accommodating the size of cannula needed, preferably one that is both visible and palpable. The junction of two veins is often a good site as the 'target' is larger and the veins tend to be less mobile

2. The vein should be allowed to dilate as this increases the success rate of cannulation. In the limb veins, this is usually achieved by using a proximal tourniquet. Further dilation can be encouraged by gently tapping the skin over the vein. When cannulating the external jugular vein, if it is safe to do so, the patient can be tipped slightly head down to encourage the vein to dilate. Turning the patient's head to the opposite side will also facilitate cannula insertion

3. The skin over the vein should be cleaned. If alcohol-based agents are used, they must be given time to work (2–3 minutes), ensuring that the skin is dry before proceeding further

4. The vein should now be immobilised in order to prevent it being displaced by the advancing cannula. This is achieved by pulling the skin over the vein tight, with the operator's free hand

5. Holding the cannula firmly, at an angle of 10–15° to the skin, it should be advanced through the skin and into the vein. Often a slight loss of resistance is felt as the vein is entered. This should be accompanied by the appearance of blood in the flashback chamber of the cannula

6. While keeping the skin taut, the angle of the cannula is reduced slightly and advance it a further 2–3 mm into the vein. This is to ensure that the first part of the plastic cannula lies within the vein. Care must be taken at this point not to push the needle out of the back of the vein
7. The needle is now withdrawn 5–10 mm into the cannula, so that the point no longer protrudes from the end. As this is done, blood will often be seen to flow between the needle body and the cannula, confirming that the tip of the cannula is within the vein
8. The cannula and needle are advanced along the vein together. The needle is retained within the cannula to provide support and prevent kinking at the point of skin puncture
9. Once the cannula is inserted as far as the hub, the tourniquet should be released and the needle completely removed and disposed of safely
10. Confirmation that the cannula lies within the vein should be made by injection of a saline flush
11. Finally, the cannula should be secured using adhesive tape or a specific cannula dressing.

Complications

Early

- Failure of cannulation
- Haematoma
- Extravasation
- Damage to local structures
- Air embolus (rare)
- Breakage of the cannula.

Late

- Infection and inflammation (thrombophlebitis)
- Irritation can be caused by high concentration drugs or fluids.

Intraosseous access

The intraosseous route allows the administration of fluids and drugs, with circulating levels of drugs being comparable with those achieved when given via a central vein.

In children, access is generally gained in the limbs, in adults the sternum and pelvis can also be used.

Sites for intraosseous access

Four peripheral sites can be used for intraosseous access:

- The anteromedial surface of the tibia, 2–3 cm below the tibial tuberosity

- The distal tibia, just proximal to the medial malleolus
- The anterior surface of the femur, 3 cm above the lateral condyle
- The humeral head at the shoulder.

These sites are relatively free of other local important structures. The most relevant feature to be borne in mind is the proximity of the epiphyses (growth plates). Damage to these could interfere with subsequent bone growth and development.

The main site for central IO access is the manubrium sterni which should only be used for adults.

Standard IO devices (hand inserted)

The needles have a short shaft, with a central solid trocar, which has a large handle for manual insertion. The trocar must be unscrewed before it can be removed from the needle. The external end of the needle has a standard Luer fitting. Some needles have a screw thread to improve their security in the bone.

Intraosseous needles come in a range of sizes:

- 6–20 gauge for children younger than 18 months
- 12–16 gauge for children older than 18 months.

Technique (conventional hand-inserted IO needle)

1. An appropriate site is chosen, taking care to avoid placing the needle in a fractured bone. Placement of a needle in a distal bone (e.g. the tibia) in the presence of a proximal fracture (e.g. of the femur) is acceptable. If the proximal tibia is used, it may help to place a firm support behind the knee
2. The skin over the site should be thoroughly cleaned. Ideally, local anaesthetic solution should be infiltrated into the skin and underlying periosteum
3. The needle is introduced at 90° through the skin to make contact with the bone and then advanced using a screwing action with threaded needles or a 'bradawl'-type action with unthreaded needles, at the same time applying firm pressure
4. A loss of resistance is felt as the cortex is penetrated by an unthreaded needle and the marrow cavity entered. The needle should feel as if it is 'gripped' by the bone and should hold its position once released
5. The trocar is unscrewed and removed and correct placement confirmed by the ability to aspirate bone marrow. This should always be used to check blood glucose levels. Further confirmation is provided by being able to flush 5 mL of saline through the needle without resistance or signs of extravasation.

> Never place an IO needle in a fractured bone.

EZ-IO® power driver

This device uses a battery powered motor to insert the intraosseous needles in a similar way to a hand-held drill.

The device is very effective and easy to use but requires the use of specially designed IO needles (pink for paediatrics; blue or yellow for adults).

A longer needle is available for use in the head of the humerus when lower limb insertion is inappropriate or has failed.

Sternal IO injection device (e.g. FAST®)

Specially designed to insert a needle into the manubrium of the adult sternum.

The device fires a spring-loaded needle through the outer table of the sternum.

The device activates when equal pressure is applied to the stabilisation points around the needle to ensure entry at 90° to the skin.

Bone injection gun

May be used in any of the conventional insertion sites IN ADULTS but NOT in the sternum. A paediatric version is available.

Intraosseous fluid administration

All drugs and fluids that can be given via peripheral intravenous cannulae can be administered via the IO route.

All IO routes will require fluids to be administered under pressure – by hand, using a pressure bag or a pressure infusion device – gravity alone will not be effective.

Forcing fluid into bone spaces under pressure is painful, often more painful than the insertion of the needle. If time is available, 2–3 mL of 1% lignocaine can be infused first to reduce the pain stimulus.

Fluid administration via an intraosseous line in children is most safely and effectively achieved by the administration of boluses by injection using a syringe and a three-way tap.

Complications

Complications, which are rare, include:

- Failure to enter the bone marrow cavity – the most common problem
- Extravasation of fluid
- Compartment syndrome
- Leakage from the hole left by a previous attempt
- Infection in the skin, abscess formation and ultimately osteomyelitis
- Damage to the growth plate of the bone could occur as a result of careless placement and in very young children (rare)
- Fracture might occur if excessive force is used (rare).

Fluid flow through cannulae and catheters

The diameter and length of the cannula as well as the viscosity of the fluid and the pressure applied combine to affect the rate at which fluid will flow through the cannula.

Table 8.1 Rate of flow through different sizes of Venflon cannulae

Colour	Diameter (mm)	Gauge	Length (mm)	Flow (mL/min)
Pink	1.0	20	32	54
Green	1.2	18	45	80
Grey	1.7	16	45	180
Brown	2.0	14	45	270

For further information, see Ch. 8 in *Emergency Care: A Textbook for Paramedics*.

CHAPTER 9

Taking a medical history

In medical illness, the history affords 70% of the information on which most diagnoses are made.

The history is thus much more important than the physical examination in establishing a diagnosis.

Assessment and correction of any problems in airway, breathing and circulation will take priority.

The aims of history-taking are to establish:

- What has happened (the history)
- What the patient feels to be wrong (the symptoms)
- The background to the current events (the past medical history)
- What medication the patient is taking
- A list of possible diagnoses (the differential diagnosis)
- Priorities for treatment
- Information that will not be available later (e.g. from the scene).

Structure of the history

However detailed or simple a medical history is being taken, a structured approach is essential. While at the scene a detailed history is not usually appropriate, a brief outline history is ample – and 'AMPLE' is a useful mnemonic to remember what constitutes an adequate history at the scene:

A – Allergies

In all emergencies other than cardiac arrest, it is important to try to establish any known allergies before drugs are administered.

M – Medicines

The presence of medications in the bloodstream may influence the response to injury or illness or to any other drugs which may be given. Knowledge of what medication the patient has been taking may indicate the severity and duration of any pre-existing illness.

P – Past medical history

The past medical history has a major bearing on responses to treatment and possible outcomes from illness or injury. It also offers vital clues as to what the current problem may be. Particular note should be made of any known cardiac disease, respiratory disease or such chronic conditions as diabetes or epilepsy.

L – Last food and drink

A full stomach is a major risk factor for regurgitation and consequent airway compromise. It is also helpful to obtain information about the patient's nutritional status and general level of self-care.

E – Events leading up to the current problem

This is the core of the history. The other elements are important but this is the key to understanding what is happening to the patient now.

Not all of the information needs to be acquired at the scene; some can be acquired *en route* to the hospital.

Often, rather than attempting to laboriously establish the drug history in detail, all medications should be gathered together and taken to the hospital with the patient.

Sources of information

The scene

There may be vital clues at the scene and in the vast majority of cases, only Ambulance service personnel will have the chance of interpreting them and carrying the information to those who will subsequently be caring for the patient.

The patient

If the patient cannot cooperate, further information can be sought from bystanders or witnesses.

The witnesses

Witnesses may help with information about the mechanism of injury. Some witnesses or bystanders may know the patient and be able to give background information.

Medical information devices

Medic-Alert® bracelets or necklaces are always worth looking for. Horse riders may carry medical information in a recess inside their crash helmet. Many patients have lists of medication on their person and the elderly often carry containers with compartments for timed administration of tablets.

Information to be gleaned at the scene

- Is the patient and are the surroundings clean and tidy?
- Are there carers present?
- Is it an environment to which the patient could return?
- Are there bottles of medication which could be taken to the hospital?
- Are there empty pill bottles indicating a possible overdose?
- Is there evidence of alcohol or drug abuse?
- If the patient is unconscious, are there any clues at the scene that might help establish the duration or cause of the unconsciousness?

The art of questioning

- Obtaining information from frightened, ill or injured patients is made easier by a positive, confident and friendly approach
- Patients who are confused or deaf may be reassured more by a smile than by the words that are spoken
- Whenever possible, practitioners should position themselves at the same level as the patient, e.g. kneeling beside a patient who is lying on the floor
- Eye contact should be maintained if possible
- Always introduce yourself
- Avoid inappropriate familiarity. Older patients appreciate the correct use of their surname and title, at the very least on first introductions
- Maintain conversation with the patient
- Establish the patient's name and age
- Questioning should begin with open questions such as: 'Tell me what the matter is'. Open questions can then be followed by questions that focus on the complaint.

Symptoms such as pain can be explored with a set of specific queries:

'What's the pain like?'
'How long have you had it?'
'Have you ever had a pain like this before?'
'What makes the pain worse?'

Classic descriptions of pain

Chest pain: 'like an iron band round my chest' is virtually specific to myocardial ischaemia.
Sudden pain: 'like a severe blow in the back of the neck' suggests subarachnoid haemorrhage.

Passing on the information

The key points of the history should be recorded with brevity and clarity. In many situations, a printed form assists recording of the history and findings at the scene.

The summary should include:

- The patient's name (if known)
- The patient's age (if known)
- The events surrounding the involvement of the emergency medical services
- Past history.

The receiving doctor or other professionals will need a brief handover initially but will generally have more time to receive information after they have completed the primary survey, which may only take a very few minutes.

It is essential that prehospital personnel are actively involved in the handover and do not leave until they have imparted all the information that they think is relevant to the case.

Good emergency departments will ensure a brief period of undivided attention to the incoming crew for the initial brief handover.

A copy of the prehospital record must accompany the inpatient notes to allow a complete picture of the injury or illness to be recorded.

For further information, see Ch. 9 in *Emergency Care: A Textbook for Paramedics*.

CHAPTER 10

Drug formulary

The Medicines Act allows ambulance paramedics to supply and administer prescription only medications in circumstances specified by local paramedic steering committees or their equivalent.

The Joint Royal Colleges Ambulance Liaison Committee (JRCALC) makes applications for exemption for the drugs listed in the formulary below.

The JRCALC National Clinical Guidelines for use by UK ambulance services provide the most up-to-date list of relevant drugs (see: www.asancep.org.uk/JRCALC/guidelines).

The names of a drug

Each drug has several 'names' as the full chemical name is usually unwieldy:

- *Chemical name:* 4-amino-5-chloro-N-[2-(dimethylamino)ethyl] 1-2-methoxybenzamide
- *Generic name:* metoclopramide
- *Trade name:* Maxolon.

Routes of administration

Enteral routes of administration:

- Oral
- Rectal
- Sublingual
- Buccal.

Parenteral routes of administration:

- Dermal patches
- Intradermal
- Intramuscular
- Subcutaneous

- Intravenous
- Inhaled or nebulised
- Intraosseous.

Half-life

This is the time it takes for the plasma concentration of a drug in the body to halve.

After one half-life, only 50% remains, after two half-lives, only 25% remains and so on.

This is important because drugs with a long half-life take a long time to be eliminated compared to those with a short half-life.

Naloxone, the antidote to morphine, has a much shorter half-life than morphine itself.

Prehospital formulary

Amiodarone

Main prehospital use

- Ventricular fibrillation (VF) or pulseless ventricular tachycardia (VT) refractors to three countershocks
- VT with chest pain, heart failure, or heart rate >150 bpm.

Action

An antiarrhythmic drug, which lengthens cardiac action potential and effective refractory period.

Preparations

30 mg/mL, 10 mL ampoule for intravenous injection.

Indications

Replaces lidocaine for:

- VF or pulseless VT
- VT with either chest pain, heart failure, or heart rate >150 bpm provided SBP >90 mmHg.

Cautions

None in cardiac arrest situations.

Contraindications

None in cardiac arrest situations.

For **VT**, **hypotension** (BP, 90 mmHg), bradycardia, heart block, thyroid dysfunction, iodine allergy, respiratory failure, congestive heart failure, decompensated cardiomyopathy, pregnancy, breast-feeding.

Side-effects

Not relevant in cardiac arrest situations.

Following treatment for VT: severe bradycardia, vasodilation and hypotension, bronchospasm, arrhythmias (*torsade de pointes*).

Dose

- **Cardiac arrest:** Following persistent VF or VT administer 300 mg IV after 3rd shock. A further 150 mg may also be used
- **VT:** 150 mg over 10 minutes (3 minutes if life-threatening). May be repeated once after 10 minutes.

Aspirin

Aspirin (acetylsalicylic acid) decreases platelet aggregation and inhibits clot formation on the arterial side of the circulation. Its use can reduce mortality associated with myocardial infarction and unstable angina. When indicated, a 300 mg tablet should be given regardless of any previous aspirin taken that day. In children under 12 years old, aspirin is associated with Reye's syndrome (acute encephalopathy and liver damage) and is contraindicated.

Main prehospital use

Acute coronary syndromes.

Other uses

- Prevention of thrombotic cardiovascular or cerebrovascular disease
- Simple oral analgesic and mild antiinflammatory.

Action

- Antiplatelet activity prevents or limits formation of clots
- Decreased perception of pain
- Antipyretic (lowers temperature).

Preparations

Dispersible tablet 300 mg.

Indications

Adults with ischaemic chest pain.

Cautions
- Asthma
- Pregnancy
- Kidney or liver failure
- Gastric or duodenal ulcer.

Contraindications
- Known hypersensitivity
- Children under 16 years
- Patients with known clotting disorders (e.g. haemophilia).

Side-effects
- Gastric irritation and bleeding
- Bronchospasm in some asthmatics.

Administration
Place on the tongue and chew or dissolved in water and drink.

Dose
300 mg single dose.

Atropine
Main prehospital use
Management of asystolic cardiac arrest and symptomatic bradycardia (heart rate <60). No longer recommended for routine use in asystole or PEA.

Other uses
Organophosphate poisoning.

Action
- Blocks vagal (parasympathetic) tone – blocks effect of vagus nerve at sinoatrial and atrioventricular nodes, thus increasing sinus automaticity and facilitating AV node conduction
- Reduces likelihood of VF triggered by hypoperfusion associated with extreme bradycardia.

Preparations
- 10 mL disposable syringe with 1 mg (100 µg/mL)
- 5mL disposable syringe with 1 mg (200 µg/mL)
- 10 mL disposable syringe with 3 mg (300 µg/mL)
- 1 mL ampoule with 600 µg/mL.

Indications

1. Symptomatic bradycardia associated with any of:
   - Shock
   - Syncope
   - Myocardial Ischaemia
   - Heart failure
2. Heart rate <60 and any indication of high risk of asystole:
   - Recent asystole
   - Mobility II AV block
   - Complete heart block with wide QRS
   - Ventricular pauses >3 seconds
3. Organophosphate poisoning.

Cautions

Give cautiously to avoid tachycardia post-myocardial infarction (increases myocardial oxygen demand and worsens ischaemia).

Contraindications

Bradycardia associated with hypothermia.

Side-effects

- Dilation of pupils and blurred vision
- Dry mouth
- Urine retention
- Confusion
- Tachycardia.

Administration

IV

Dose

- 0.5–3 mg IV for symptomatic bradycardia or high risk of asystole
- Children, 20 µg/kg (maximum cumulative dose 0.1 mg, minimum 100 µg)
- Organophosphate poisoning, 2 mg IV repeated as required until skin becomes flushed and dry, pupils dilate and tachycardia develops.

Benzylpenicillin

Benzylpenicillin is one of the penicillin group of drugs. It interferes with bacterial cell wall production and kills a range of bacteria which include those commonly responsible for meningococcal septicaemia and meningitis. Although the most important side-effect of benzylpenicillin is an allergic reaction, very few patients are at risk of anaphylaxis. Many patients think that they may be allergic to penicillin because of transient rashes or an episode of diarrhoea. If a patient is suspected of having meningococcal septicaemia, only a genuine (proven) history of penicillin allergy should stop benzylpenicillin being given.

Main prehospital use

The treatment of meningococcal septicaemia.

Other uses

None prehospital.

Action

Bactericidal by interfering with bacterial cell wall synthesis.

Preparations

Ampoule containing 600 mg of penicillin G (benzylpenicillin) in powder form.

Indications

- Meningococcal septicaemia
- Meningitis.

Cautions

- Previous side-effects after penicillin
- Renal impairment.

Contraindications

Genuine penicillin allergy.

Side-effects

- Rare in context of severe infection
- Hypersensitivity reactions (e.g. urticaria)
- Anaphylaxis (rare)
- Convulsions in high doses
- Hypotension (due to action of drug in releasing toxins. Manage with IV fluid challenges).

Administration

IV or IM.

Dose

Dissolve each 600 mg in 10 mL sterile water for IV use, and 2 mL sterile water for IM use. Give:

- Adult and child older than 9 years – 1200 mg (20 mL IV, 4 mL IM)

- Child 1–9 years – 600 mg (10 mL IV, 2 mL IM)
- Infant – 300 mg (5 mL IV, 1 mL IM).

Chlorpheniramine

Chlorpheniramine is used as a second-line drug in the management of anaphylactic reactions, and as the first-line treatment of less severe allergic reactions, such as severe itching.

Main prehospital use

Management of anaphylactic and allergic reactions.

Other uses

None in the prehospital setting.

Action

Chlorpheniramine blocks the action of histamine released as part of the body's response to allergens.

Preparation

10 mg/mL, 1 mL ampoule.

Indications

- Severe anaphylactic reactions (after administration of adrenaline)
- Allergic reactions causing distress (e.g. severe itching).

Cautions

- Hypotension
- Epilepsy
- Glaucoma
- Hepatic disease.

Contraindications

- Hypersensitivity
- <1 year of age.

Side-effects

Hypotension if administered rapidly.

Administration

Slow IV injection over 1 minute.

Dosage
- Adult >12 years 10 mg
- Child 6–12 years 5 mg
- Child 1–5 years 2.5 mg.

Compound sodium lactate (hartmann's/ ringers lactate)
Main prehospital uses
Fluid replacement therapy.

Other uses
None.

Action
As an infusion, transiently increases intravascular volume.

Preparations
- 500 and 1000 mL bags
- 5 and 10 mL ampoules.

Indications
- Status asthmaticus (to limit formation of dry mucous plugs)
- Hypovolaemic shock in the absence of a radial pulse
- Burns
- Anaphylaxis
- Hyperthermia
- Dehydration.

Cautions
None.

Contraindications
- Hyperglycaemic ketoacidosis
- Crush injury.

Side-effects
- Fluid overload in patients with uncontrolled haemorrhage can cause clot disruption and increased bleeding
- Fluid overload causing heart failure (particularly in the elderly)
- Exacerbation of pre-existing acidosis.

Administration

IV infusion or bolus.

Dose

Adults with dehydration, status asthmaticus, hyperthermia:

- Give 500 mL infusion in 20 minutes repeated to effect (maximum dose 2000 mL).

  Children with dehydration, status asthmaticus, hyperthermia:

- Give 20 mL/kg bolus repeated once to effect.

Adults and children with hypovolaemic shock or burns, see Figure 10.1.

Do *not* give compound sodium lactate to patients with crush syndrome.

Diazepam

Diazepam is the benzodiazepine that has been most commonly used in the management of seizures and status epilepticus. It is ideally given intravenously in someone who is actively fitting at the scene or is having repeated fits. It is given IV as the emulsion Diazemuls to reduce the risk of venous thrombophlebitis. Rectal diazepam is given when IV access cannot be obtained.

Main prehospital use

Management of seizures.

Other uses

Cocaine toxicity.

Action

CNS depressant and anticonvulsant.

Preparations

- Rectal tubes containing 5 mg or 10 mg
- 2 mL ampoule (diazepam emulsion) containing 10 mg (5 mg/mL).

Indications

Prolonged or repeated seizures such as may occur in:

- Status epilepticus
- Convulsions secondary to infections

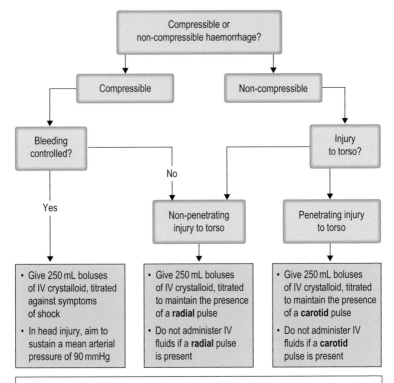

Figure 10.1 Intravenous fluid therapy in hypovolaemic shock, burns and crush injury.

Notes:

- For isolated burns >25% body surface area and/or >1 hour from hospital, give a 1 litre crystalloid fluid challenge (500 mL for child 10–15 years; 250 mL for child 5–10 years; no fluids under 5 years)
- For crush syndrome without significant non-compressible haemorrhage, give 2 litres of n/saline IV prior to extrication, followed by 1.5 litres of n/saline per hour (20 mL/kg boluses in children)

- Alcohol withdrawal seizures
- Convulsions due to poisoning
- Eclampsia
- Head injury (rule out hypoxia).

Symptomatic cocaine toxicity

- Severe hypertension
- Chest pain
- Fitting.

Cautions

- Respiratory disease/depression
- History of drug or alcohol abuse
- Reduce dose in elderly and debilitated
- Facilities for ventilatory support should be immediately available
- Consider doses previously administered by carers
- Use of CNS depressants.

Contraindications

- Known hypersensitivity
- Respiratory failure.

Side-effects

- Respiratory depression (especially with opioids and alcohol)
- Apnoea
- CNS depression and loss of consciousness
- Cardiovascular depression and postural hypotension
- Amnesia.

Administration

- IV through a large proximal vein at a rate of 3 mg/min
- Rectal via a tube which should be inserted no more than 2 cm in children and 3–4 cm in adults (tubes have markers)
- Rectal tubes should be held in place for a few moments after expelling the contents and the patient's buttocks held together to reduce seepage from the rectum.

Dose

If a single dose of diazepam has been given rectally, the second dose may be given IV.

Table 10.1 Diazepam dosage per age		
Age (years)	**IV**	**Rectal**
>12	10 mg, repeated once	10 mg repeated once
6–12	300 µg/kg	10 mg repeated once
1–5	300 µg/kg	5 mg repeated once
<1	300 µg/kg	2.5 mg repeated once

Entonox

Nitrous oxide is an anaesthetic gas, which is rapidly absorbed by inhalation. A mixture of nitrous oxide and oxygen containing 50% of each gas (Entonox) is used in prehospital care to gain rapid control of pain without loss of consciousness. It is administered by the casualty via a demand valve. Slow, deep breaths are required. The casualty must be conscious, cooperative and have sufficient respiratory excursion to operate the demand valve. Nitrous oxide is extremely soluble and will diffuse rapidly into any gas-filled cavity; it may thus increase the size of a pneumothorax. At temperatures below $-7°C$, nitrous oxide may liquefy and the oxygen and nitrous oxide will separate. The patient may then inhale pure oxygen followed by pure nitrous oxide. It is not adequate to simply shake the cylinder in these situations. Cylinders need to be kept at temperatures above freezing.

Main prehospital use

Rapid control of pain
May be used whilst preparing to give opiates.

Action

Anaesthetic agent.

Preparations

A mixture of 50% nitrous oxide and 50% oxygen in a blue cylinder with a white shoulder.

Indications

Acute pain.

Cautions

- Chest injuries
- Head injuries

- Cold weather
- Alcohol/drug intoxication
- Sickle cell crisis
- >50% oxygen indicated.

Contraindications

- Pneumothorax
- Gastrointestinal obstruction
- Recent diving activity
- Reduced Glasgow coma scale (GCS)
- Disturbed psychiatric patients.

Side-effects

- Decreased level of consciousness
- Nausea and vomiting
- Confusion ± distress.

Administration

Inhalation via demand valve with onset of action within 3–5 minutes.

Dose

As required to relieve pain.

Epinephrine (adrenaline)

Epinephrine is a sympathomimetic drug which stimulates both a and β receptors. a receptor activity increases peripheral vascular resistance without constricting coronary and cerebral vessels. This raises systolic and diastolic pressures during CPR, which makes CPR more effective; β receptor activity increases myocardial contractility in cardiac arrest and relieves bronchospasm in acute severe asthma. Epinephrine also reverses the allergic manifestations of acute anaphylaxis. If epinephrine has already been self-administered by the patient (e.g. EpiPen 0.3 mg for adults or 0.15 mg for children), this should be taken into account when determining the timing and dosage for administration.

Main prehospital use

- Cardiac arrest
- Acute anaphylaxis
- Life threatening asthma with failing ventilation and continued deterioration despite nebuliser therapy.

Other uses

Nebulised in severe croup.

Action

- Increases heart rate
- Increases blood pressure
- Increases myocardial contraction force
- Bronchodilation
- Vasoconstriction.

Preparations

- 10 mL disposable syringe with 0.1 mg/mL (1:10 000)
- 1 mL disposable syringe or ampoule with 1 mg/mL (1:1000).

Indications

- Cardiac arrest
- Acute anaphylaxis
- Severe croup.

Cautions

Hypothermia (give single dose only).

Contraindications

None in cardiac arrest.

Side-effects

- Tachycardia
- Angina and arrhythmias
- Hypertension
- Anxiety
- Headache.

Administration

- IV, IM, intraosseous, nebulised or subcutaneous
- IV administration is far better in cardiac arrest
- IM administration should be used in anaphylaxis.

Dose

- In cardiac arrest, 1 mg (10 mL of 1:10 000) every 3–5 minutes
- In children, initial dose 0.01 mg/kg IV (0.1 mL/kg of 1:10 000) repeated every 3–5 minutes. Use 0.1 mg/kg via ET tube (0.1 mL/kg of 1:1000) in children if IV or IO access cannot be gained quickly. This is the least satisfactory route. In anaphylaxis, if stridor, wheeze, respiratory distress, upper airway or oral swelling or hypotension are present:

- Adults (>12 years of age) 500 micrograms (0.5 mg) IM (0.5 mL of 1:1000) repeated after 5 minutes if necessary (halve dose in prepubertal children)
- Child 6 years – <12 years 250 micrograms IM (0.25 mL of 1:1000) repeat after 5 minutes if necessary
- Child 6 months–<6 years 120 micrograms IM (0.12 mL of 1:1000) repeat after 5 minutes if necessary
- Child <6 months 50 micrograms (0.05 mL of 1:1000) repeat after 5 minutes if necessary.
  In *severe* croup:
  - 1 mg (1 mL of 1:1000 diluted to 5 mL with normal saline) via nebuliser.

Frusemide (Furosemide)

Furosemide is a potent loop diuretic with a rapid onset used in pulmonary oedema due to left ventricular failure. IV administration produces rapid relief of breathlessness.

Main prehospital use

Acute left ventricular failure.

Action

- Reduces preload
- Inhibits reabsorption from the ascending limb of the loop of Henle in the kidney.

Preparations

- 5 mL ampoule with 50 mg (10 mg/mL)
- 2 mL ampoule with 40 mg (20 mg/mL)
- Minijet containing 80 mg in 8 mL (10 mg/mL).

Indications

Pulmonary oedema due to left ventricular failure.

Cautions

- Patients with long-standing heart failure
- Pregnancy
- Hypokalaemia.

Contraindications

- Liver failure with pre-comatose state
- Renal failure with anuria.

Side-effects
- Hypotension
- GI disturbance.

Administration
Slow IV injection over 2 minutes.

Dose
- 40 or 50 mg initially
- Repeat to a maximum of 120 mg (3 × 40 mg) or 100 mg (2 × 50 mg).

Glucagon

Glucagon is an alternative to IV glucose in hypoglycaemia. It increases plasma-glucose concentration by mobilising glycogen stored in the liver. It is therefore less effective in hypoglycaemia associated with malnutrition and chronic illness. It can be injected IM in a dose of 1 mg (1 unit) in circumstances when IV glucose would be difficult or impossible to administer. Note that IV glucose is the preferred treatment.

Main prehospital use
Treatment of hypoglycaemia.

Other uses
Poisoning with ß-blockers.

Action
- Breaks down glycogen (a reserve form of glucose found in the liver and other tissues)
- Increases heart rate
- Increases myocardial contractility.

Preparations
Vial with 1 mg powder for reconstitution with sterile water.

Indications
- Blood glucose level is <3.0 mmol/L *or*
- Suspected hypoglycaemia where oral glucose cannot be administered *or*
- Unconscious patient, where hypoglycaemia cannot be excluded.

Cautions

- Starvation and malnutrition (ineffective)
- Adrenal insufficiency
- Chronic alcoholism (ineffective).

Contraindications

None.

Side-effects

- Nausea and vomiting
- Hypersensitivity reactions.

Administration

- IM
- The IV route should *not* be used because it is associated with nausea and vomiting.

Dose

- 1 mg in adult and child over 20 kg, 0.5 mg in children under 20 kg, age <1 month 100 µg
- If not effective in 10 minutes, IV glucose should be given
- Any patient receiving glucagon must be given oral carbohydrates when they are fully conscious. If this is not possible the patient must be hospitalised as blood sugar levels will fall significantly.

Glucose

Main prehospital use

Hypoglycaemic states.

Action

Reverses hypoglycaemia.

Preparations

500 mL bags of 10% (100 mg/mL) glucose solution.

Indications

- Blood glucose level <3.0 mmol/L *or*
- Suspected hypoglycaemia where oral glucose cannot be administered *or*
- Unconscious patient, where hypoglycaemia cannot be excluded.

Cautions

Use large-bore cannula in largest available vein to minimise risk of thrombo-phlebitis.

Contraindications

None.

Side-effects

Tissue necrosis following extravasation.

Administration

IV via a large-bore, free-flowing proximal vein.

Dose

- 5 mL/kg of 10% glucose solution in children (max. 50 mL bolus at once)
- 50 mL of 10% glucose solution (5 g) in adults repeated at 5 minute intervals to effect.

Glyceryl trinitrate

Glyceryl trinitrate may be given as tablets to be dissolved under the tongue (sublingual), modified-release tablets to be dissolved inside the lip (buccal) or as an aerosol spray. The spray has a much longer shelf-life and is therefore more often carried by patients with angina for use when they have symptoms. It is one of the most effective drugs for rapid relief of angina.

Main prehospital uses

Management of ischaemic chest pain associated with acute coronary syndromes
Acute cardiogenic pulmonary oedema.

Other uses

None in the prehospital setting.

Action

Vasodilator which dilates coronary arteries and reduces cardiac preload by dilating systemic veins.

Preparations

- Sublingual tablets, 300 µg
- Aerosol spray, 400 µg/metered dose
- Modified-release buccal tablets 2 mg and 5 mg (Suscard).

Indications

- Cardiac chest pain due to angina and myocardial infarction
- Severe breathing difficulty due to left ventricular failure (acute cardiogenic pulmonary oedema).

Cautions

None.

Contraindications

- Hypotension – do not give if systolic BP <90 mmHg
- Concomitant use of Viagra (sildenafil) or similar drugs. Risk of profound hypotension – do not give within 24 hours
- Hypovolaemia
- Head trauma
- Cerebral haemorrhage.

Side-effects

- Postural hypotension (remove tablet and flush mouth with water)
- Headache
- Flushing
- Dizziness
- Tachycardia.

Administration

Sublingual or buccal.

Dose

- Sublingual tablet, 300 µg repeated as required
- Aerosol, 1–2 sprays under the tongue or into the open mouth, and then close the mouth. Repeat after 5 minutes if required
- Buccal tablet, 2 mg between gum and inner cheek replaced by 5 mg if symptoms not relieved in 3–5 minutes.

HEPARIN (unfractionated heparin)

Main prehospital uses

Given with thrombolytic agents in ST segment elevation myocardial infarction to prevent thrombus reforming (thrombolytic agents are also platelet activators).

Other uses

None in the prehospital setting.

Action

Heparin is a short-acting anticoagulant.

Preparations
1000 units/mL, 5 mL ampoule.

Indications
Immediately following administration of tenecteplase or first bolus of reteplase.

Cautions
- Hepatic and renal impairment
- Pregnancy.

Contraindications
- Haemophilia and other bleeding disorders
- Thrombocytopenia
- Peptic ulcer
- Recent cerebral haemorrhage
- Severe hypertension
- Recent major trauma or surgery
- Recent spinal or epidural anaesthesia
- Hypersensitivity to heparin.

Side-effects
- Haemorrhage
- Skin necrosis
- Thrombocytopenia
- Hyperkalaemia
- Hypersensitivity reactions.

Administration
IV bolus.

Dose
- With Tenecteplase: 4000 units
- With Reteplase: 5000 units.

> A Patient Group Directive is required for paramedics to administer heparin.

Hydrocortisone

Hydrocortisone is administered to help prevent the response to secondary mediators in anaphylaxis of severe asthma. Although its onset of action may be delayed by several hours, it should be given as a second-line treatment in prehospital care to avoid unnecessary delays.

Main prehospital use
- Severe/life-threatening asthma
- Anaphylaxis.

Other uses
None in prehospital care.

Action
Limits the effect of secondary mediators (such as kinins) and atopic response.

Preparations
Ampoule with 100 mg in 1 mL.

Indications
- Severe or life-threatening asthma
- Anaphylaxis.

Cautions
None for these indications/doses.

Contraindications
Allergy to the diluent.

Side-effects
- Burning or itching sensation in the groin
- Hypotension if administered quickly.

Administration
Slow IV injection over 2 minutes.

Dose
- Adult/child >12 years 200 mg
- Child 1 month–12 years 4 mg/kg
- Child <1 month 2.5 mg/kg.

Hypostop
Hypostop is a 40% glucose gel containing 23 g of glucose per dose.

Main prehospital use
Management of conscious hypoglycaemic patients able to cooperate and with intact swallow and gag reflexes.

Other uses

None.

Action

Reverses hypoglycaemia.

Preparations

Box containing three single dose tubes of 40% glucose (23 g per tube).

Indications

- Hypoglycaemia in conscious cooperative patients with intact swallow and gag reflexes
- May be used following glucagon administration when GCS is normal.

Cautions

None.

Contraindications

Reduced level of consciousness.

Side-effects

- Aspiration
- Airway obstruction.

Administration

Smear on to gums for most rapid effect.

Dose

Titrated to effect against blood glucose measurements – no upper limit, but if ineffective use 10% glucose IV.

Ipratropium bromide

Main prehospital uses

- Management of acute severe or life-threatening asthma in adults
- Management of acute asthma unresponsive to β2 agonist therapy in children
- Management of acute exacerbations of COPD.

Other uses

Short-term relief of chronic reversible airways obstruction.

Action

Ipratropium is an antimuscarinic (atropine-like) drug that causes bronchodilation.

Preparations

Ipratropium bromide nebuliser solution presented in vials of 250 µg in 1 mL or 500 µg in 2 mL.

Indications

- Life-threatening asthma in adults (mix with first dose of salbutamol)
- Acute severe asthma in adults (mix with first dose of salbutamol)
- Acute exacerbation of COPD in adults that is unresponsive to the first dose of salbutamol (mix with second dose of salbutamol)
- Acute episode of asthma in children that is unresponsive to the first dose of salbutamol (mix with second dose of salbutamol).

Cautions

- Glaucoma (protect patient's eyes from nebuliser mist)
- Prostatic hyperplasia and bladder outflow obstruction.

Contraindications

None.

Side-effects

- Dry mouth
- Nausea
- Headache
- Acute angle-closure glaucoma (see Cautions, below)
- Constipation
- Tachycardia and atrial fibrillation (rare)
- Paradoxical bronchospasm (rare).

Administration

Via nebuliser.

Dose

- Adults and children >5 years: 500 µg, once only
- Children 1–5 years: 250 µg once only
- Infants (<1 year): 125 µg once only.

Lidocaine (lignocaine)

Lidocaine is a local anaesthetic drug used in the management of wide-complex tachycardia and ventricular fibrillation. It is effective in suppressing ventricular tachycardia and reducing the risk of ventricular fibrillation (especially after myocardial infarction). It has not been shown to reduce mortality when used prophylactically in myocardial infarction.

Main prehospital use

Treatment of refractory VF, pulseless VT, or symptomatic VT (Amiodarone is now the preferred treatment).

Other uses

Local anaesthetic.

Action

- Suppresses ventricular ectopic activity and decreases ventricular automaticity
- Raises threshold for VF (by depressing conduction in ischaemic areas or improving conduction in normal areas)
- Slows conduction of impulses through the Purkinje system
- Raises defibrillation threshold.

Preparations

10 mL disposable syringe containing 100 mg (10 mg/mL).

Indications

- Ventricular fibrillation or pulseless VT refractory to three shocks especially after myocardial infarction, if amiodarone is not available
- Symptomatic ventricular tachycardia.

Cautions

Reduce dose in congestive cardiac and liver failure.

Contraindications

- Patients in heart block
- Premature ventricular contraction with bradycardia
- SBP <90 mmHg (VT with a pulse)
- Known allergy
- If amiodarone has already been administered.

Side-effects
- Central nervous system toxicity with confusion, nausea, vomiting, drowsiness, seizures
- Dizziness and paraesthesia (if injection too rapid)
- Hypotension and bradycardia.

Administration
IV and intraosseous.

Dose
- VF/pulseless VT, 100 mg IV bolus, repeated once if necessary.

Metoclopramide
Metoclopramide is an antiemetic drug which is currently used to reduce the risk of nausea and vomiting following intravenous morphine and to treat severe nausea and vomiting.

Main prehospital use
Reduce risk of nausea and vomiting following administration of morphine sulphate.

Action
- Central effects on chemoreceptor trigger zone
- Peripheral effects on gut.

Preparations
2 mL ampoule with 10 mg (5 mg/mL).

Indications
- Nausea or vomiting in adults
- Concomitant administration with morphine sulphate and other opiates.

Cautions
- Hepatic and renal impairment
- Elderly.

Contraindications
- Avoid in first 12 weeks of pregnancy

- Renal failure
- Patients under age of 20
- Gastrointestinal obstruction
- Phaeochromocytoma.

Side-effects
- Acute dystonic reactions with facial and skeletal muscle spasms. These are more common in the young (especially girls and young women) and the very old.
- Drowsiness
- Rarely, cardiac dysrhythmias.

Administration
- IV over 2 minutes or IM
- Monitor ECG, pulse and BP before, during and after administration.

Dose
10 mg.

Morphine sulphate

Morphine sulphate is the standard opioid analgesic against which all others are judged. It is used for the treatment of severe pain including myocardial infarction, major limb injuries or burns. It produces sedation and euphoria as well as its analgesic effect. Onset of action is within 2–3 minutes if given intravenously with the peak effect in 10–20 minutes. In medical cases, smaller doses may be effective (2.5–5 mg), whereas in injured patients, much larger doses may be needed to achieve effective analgesia.

Prehospital use of opioids has been shown to be safe and effective when used appropriately and titrated to effect according to pain scores. Nevertheless, prehospital practitioners must be able to recognise and deal with the three most important side-effects: respiratory depression, systemic vasodilation and nausea and vomiting. Naloxone should always be available whenever opioids are used.

Morphine is a controlled drug under Schedule 2 of the Misuse of Drugs Regulations 1985. It must be stored and its use documented in accordance with these regulations.

Main prehospital use
Severe pain associated with myocardial infarction, fractures and burns, and other causes.

Other uses
Left ventricular failure.

Action

Acts on µ opioid receptors in the spinal cord and brain.

Preparations

1 mL ampoule with 10 mg (10 mg/mL).

Indications

Severe pain.

Cautions

- Recent alcohol use
- Respiratory depression/disease
- Chest injuries
- Hypotension
- Elderly and debilitated
- Antidepressant use
- Pregnancy.

Contraindications

- Acute respiratory depression (adult <10 bpm)
- Coma or impaired level of consciousness (GCS <12)
- Infants <1 year
- MAOIs
- Phaeochromocytoma
- Hypersensitivity
- Hypotension:SBP
- Adults <90 mmHg
- 5–16 years <80 mmHg
- 1–4 years <70 mmHg.

Side-effects

- Respiratory depression
- Cardiovascular depression
- Nausea and vomiting
- Pupillary constriction.

Administration and dose

- Adults: IV bolus of 2.5–5 mg followed by 1 mg increments titrated against pain score over 10 minutes. Give further 5 mg increments at 5 minute intervals, titrated to effect (max. dose 20 mg)

- Best achieved by diluting 10 mg (1 mL) in 9 mL of water or 0.9% saline to make a 1 mg/mL solution
- Children: use 10 mg in 10 mL solution to administer 0.05 mg/kg (0.05 mL/kg) over 2–3 minutes. Repeat dose at 5–10 minute intervals titrated to effect (max. dose 0.2 mg/kg).

Naloxone

Naloxone is the specific antidote to opioid-induced coma or respiratory depression. Since naloxone has a shorter duration of action than many opioids, close monitoring and repeated injections are necessary according to the respiratory rate and depth of coma.

Main prehospital use

Reversal of respiratory depression associated with opioid excess.

Action

- Competitive antagonist at opioid μ receptors
- In the context of opioid excess, will increase respiratory rate and level of consciousness.

Preparations

1 mL ampoule with 400 μg.

Indications

- Reversal of opioid-induced respiratory, cardiovascular and CNS depression
- Overdose with opioids and opioid-containing medicines
- Unconsciousness associated with respiratory depression or arrest where opiate or opioid overdose is a possibility.

Cautions

- Pain
- Short duration of action
- May precipitate a withdrawal syndrome in those dependent on opiates
- May precipitate fits in patients with epilepsy.

Contraindications

- Known hypersensitivity
- Neonates with opioid-dependent mother.

Side-effects

- Nausea and vomiting
- Tachycardia
- Withdrawal symptoms in opioid dependency.

Administration

- IV or IM
- Where rapid reversal is undesirable (e.g. acute pain or risk of withdrawal), then dilute 2 mL (0.8 mg) in 8 mL of water or 0.9% saline and titrate to effect.

Dose

- 0.4 mg repeated every 2–3 minutes up to a maximum of 10 mg in adults
- 0.01 mg/kg in children followed once by 0.1 mg/kg
- 0.1 mg (0.25 mL) in neonates IM once only.

Patients who are opioid-dependent are at risk of absconding on recovery. Because IV naloxone has shorter half-life than most opioids, respiratory depression may recur. Consider giving a 'depot' IM injection of 0.8 mg in this group before any IV dose.

Normal saline

Main prehospital uses

Fluid replacement.

Other uses

- Flush to keep intravenous cannula patent
- Flush to 'push' IV drugs into the circulation.

Action

As an infusion, transiently increases intravascular volume.

Preparations

- 500 and 1000 mL bags
- 5 and 10 mL ampoules.

Indications

- Hyperglycaemic ketoacidosis
- Hypovolaemic shock in the absence of a radial pulse
- Burns
- Crush injury
- Anaphylaxis
- Hyperthermia
- Dehydration
- Post-cannulation flush
- Post-IV drug administration flush.

Cautions

None.

Contraindications

None.

Side-effects

- Fluid overload in patients with uncontrolled haemorrhage can cause clot disruption and increased bleeding
- Fluid overload causing heart failure (particularly in the elderly).

Administration

IV infusion or bolus.

Dose

- As a post-drug flush: 10–20 mL (adults and children)
- As a post-cannulation flush: 2 mL (adults and children)
- Adults with dehydration, status asthmaticus, diabetic ketoacidosis, hyperthermia:
    Give 500 mL infusion in 20 minutes repeated to effect (maximum dose 2000 mL)
- Children with dehydration, status asthmaticus, diabetic ketoacidosis, hyperthermia:
    Give 20 mL/kg bolus repeated once to effect
- Adults and children with hypovolaemic shock, burns, or crush injury.

Oxygen

Regardless of whether a patient is known to have COPD, if they are acutely unwell (pulse oximetry under 90% on room air or low respiratory rate, severe dyspnoea and abnormal respiratory pattern), they should be given high-concentration oxygen via a non-rebreathing mask with a flow rate set at 10–15 L/min.

Main prehospital use

Supplemental oxygen in trauma and acute medical emergencies.

Action

- Essential component of the chemical reaction that occurs in all cells and supports life
- Combines with glucose to liberate energy and carbon dioxide.

Preparations

- Oxygen cylinders are black with a white shoulder
- New light-weight cylinders do not follow this convention.

Indications

- Hypoxia from any cause
- Cardiorespiratory arrest
- Significant trauma
- Pulmonary disease.

Cautions

Patients with COPD.

Contraindications

Paraquat poisoning.

Side-effects

- Respiratory depression in COPD
- Dry mouth.

Administration

Inhalational via non-rebreathing or fixed concentration masks.

Dose

- 100% (in practice approximately 85%) via non-rebreathing reservoir masks usually 10–15 L/min: A sufficient flow rate should be used to keep the reservoir bag inflated in all acutely hypoxic or injured patients
- 24–40% via fixed flow mask in patients with COPD who are not acutely hypoxic (may require more to maintain pulse oximetry in the region of 88–92%).

Paracetamol

Paracetamol is a simple and safe pain-relieving and temperature-reducing drug, which is widely available. In prehospital emergency care, administration of paracetamol in children can control pain and rapidly reduce temperature.

Main prehospital use

Pain relief and temperature control in children.

Action

Simple analgesic and antipyretic (temperature-reducing) drug.

Preparations

Syrup containing 120 mg/5 mL of solution or 250 mg/5 mL of solution. 500 mg tablets.

Indications

- Mild to moderate pain
- Pyrexia.

Cautions

Hepatic and renal impairment.

Contraindications

- Paracetamol overdose
- Previous administration. Within 4 hours or maximum. Cumulative dose given.

Side-effects

Rare.

Administration

Orally as a single dose using a 5 mL syringe without needle or a measuring spoon.

Dose

- 3 months–1 year: 60–125 mg (repeat at 4 hourly intervals to max. 500 mg)
- 1–5 years: 120–250 mg (max. dose in 24 hours = 1 g)
- 6–12 years: 250–500 mg (max. dose in 24 hours = 2 g)
- Adult: 1 g (max. dose in 24 hours = 4 g).

Each dose repeated every 4–6 hours as necessary (max. 4 doses in 24 hours).

Salbutamol

Salbutamol is used in the management of uncontrolled, acute severe and life-threatening asthma and other causes of reversible airways obstruction.

Main prehospital use

Treatment of acute asthma.

Other uses

Bronchospasm from any other cause (COPD, anaphylaxis, LVF).

Action

- Sympathomimetic
- Selective ß2-adrenoreceptor stimulant which reverses bronchospasm.

Preparations

- Nebules containing either 2.5 mg or 5 mg
- Metered dose inhaler (various doses).

Indications

- Acute asthma attack where normal inhaler therapy has failed to relieve symptoms
- Wheezing associated with allergy, anaphylaxis or smoke inhalation
- Exacerbation of COPD
- Second-line treatment for LVF.

Cautions

- Hypertension
- Angina
- Hyperthyroidism
- Late pregnancy.

Contraindications

None.

Side-effects

- Tremor
- Palpitations
- Tachycardia
- Headache
- Peripheral-vasodilation.

Administration

Inhaled as nebulised solution or as an aerosol via a spacer device if the patient has one.

Dose

- Adults and children >5 years: 5 mg via nebuliser repeated to effect or side-effects are intolerable

- 12 months–5 years: 2.5 mg repeated to effect at 15 minute intervals
- <12 months: 2.5 mg once only.

In severe or life-threatening asthma, continuous nebulisation is required.

Syntometrine

Oxytocic (uterus-stimulating) drugs are used to minimise blood loss from the placental site during the routine management of the third stage of labour. The combination of ergometrine 500 µg with oxytocin 5 units is given by IM injection with or after delivery of the shoulders.

Main prehospital use

Management of third stage of labour.

Other uses

- Postpartum haemorrhage within 24 hours of delivery
- Control of bleeding in incomplete miscarriage.

Action

Stimulates contraction of the uterus within 7 minutes of IM injection.

Preparations

1 mL ampoule containing ergometrine 500 µg and oxytocin 5 units.

Indications

- Active management of the third stage of labour
- Following delivery of the placenta to prevent or treat postpartum haemorrhage
- Control of bleeding in incomplete miscarriage.

Cautions

- Cardiac disease
- Hepatic and renal impairment.

Contraindications

- Known hypersensitivity
- First or second stage of labour
- Severe cardiac, liver or kidney disease
- Hypertension
- Eclampsia/pre-eclampsia

- Multiple pregnancy (fetus still *in utero*).

Side-effects

- Nausea and vomiting
- Abdominal pain
- Headache
- Hypertension
- Cardiac arrhythmias (bradycardia)
- Chest pain
- Anaphylactic reactions (rare).

Administration

IM with or after delivery of the shoulders.

Dose

1 mL.

Tenecteplase and reteplase

Tenecteplase and reteplase are thrombolytic drugs which are indicated for myocardial infarction due to their ability to break up thrombus and permit return of blood supply. The benefits of treatment must be considered to outweigh the risks (hence the specific indications and contraindications given below). Trials have shown that the benefit is greatest in those with ECG changes that include ST segment elevation (especially in those with anterior infarction) and in those with *new* bundle brand block.

Main prehospital use

Treatment of acute myocardial infarction with pain of >15 minutes and <6 hours duration.

Other uses

None prehospital.

Action

Activates the fibrinolytic system, inducing the breaking up of intravascular thrombi and emboli.

Preparations

Tenecteplase

Powder for reconstitution 40 mg (8000 units), or 50 mg (10 000 units).

Reteplase
Powder for reconstitution 10 units to be dissolved in 10 mL of water for injection
   Both with prefilled syringe of water for injection.

Indications

- Acute myocardial infarction, where pain has been present continuously for at least 15 minutes and less than 6 hours
- Patient must fulfill all JRCALC guideline criteria
- JRCALC criteria for paramedic-administered thrombolysis (version 3).

Primary assessment

1. Can you confirm that the patient is conscious, coherent and able to understand that clot-dissolving drugs will be used?
2. Can you confirm that the patient is aged 75 or less?
3. Can you confirm that the patient has had symptoms characteristic of a heart attack (i.e. continuous pain in a typical distribution and of 15 minutes duration or longer)?
4. Can you confirm that the symptoms started less than 6 hours ago?
5. Can you confirm that the pain built up over seconds and minutes rather than starting totally abruptly?
6. Can you confirm that breathing does not influence the severity of the pain?
7. Can you confirm that the heart rate is between 50 and 140 bpm?
8. Can you confirm that the systolic blood pressure is more than 80 mmHg and less than 160 mmHg and that the diastolic blood pressure is below 110 mmHg?
9. Can you confirm that the electrocardiogram shows abnormal ST segment elevation of 2 mm or more in at least two standard leads or in at least two adjacent precordial leads, not including V_1 (ST elevation can sometimes be normal in V_1 and V_2)?
10. Can you confirm that the QRS width is 0.16 mm or less, and that left bundle branch block is absent from the tracing? (*Note*: RBBB permitted only with qualifying ST segment elevation.)
11. Can you confirm that there is NO atrioventricular block greater than 1st degree? (If necessary after treatment with IV atropine.)

Secondary assessment

12. Can you confirm that the patient is not likely to be pregnant, nor has delivered within the last 2 weeks?
13. Can you confirm that the patient has not had a peptic ulcer within the last 6 months?
14. Can you confirm that the patient has not had a stroke of any sort within the last 12 months and does not have permanent disability from a previous stroke?

15. Can you confirm the patient has no diagnosed bleeding tendency; has had no recent blood loss (except for normal menstruation); and is not taking warfarin (anticoagulant) therapy?
16. Can you confirm the patient has not had any surgical operation, tooth extractions, significant trauma, or head injury within the last 4 weeks?
17. Can you confirm that the patient has not been treated within the last 3 months for any other serious head or brain condition? (This is intended to exclude patients with cerebral tumours.)
18. Can you confirm that the patient is not being treated for liver failure, renal failure, or any other severe systemic illness?

Contraindications

Does not meet JRCALC guideline criteria.

Side-effects

- Elevation of body temperature
- Nausea and vomiting
- Haemorrhage, including stroke
- Hypotension
- Reperfusion arrhythmias
- Anaphylaxis (rare)
- Allergic responses including urticarial rash and low back pain.

Administration

- Tenecteplase: slow IV bolus
- Reteplase: slow IV bolus repeated after 30 minutes.

Dose

Tenecteplase

Single intravenous dose according to the patient's weight

- <60 kg 6000 μ
- 60–69 kg 7000 μ
- 70–79 kg 8000 μ
- 80–89 kg 9000 μ
- >90 kg 10 000 μ

Reteplase

10 units repeated exactly 30 minutes later.

Tetracaine 4% gel (AMETOP)

Main prehospital uses

Use to provide local anaesthesia prior to non-urgent venepuncture.

Other uses

None in the prehospital setting.

Action

Local anaesthetic agent designed to penetrate intact skin to provide local numbing prior to venepuncture.

Preparations

1.5 g tubes of white semitransparent gel.

Indications

Patient requiring non-urgent venepuncture after 30–45 minutes and at risk of distress from the procedure.

Cautions

Check for allergy to occlusive dressing of choice.

Contraindications

- Venepuncture required in less than 30–45 minutes
- Do not apply to open wounds, broken skin, lips mouth, eyes, ears, anal or genital region or mucous membranes
- Known allergy to tetracaine, any of its constituents or other local anaesthetic agents. Infants less than 1 month old
- Pregnancy or breast-feeding.

Side-effects

- Inappropriately rapid absorption from mucous membranes, wounds or inflamed tissue
- Hypersensitivity reactions.

Administration

Topical application at proposed venepuncture site(s). Cover with transparent occlusive dressing. Wait for 30–45 minutes before removing dressing and cream and attempting venepuncture.

Dose

- Apply sufficient cream to cover intended venepuncture site(s)

For further information, see Ch. 10 in *Emergency Care: A Textbook for Paramedics*.

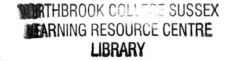

CHAPTER 11

Respiratory emergencies

Respiratory emergencies are a frequent part of the workload of a pre-hospital clinician. The following definitions are important in managing patients with respiratory problems:

- Hypoxaemia – inadequate oxygenation of the blood
- Hypoxia – inadequate oxygenation of the body
- Hypercarbia – high level of carbon dioxide in the blood, leads to acidaemia
- Acidaemia – where the blood becomes excessively acid (low pH), the body's immediate response is to increase the respiratory rate (tachypnoea)
- Tachypnoea – a raised respiratory rate (usually >30 breaths/min)
- Hyperventilation – excessive breathing rate. In the absence of acidaemia will cause symptoms such as tingling around the lips and carpo-pedal spasm (seen in panic attacks).

Asthma

Approximately 1000 people die in the UK each year from this condition, so never underestimate the severity of an asthma attack. Individuals susceptible to other atopic disorders such as eczema, are more prone to developing asthma. There also appears to be a familial element.

Generalised airway obstruction is caused by:

- Inflammation of the airway passages, leading to oedema and swelling
- Increased production of thick mucus, leading to plugging of bronchioles
- Generalised bronchial smooth muscle constriction, leading to bronchospasm.

Precipitating causes of an acute exacerbation of asthma include:

- Exercise

- Infection
- Allergy to drugs or other substances
- Emotional upset.

Be especially cautious with patients who have a previous history of near-fatal asthma, with previous hospital admission or even a previous stay on intensive care for their asthma. These patients are sometimes referred to as 'brittle' asthmatics.

> Life-threatening deterioration of an asthma attack may be very rapid.

Use of the peak flow meter

The patient's peak expiratory flow rate (PEFR) is a useful predictor of the severity of an attack, particularly if the patient knows the value of their usual/normal PEFR. A predicted PEFR can be calculated if necessary, although the patient or parent (if the patient is a child) will often know it.

Table 11.1 Features of severe asthma	
Adults	**Children**
Cannot complete sentences	Cannot talk or feed
Pulse >110 bpm	Pulse >140 bpm
Respiratory rate ≥25 breaths/min	Respiratory rate >50 breaths/min
Peak flow rate 33–50% of predicted	

In rare cases, asthmatic patients develop spontaneous pneumothorax as a result of a ruptured bulla (lung cyst). They may also develop subcutaneous emphysema in the neck and anterior chest wall.

The differential diagnosis of a severe asthma attack includes pulmonary oedema, anaphylaxis, pneumothorax and airway obstruction.

> Beware the asthma patient with a silent chest.

Management of asthma

- Maintain an air of calm
- Take a rapid history, including recent episodes and current treatment
- If the patient is unable to give a history, do not delay transfer to hospital
- Measure a PEFR if possible
- If severe or life-threatening features are present, or the patient does not respond to treatment, then warn the receiving hospital of your impending arrival.

Patients with severe or life-threatening asthma may not appear distressed or have all of these features. Make the diagnosis if any feature is present.

Table 11.2 Features of life-threatening asthma

Adults	Children
Exhaustion	Reduced conscious level
Cyanosis	Agitation
Bradycardia	Cyanosis
Hypotension	Silent chest
Silent chest	Coma
Peak flow <33% of predicted	
Coma	
SpO_2 <92% on air/95% on oxygen	
Reduced respiratory effort	

Prehospital treatment of severe and life-threatening asthma

The aim of emergency treatment is to reverse hypoxia with oxygen and reduce bronchospasm using β2-adrenoreceptor agonists. Oral or intravenous steroid therapy has no effect for at least 4 hours.

Adults

- Oxygen, high flow via a reservoir mask (10–15 L/min)
- Salbutamol 5 mg via an oxygen-driven nebuliser, repeated as necessary
- Intravenous access (consider crystalloid infusion if dehydrated)
- Hydrocortisone 200 mg IV
- ECG monitoring
- Immediate evacuation to hospital.

If the asthma is severe or life-threatening, ipratropium 0.5 mg should be added to the nebuliser.

Children

- Oxygen, high flow via a reservoir mask (10–15 L/min)
- Salbutamol 5 mg via an oxygen-driven nebuliser (the dose should be halved in children under 6 years old), repeated as necessary
- Intravenous access (consider crystalloid infusion if dehydrated)
- Hydrocortisone 200 mg IV
- ECG monitoring
- Immediate evacuation to hospital.

If the attack is severe or life-threatening, ipratropium 0.25 mg should be added to the nebuliser (0.125 mg in children under 1 year).

Unnecessary time should not be lost, in either adults or children, while intravenous access is obtained.

Transport to hospital

It is essential that time is not wasted in repeatedly attempting to perform clinical interventions that are not going according to plan. If problems are encountered, the patient should be immediately transferred to hospital. All of the above procedures can be carried out in the back of a moving ambulance. It is important to be prepared to intubate the patient if respiratory arrest occurs; airway pressures are likely to be high and ventilation will therefore be difficult. Cardiac arrest may ensue and the standard protocols should be followed.

Paramedics are well placed to deal with severe and life-threatening asthma, but they must act with speed and foresight to ensure a satisfactory outcome.

Pulmonary oedema

Pulmonary oedema is usually caused by acute left ventricular failure (LVF) and is common in the elderly. Heart failure leads to fluid collection in the alveoli of the lungs. The causes of 'pump failure' include:

- Acute myocardial infarction
- Dysrhythmias
- Antiarrhythmic drug overdose
- Inadequate heart rate (β-blocking drugs or post-infarction)
- Chronic valvular heart disease (usually aortic or mitral valve)
- Cardiac tamponade
- Fluid overload.

Symptoms of pulmonary oedema

- Breathlessness on exertion
- Paroxysmal nocturnal dyspnoea (waking at night with severe shortness of breath)
- Orthopnoea (breathlessness on lying down)
- Wheeze and cough are often reported
- Acute respiratory distress
- Coughing up pink froth or blood
- Chest pain may be present if an acute MI is the underlying cause.

Signs of pulmonary oedema

- Anxiety
- Pale, cold, clammy patient

- Cyanosis, tachypnoea, tachycardia
- Hypotension
- ECG monitoring may reveal an MI or a dysrhythmia
- Auscultation of the chest may reveal fine crepitations or a wheeze.

Management of pulmonary oedema

Treatment is aimed at improving oxygenation, reducing the volume of blood returned to the left ventricle and treating the underlying cause. Definitive treatment of acute pulmonary oedema requires hospital admission.

- Sit the patient up. This is vital and often forgotten
- Take a rapid history, noting the patient's current medication
- Give high flow oxygen via a reservoir mask
- If systolic blood pressure is >90 mmHg, then give two puffs of glyceryl trinitrate (GTN) spray under the patient's tongue
- Obtain intravenous access and give IV frusemide (a diuretic)
- Put the patient on ECG monitoring (treat any life-threatening dysrhythmia promptly)
- Consider morphine and Aspirin 300 mg if chest pain is present
- Transfer the patient to hospital
- Take a 12-lead ECG recording *en route*.

Anaphylaxis

- Anaphylaxis is an acute hypersensitivity (allergic) reaction to foreign protein (the allergen)
- Reactions worsen with repeated exposures to the allergen
- Common protein allergens include: antibiotics (particularly the penicillins), insect stings, shellfish, strawberries and nuts (e.g. peanuts)
- Colloid intravenous fluids (such as Hemaccel and Gelofusine) are rare causes of anaphylaxis
- The allergen is often never identified
- Some patients carry their own adrenaline for self-administration (such as the EpiPen®).

Allergic responses vary in severity, from a simple urticarial rash ('nettle rash') to a full-blown acute anaphylactic reaction with cardiorespiratory arrest. The speed of onset is variable and patients with marked sensitivity can progress to a severe reaction in a matter of minutes.

Symptom progression in anaphylaxis

- Urticarial rash ('nettle rash')
- Itchy skin
- Running eyes and nose
- Swelling of the face, eyes and lips, and occasionally the tongue
- Laryngeal oedema leading to airway obstruction

- Bronchospasm
- Tachycardia
- Tachypnoea
- Hypotension (shock)
- Cardiac arrest.

Management of anaphylaxis

- Try to reassure the patient and keep them calm
- Establish the history and if possible, the precipitating cause
- Oxygen 100%, 15 L/min via a reservoir mask, should be administered
- Establish intravenous access and give IV crystalloid fluids rapidly according to the patient's requirements and local protocols
- If bronchospasm is present, this should be treated as asthma (see above)
- Hydrocortisone 200 mg IV (children 4 mg/kg) and chlorpheniramine 10 mg IV should be given.

Adrenaline

Severe cases must be treated with adrenaline 1:1000, 0.5 mL IM immediately. It may be necessary to repeat this. Airway obstruction must be treated promptly with basic and advanced techniques, and if necessary a surgical cricothyroidotomy.

Table 11.3 Paediatric doses of adrenaline solutions (1:1000 contains 1 mg/mL)

Age	Adrenaline 1:1000 (mL)
<6 months	0.05
6 months–5 years	0.12
6–11 years	0.25
>12 years	0.5

Paediatric doses of adrenaline should be drawn up in small volume syringes and must be double checked with another practitioner before use. *Note*: Anaphylaxis is extremely rare in patients under the age of 2 years.

Chronic obstructive pulmonary disease

- Chronic obstructive pulmonary disease (COPD) was previously referred to as chronic obstructive airways disease (COAD) and includes chronic bronchitis and emphysema
- Chronic bronchitis is defined as the production of sputum for at least 3 months each year in two consecutive years. It causes obstruction by

plugging the airways (bronchioles) with mucus, and by inflammation and thickening of the airway mucosa

- Emphysema is the dilation of alveolar airspaces by the destruction of their walls. The elastic recoil that holds the airways open in expiration is lost and obstruction to airflow occurs
- The main cause of COPD is smoking, although some cases are attributable to a rare inherited enzyme (α1-antitrypsin) deficiency
- The majority of patients demonstrate features of both bronchitis and emphysema
- Patients often present with recurrent pneumonias (lower respiratory tract infections)
- Patients with COPD rely on hypoxia as their drive to breathe because their respiratory centre, driven by a high carbon dioxide concentration in people without this condition, becomes relatively insensitive to carbon dioxide due to chronic exposure to elevated levels
- Patients often have wheeze, an element of their disease that may respond to the use of nebulisers.

Management of COPD

Patients with acute exacerbations of COPD are hypoxic. Emergency treatment is aimed at general supportive measures and relief of hypoxia. Rapid transport to hospital is mandatory. The preemptive siting of an IV cannula may be helpful in case of cardiorespiratory arrest.

> HYPOXIA KILLS.

Patients with acute respiratory decompensation need supplemental oxygen. However, it is potentially dangerous to give supplemental oxygen to these patients unless they are carefully observed and the paramedic is prepared to assist ventilation if required. It is possible that administering oxygen will raise the oxygen concentration in the blood (PO_2) to a level at which the hypoxic drive is switched off, resulting in hypoventilation or apnoea. Patients can be verbally instructed to take additional breaths and can be assisted with a bag and mask with oxygen reservoir if necessary. The risk of shutting off hypoxic drive can be minimised by adjusting oxygen delivery to maintain SpO_2 at the patient's usual level or at 90–92% if unknown.

> NEVER WITHHOLD OXYGEN FROM A PATIENT WHO NEEDS IT.

Patients who die, do so from hypoxia, either because oxygen therapy is withheld or because practitioners fail to identify and support ventilation when the hypoxic drive is lost.

- HYPOXIA KILLS QUICKLY
- HYPERCARBIA KILLS SLOWLY

So give oxygen and support ventilation if the 'hypoxic drive' is lost.

If the patient has a wheeze, then give salbutamol 5 mg via nebuliser, repeated to effect. Mix 500 mg ipratropium with first dose of salbutamol.

For further information, see Ch. 11 in *Emergency Care: A Textbook for Paramedics.*

CHAPTER 12

The cardiovascular system and the ECG

Blood

The normal circulating blood volume is variable, but in a 70 kg adult it is about 5 L (equivalent to about 70 mL/kg body weight).

Table 12.1 Circulating blood volume in relation to age	
Age group	**Blood volume (mL/kg body weight)**
Adult	70
Child	80
Neonate	90

Cardiac cycle

- The adult human heart beats about 70 times/min at rest
- One heartbeat within a single cardiac cycle therefore lasts about 0.8 seconds or 800 milliseconds (ms)
- The phase of contraction is called systole, the phase of relaxation is called diastole.

Cardiac output

Cardiac output is defined as the volume of blood ejected by each ventricle per minute. Cardiac output is calculated by multiplying the heart rate by the stroke volume (volume ejected per heart beat).

Cardiac output = stroke volume × heart rate

Stroke volume

Three factors determine stroke volume:

1. Preload – the filling of the heart during diastole
2. Afterload – the resistance in the arterial circulation against which the heart has to pump
3. Contractility – the intrinsic performance of the heart muscle at a given preload and afterload.

Regulation of heart rate

- Heart rate <60 bradycardia
- Heart rate >100 tachycardia.

The parasympathetic system, via the vagus nerve, slows the heart rate down. Atropine blocks the vagus nerve thereby increasing the heart rate.

The sympathetic nervous system tends to speed heart rate up and β-blocking drugs (e.g. propranolol or atenolol) prevent tachycardia by blocking the sympathetic nerves.

Adrenaline and noradrenaline are released from the adrenal glands and increase both heart rate and contractility.

Blood pressure

Blood pressure is determined by the cardiac output and the peripheral vascular resistance. The vascular resistance will fall in conditions such as severe anaphylaxis.

Table 12.2 Normal blood pressure in healthy, young adults

	Normal blood pressure		
	(mmHg)	(kPa)	Range
Systolic	120	16	±10%
Diastolic	80	11	±10%

Electrocardiography

The ECG gives information about the electrical activity of the heart and can predict problems such as myocardial infarction. It does not enable any conclusions to be made about mechanical activity of the heart such as force of contraction or blood pressure.

Electrocardiograms are conventionally recorded from 12 leads. This is achieved by placing electrodes on the right arm, left arm and left leg, as well as six electrodes in predefined locations on the chest and a ground reference on the right leg. The position of these leads is described in degrees clockwise from lead I (0°); thus lead aVF is 90°, lead III is 120° and lead aVR is 210°. It is apparent, therefore, that leads II, III and aVF 'look at' the undersurface of the heart – these are the inferior leads. Lead aVL 'looks at' the heart from 'above' (i.e. from the left shoulder).

ECG recording paper

- The ECG machine, or the printer of a defibrillator or ECG monitor, runs with a paper speed of 25 mm per second
- The graph paper is divided into small squares of side 1 mm. A large square consists of five small squares and measures 5 mm × 5 mm
- At the standard paper speed, each small square (1 mm) represents 0.04 seconds and each large square (5 mm) represents 0.20 seconds
- The amplitude of the electrical impulse is indicated along the vertical axis. A 10 mm deflection (two large squares) represents a 1 mV electrical signal provided that the ECG machine is properly calibrated.

- The horizontal axis of the ECG trace is time
- One small square equals 0.04 seconds
- One large square equals 0.20 seconds.

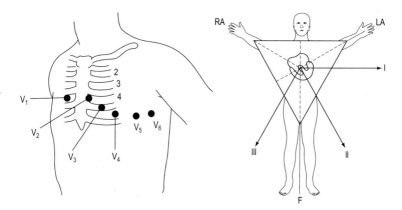

Figure 12.1 Chest and limb lead placement.

Components of the ECG

P wave

The P wave represents depolarisation of the atria and in lead II is a small positive (upward) deflection which precedes each QRS complex.

QRS complex

The QRS complex represents depolarisation of the ventricles. It consists of one or more waves.

- R wave: any positive deflection
- Q wave: any negative deflection preceding an R wave
- S wave: any negative deflection following an R wave.

The duration of a normal QRS complex is less than 0.12 seconds (less than three small squares) in adults. The height or amplitude is variable from 2 mm to 15 mm. The QRS complex in lead II usually shows a large positive (upward) R wave.

T wave

The T wave represents repolarisation of the ventricles and is positive (upright) in lead II. Its duration is variable (0.10–0.25 second) and its amplitude is less than 5 mm.

PR interval

The PR interval represents the time it takes for an electrical impulse generated in the SA node to reach the ventricles via the AV node and bundle branches.

The PR interval begins with the onset of the P wave and terminates at the onset of the QRS complex. The duration of the PR interval is normally 0.12–0.20 seconds (3–5 small squares). A normal PR interval indicates that no conduction delay has occurred between the SA node through the AV node and bundle of His.

ST segment

The ST segment represents the interval between ventricular depolarisation and repolarisation of the ventricles. It stretches from the end of the S wave or QRS complex to the beginning of the T wave. Normally, the ST segment is flat or identical with the isoelectric line.

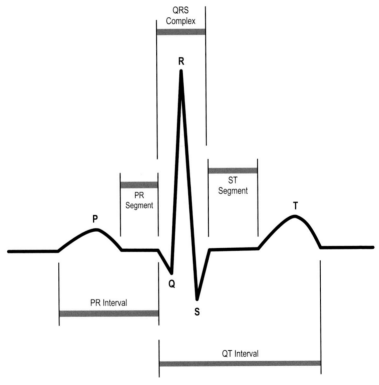

Figure 12.2 The P wave and QRS complexes and the PR interval.

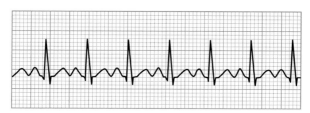

Figure 12.3 Sinus tachycardia.

Systematic analysis of the ECG

Step 1: Determine the heart rate

The heart rate is most easily calculated by dividing 300 by the number of large squares between two consecutive R waves of QRS complexes, the RR interval.

Step 2: Determine the heart rhythm

The heart rhythm is determined by comparing the length of several RR intervals on a sufficiently long strip of the ECG trace. The heart rhythm is regular if the distances between R waves counted in large or small squares are equal. Irregular rhythms can be either 'regularly irregular' or 'irregularly irregular'. The latter describes a rhythm where the QRS complexes occur in totally haphazard fashion.

Step 3: Analyse the P waves

In sinus rhythm, there is a P wave before each QRS complex. In atrial fibrillation, P waves are absent. In atrial flutter the P wave rate is about 300/min and appears as a 'saw-tooth' pattern. If there are more P waves than QRS complexes, an atrioventricular block may be present.

Step 4: Analyse the QRS complex

The QRS complex may exhibit up to three waveforms (see above) and normally lasts less than three small squares or 0.12 second. If the QRS duration is greater than this, conduction through the ventricle is abnormally slow, either because one of the bundles of His is not functioning or because the origin of depolarisation is within the ventricle.

Step 5: Measure the PR interval

If the PR interval is less than 0.12 seconds (three small squares), the electrical impulse has not progressed from the atria to the ventricles via the normal conduction pathway. A prolonged PR interval, greater than 0.2 seconds (five small squares), occurs in 'first-degree' heart block.

Step 6: Analyse the T wave

A normal T wave is upright and oriented in the same direction as the R wave of the QRS complex in that lead. Inversion of the T wave may indicate that an acute myocardial infarction has occurred in the past or that the myocardium is currently ischaemic. The T wave appears tall and symmetrically peaked if the patient has a high serum potassium level (hyperkalaemia).

Step 7: Analyse the ST segment

ST segment abnormalities are seen in acute coronary syndromes, pericarditis, ventricular hypertrophy and as an effect of some drugs (e.g. digoxin). Elevation of the ST segment can signify an acute myocardial infarction, especially if it is greater than two small squares above the isoelectric line. An ST segment depression can occur in acute cardiac ischaemia but should only confidently be diagnosed on a 12-lead ECG. In terms of treatment, ST segment elevation is particularly important because it is an indication for administration of thrombolytic therapy or conveying for primary angioplasty in cases of suspected acute myocardial infarction.

Analysis of rhythm

Heart rhythms can be divided into three groups:
1. Normal sinus rhythm
2. Slow rhythms (bradyarrhythmias)
3. Fast rhythms (tachyarrhythmias).

Sinus rhythm

Sinus rhythm is defined as a rhythm where each P wave is followed by a QRS complex, with an equal number of P waves and QRS complexes.

Tachycardias

Any rhythm with a rate exceeding 100 beats/min is a tachycardia. Such rhythms can be simply described in terms of their regularity and the width of the QRS complex. The warning signs of an immediately life-threatening tachycardia include:

- Chest pain
- Systolic blood pressure <90 mmHg
- Unconsciousness
- Signs of heart failure.

If these warning signs are seen, apply advanced life support treatment and consider the need for defibrillation.

Box 12.1 **Summary of tachycardias**

Narrow complex and regular (supraventricular tachycardia – SVT)

- Sinus tachycardia (causes: anxiety, blood loss, fever, pain)
- True atrial tachycardia
- AV nodal reentrant (junctional) tachycardia
- Atrial flutter with fixed AV relationship (e.g. 2:1, 3:1 conduction)
- AV re-entrant tachycardia (accessory pathway).

Narrow complex and irregular

- Atrial fibrillation (no P waves, increasingly common with age)
- Atrial flutter with variable conduction (saw-tooth appearance of P waves)
- Frequent atrial ectopic beats.

Broad complex and regular

- Any cause of SVT with co-existing bundle branch block
- Ventricular tachycardia (check your patient!).

Broad and irregular

- Atrial fibrillation with bundle branch block
- Polymorphic ventricular tachycardia (torsades de pointes).

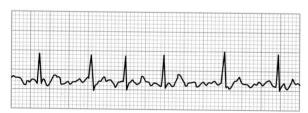

Figure 12.4 Atrial fibrillation.

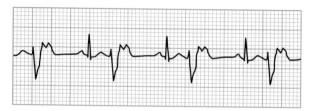

Figure 12.5 Ventricular ectopic beats.

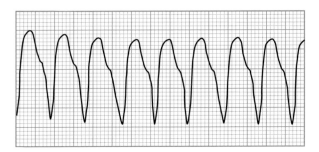

Figure 12.6 Ventricular tachycardia.

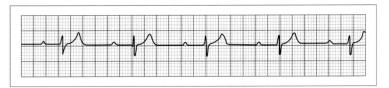

Figure 12.7 First-degree heart block.

Bradycardia and heart block

- Sinus bradycardia occurs when the pulse is less than 60 bpm, but the ECG is otherwise normal
- When sinus rhythm is present but the PR interval is longer than 0.2 seconds, it is termed first-degree heart block. Treatment is rarely required
- If some waves of atrial depolarisation fail to be transmitted to the ventricles, second-degree heart block has occurred. Because atrial depolarisation has occurred normally, the P wave is normal whether or not it is followed by a QRS complex
- Second-degree (Mobitz) type I heart block (also known as the Wenckebach phenomenon) occurs when there is progressive prolongation of the PR interval, until a P wave occurs without a following QRS complex
- Alternatively, the PR interval may remain constant with occasional depolarisations failing to transmit to the ventricles. The missed (or dropped) beat may be regular (e.g. every third or fourth beat) or irregular (random). This is (Mobitz) type II second-degree heart block. This is a more significant abnormality and may progress to complete heart block or ventricular standstill. Causes include ischaemia, fibrosis of the AV node, connective tissue disorders and some drugs

- The most serious form of heart block is third-degree or complete heart block. The ventricular rhythm and pulse, are slow and usually regular. P waves and QRS complexes appear independently on the ECG, with some P waves hidden by QRS complexes. Because there is no relationship between the electrical activity of the atria and the ventricles, this is also known as complete atrioventricular dissociation.

For further information, see Ch. 12 in *Emergency Care: A Textbook for Paramedics.*

CHAPTER 13

Assessment and monitoring

Colour

- Pallor: very pale appearance, best visualised in the conjunctivae or the mouth. Usually a sign of anaemia but may also be seen in vasoconstriction due to hypotension, hypothermia or severe pain
- Flushing or redness of the skin is caused by vasodilation and may be a sign of fever, extreme exertion or superficial burns
- Cyanosis refers to bluish-grey discolouration of skin or mucous membranes caused by an excess of deoxygenated haemoglobin:
    Central cyanosis – imperfect oxygenation of the blood by the lungs or where deoxygenated blood bypasses the lungs for example in congenital heart defects.
    Peripheral cyanosis – where slow blood flow leads to increased deoxygenation of the haemoglobin in the peripheries. May be a normal finding for example in patients who are cold.

Pulse

- In the collapsed patient, palpate for a pulse at the carotid or the femoral artery
- The brachial pulse is recommended for palpation in cardiac arrest in infants
- Consider the rate, strength and character of the pulse
- Heart rate can also be documented by the ECG or the pulse oximeter.

Respiratory rate

- Always measure the respiratory rate in breaths per minute
- Neonates have the highest normal respiratory rate and it falls progressively up to the adult range of 12–18 breaths/minute

- A rapid respiratory rate is known as *tachypnoea*. Rates >30 breaths/minute are usually a sign of serious illness
- Conscious patients may be using their accessory muscles of respiration, e.g. in severe asthma
- A low respiratory rate is *bradypnoea*, sometimes caused by opiate use
- Some patients with heart failure, neurological disease or drug intoxication demonstrate varying respiratory rate and depth known as *Cheyne–Stokes respiration.*

Blood pressure

- Accurate blood pressure measurement is important and allows successive readings to be compared to allow monitoring of the patient's progress and response to treatment
- Most portable monitors now provide automatic blood pressure monitoring
- Anaeroid sphygmomanometers are used if electronic devices fail or are unavailable
- Where possible the patient should be seated comfortably, with the upper arm at the level of the heart
- The cuff must be correctly sized to the patient – small cuffs for children and large cuffs for the obese adult
- The ideal size of cuff is equal in width to approximately two-thirds of the length of the upper arm
- The blood pressure cuff is applied to the upper arm, in the absence of intervening clothing. Most modern cuffs have a method of indicating the correct position of the cuff over the brachial artery
- Portable monitors usually allow the interval between blood pressure measurements to be adjusted depending on the patient's requirements
- Systematic errors are often seen when the pulse is irregular, such as in atrial fibrillation.

Intra-arterial blood pressure monitoring

Intra-arterial measurement is performed when continuous monitoring of arterial pressure is required, most often in the operating theatre or intensive therapy unit. A catheter is inserted directly into an artery and the pressure wave is monitored by a transducer connected to the catheter. Such intra-arterial monitoring lines may be *in situ* when a patient is transferred between hospitals; paramedics should be aware of their presence and clarify any precautions necessary during the journey with the appropriate staff.

Pulse oximetry

- Pulse oximetry is the most convenient non-invasive method of monitoring arterial oxygen saturation and is presented in percentage terms

- Oxygenated and deoxygenated haemoglobin absorbs or attenuates differing wavelengths of light. The probe emits rapid bursts of red light which are picked up by a photodetector on the other side of the probe
- The probe can be used on any digit or earlobe or especially in children, the forehead
- Pulsatile blood flow is required so reading may be difficult if the patient is shocked or peripherally shut-down
- Rapid fluctuations in ambient light levels may produce false signals and movement during patient transport may also cause inaccurate readings. Other causes of inaccurate readings include:
  - Poor circulation
  - Fluctuating light levels
  - Carbon monoxide poisoning
  - Skin, dirt and grease
  - Nail varnish (dark and metallic colours only)
- Carbon monoxide poisoning may cause a pulse oximeter to overestimate the true oxygen saturation: the pulse oximeter will measure the total percentage saturation of haemoglobin with oxygen (oxyhaemoglobin) and carbon monoxide (carboxyhaemoglobin)

Box 13.1 **Arterial oxygen saturation values on air**	
Normal range:	97–100%
Mild hypoxia:	90–97%
Moderate hypoxia:	85–90%
Severe hypoxia:	<85%

- The relationship between arterial oxygen tension (PaO_2) and arterial oxygen saturation is described by the oxyhaemoglobin dissociation curve

> Pulse oximetry does not measure carbon dioxide.

- Because pulse oximetry cannot measure carbon dioxide levels, it does not give a complete picture of ventilation. Inadequate ventilation may give rise to hypercarbia in the present of normal oxygen saturations
- Anaemia or blood loss will not be picked up by pulse oximetry. The patient may have lost a significant proportion of their blood volume but they can continue to have 100% oxygen saturation of the haemoglobin that is left.

Electrocardiographic monitoring

Electrocardiographic (ECG) monitoring is undertaken to define the cardiac rhythm. Accurate rhythm monitoring and interpretation are especially important in the management of cardiac arrest. Manual defibrillators and cardiac monitors feature a screen for displaying the cardiac rhythm and usually incorporate an arrangement for obtaining a printout of the ECG. Automated external defibrillators (AEDs) often store the ECG electronically and a hard copy is obtained from the appropriate playback device. Many cardiac monitors incorporate a heart rate meter which is triggered by the QRS complex of the ECG. An alarm will sound automatically should the heart rate fall outside preset limits; lights and audible signals may also provide additional indications of the heart rate.

Monitoring electrodes

- ECG monitoring requires the attachment of adhesive electrodes to the patient's chest
- The monitor will interpret the signals to provide records that approximate to leads I, II or III of the conventional ECG
- Lead II normally allows for the best evaluation of the P wave and QRS complex
- Occasionally, hair will need to be shaved to allow electrode placement
- Muscle movement will create artefact waveforms – keep the patient warm and ask the patient to remain still
- Monitoring can be achieved through adhesive defibrillation pads to allow prompt treatment of VT or VF. The monitor/defibrillator may require changing from displaying the monitor leads to the defibrillator pads and vice versa.

Diagnosis from cardiac monitors

The printout of the ECG should be inspected carefully to diagnose the cardiac rhythm and retained for transfer to the patient's records on arrival at hospital. The time when the trace is recorded is essential information and should be added manually at the start of the record if this is not done automatically by the monitor. It is also good practice to write on the printed rhythm strip other relevant clinical information such as symptoms or blood pressure. Some monitors allow this information to be entered electronically.

Defibrillators

During defibrillation sufficient electrical energy is delivered to the surface of the chest to enable a current of electricity to depolarise a critical mass of the fibrillating myocardium, in the hope that orderly cardiac depolarisation ensues. Most defibrillators deliver a predetermined energy, measured in joules (J).

'Hands-free' defibrillation via adhesive pads is now standard across all models.

Types of defibrillator:
- Manual
- Semi-automatic (advisory)
- Fully automated.

- **Manual Defibrillators:** the operator interprets the cardiac rhythm, decides whether a defibrillatory countershock is required, charges the machine and administers the shock. Experience in ECG interpretation is required and training in the use of such devices is therefore more prolonged
- **Semi-automatic defibrillator:** the processes of rhythm recognition and charging for defibrillation are automated. All that is required of the operator is to recognise that cardiac arrest may have occurred, to attach two electrodes to the patient's chest and to follow the instructions from the defibrillator if these seem appropriate. During the analysis period (which in most models is less than 10 seconds), no contact must be made with the patient to avoid the chance of movement artefact. Many models incorporate written on-screen instructions and some models also feature synthesised voice instructions to guide the operator
- **Automated external defibrillators** (AED) are accurate in the interpretation of shockable rhythms and only rarely is a DC shock advised inappropriately. An override key can be used to convert an automated external defibrillator into a manual one.

All prehospital defibrillators will run off batteries. Monitors that incorporate blood pressure monitoring will tend to use battery power quicker. Batteries should always be checked at the beginning of a shift and spares should be carried where possible. Biphasic defibrillators use less power and achieve more successful defibrillation. These are gradually replacing the older monophasic devices. Lower energy requirements are sometimes recommended – consult the manufacturer's instructions.

Defibrillator safety

- It is essential that no part of the operator or any assistant is in electrical contact with the patient when the shock is administered
- The operator must shout 'Stand clear! Shocking!' and visually check that no person is touching the patient
- Intravenous fluid giving sets may act as a potential conductor and helpers should not be holding these while a shock is administered
- Defibrillation in the rain is normally safe, providing the chest is wiped dry first

- Patients lying in a pool of water should be moved before defibrillation and the carers must ensure they are not connected to the patient by standing in water
- Nitrate patches should be removed to reduce the risk of them igniting and causing severe burns
- Any oxygen source (e.g. bag-valve-mask) should be removed from the patient before administering each shock
- Patients with pacemakers should still be defibrillated – however, do not place the adhesive pad directly over the pacemaker box.

For further information, see Ch. 13 in *Emergency Care: A Textbook for Paramedics*.

CHAPTER 14

Cardiac arrest in adults: Advanced life support

The chances of surviving an out of hospital cardiac arrest are 1:100. The paramedic has two challenges:

1. To recognise and intervene appropriately in the care of the critically ill patient in order to prevent a cardiac arrest occurring
2. To respond promptly and skillfully to patients in cardiac arrest in order to optimise their chance of survival.

Defining cardiac arrest

- Cardiac arrest may be defined as the absence of a palpable pulse in an unresponsive patient. The pulse check is an unreliable sign if used in isolation from the clinical setting
- Lay rescuers are no longer taught to use a pulse check to verify cardiac arrest. Instead, they start chest compressions if there are no signs of circulation (such as normal breathing, coughing or movement)
- Paramedics should not rely solely on the pulse check to diagnose cardiac arrest, but should look for other indicators that the circulation has failed.

Cardiac arrest rhythms

Electrocardiogram (ECG) monitoring in cardiac arrest will establish the initial rhythm, which will be one the following:

> Box 14.1 **Risk factors for cardiac arrest**
>
> - Obstructed airway
> - Myocardial infarction, unstable angina
> - Peri-arrest arrhythmia
> - Status asthmaticus
> - Status epilepticus
> - Uncontrolled haemorrhage
> - Anaphylaxis.

1. Ventricular fibrillation (VF)
2. Pulseless ventricular tachycardia (VT)
3. Asystole
4. Pulseless electrical activity (PEA).

For treatment purposes, these rhythms are divided into:

- Shockable (VF/pulseless VT)
- Non-shockable (PEA or asystole).

The initial rhythm of a patient in cardiac arrest will determine which treatment algorithm is used first.

Chain of survival

The aim is a return of spontaneous circulation (ROSC). Factors that are likely to result in a successful ROSC are:

1. Immediate basic life support including effective CPR. This means the patient stays in a shockable rhythm for longer
2. Fast defibrillation. Automatic external defibrillators are increasingly available in public areas for this reason
3. Early advanced life support. Successful intubation, oxygen and adrenaline will improve patient outcomes
4. Transfer to hospital. The underlying cause needs to be identified and treated.

The advanced life support approach

- SAFE approach
- Establish unresponsiveness
- Open the airway

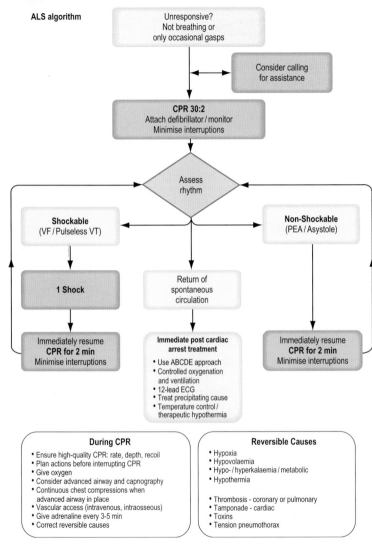

Figure 14.1 The adult advanced life support algorithm (Resuscitation Council UK). The authors are aware of impending changes in resuscitation guidelines (late 2010). Refer to: www.resus.org.uk for further up-to-date information.

- Assess breathing
- Attach monitor and assess the circulation.

Continue CPR with as few interruptions as possible. If good-quality bystander CPR is in progress, then encourage them to continue until the paramedic team is ready to take over. Apply defibrillating gel pads immediately to identify a shockable rhythm.

Once the patient is confirmed to be in cardiac arrest, he should be treated according to the initial rhythm.

Shockable (VF or pulseless VT)

Precordial thump

If a cardiac arrest is witnessed and monitored then a precordial thump may be administered. It should not delay, however, calling for help or accessing a defibrillator. This is equivalent to a low-energy defibrillatory shock and may revert a patient in the early stages of VF or VT to a perfusing rhythm. The thump should be given in the normal position for chest compression from a height of approximately 20 cm above the chest, using a closed fist.

Defibrillation

- VT without cardiac output will rapidly degenerate into ventricular fibrillation
- Defibrillation is the same for both conditions
- Success is greatest if a shock is applied within the first 90 seconds of the arrest
- Chances of successful defibrillation decline by about 10% per minute thereafter
- Single shocks are delivered and CPR is continued for 2 minutes. Only after one cycle (2 minutes) are checks made for a cardiac output. This is because even after successful defibrillation the heart will not function effectively for the first minute (myocardial stunning/cardiac standstill).

Adrenaline

- Adrenaline is the first-line drug in cardiac arrest in the UK. In cardiac arrest, its greatest effect is through peripheral vasoconstriction which raises the systemic vascular resistance, hence increasing cerebral and coronary perfusion during CPR
- When treating VF/VT cardia arrest, adrenaline 1 mg is given once chest compressions have restarted after the third shock
- 1 mg doses should be administered IV every other cycle (every 3–5 minutes), preferably not at the exact same time as a defibrillation shock
- Adrenaline can be administered by the intraosseous route if peripheral cannulation is unsuccessful
- Higher doses of adrenaline are not recommended.

Amiodarone

- If three unsuccessful shocks have been administered and the patient remains in VF or pulseless VT, then amiodarone should be given
- Amiodarone 300 mg IV bolus followed by a 20 ml IV flush whilst performing CPR
- A further dose of 150 mg IV can be given for recurrent or refractory VF/VT followed by an in-hospital infusion of 900 mg over 24 hours
- Do not abandon resuscitation in the face of VF/VT as these are potentially reversible.

Non-shockable (PEA/asystole)

The management of a PEA or asystolic cardiac arrest shifts from rapid defibrillation to undertaking good quality CPR, endotracheal intubation and intravenous adrenaline while seeking to identify and treat any reversible causes of the cardiac arrest. Adrenaline is administered every 3–5 minutes.

Pulseless electrical activity

- PEA may be defined as the presence of an ECG trace compatible with but not producing any detectable cardiac output
- Consider the four 'Hs' and the four 'Ts' (see below).

Asystole

- Asystole tends to be the terminal stage of primary cardiac arrest
- When asystole is secondary to other causes such as respiratory arrest or drug intoxication, the prognosis may be more favourable
- The diagnosis of asystole is confirmed by the presence of an almost flat ECG trace in a pulseless patient
- A rapid check must be made to confirm that:
  1. The leads are connected correctly
  2. The defibrillator is set to read through the leads
  3. The chest electrodes remain attached
  4. The amplitude setting (gain) on the monitor has not been set too low.
- Fine VF should be managed as for non-VF/VT. A shock is likely to be unsuccessful at this stage but good quality CPR may improve the amplitude of the ventricular fibrillation.

Reversible causes of cardiac arrest

There are a number of potentially reversible causes of cardiac arrest which should be excluded or identified whenever possible, especially in patients with non-VF/VT rhythms.

- These include the four 'Hs':
  - Hypoxia
  - Hypovolaemia
  - Hypothermia
  - Hypo/hyperkalaemia, hypocalcaemia, acidaemia, and other metabolic disorders
- and the four 'Ts':
  - Tension pneumothorax
  - Cardiac Tamponade
  - Thromboembolics (pulmonary or coronary)
  - Toxic (drug overdose or intoxication).

Resuscitation in special circumstances

Hypothermia

Severe hypothermia may cause significant bradycardia and reduced respiratory effort. Patients with a core temperature <30°C are unlikely to respond to defibrillation.

Distinguish patients in cardiac arrest due to hypothermia from those that have died and subsequently become cold. Do not declare hypothermic patients

---

Box 14.2 **Treatable causes of cardiac arrest**

Hypoxia
- **Recognition:** Obstructed airway, severe asthma, drowning
- **Treatment:** Endotracheal intubation and ventilation with high-concentration oxygen

Hypovolaemia
- **Recognition:** History/evidence of trauma, internal or external bleeding
- **Treatment:** Control external bleeding, fluid protocols for shock. Aggressive fluid therapy is likely to be needed

Tension pneumothorax
- **Recognition:** History of asthma or penetrating chest injury, high inflation pressures required to ventilate the patient, trachea deviated away from the pneumothorax, reduced breath sounds on the side of the pneumothorax
- **Treatment:** Needle thoracocentesis

Cardiac tamponade
- **Recognition:** penetrating chest injury, tension pneumothorax excluded, dilated neck veins
- **Treatment:** need a prehospital care team capable of performing open thoracotomy. Success only likely if within 10 min of the arrest.

---

dead on-scene but continue life support measures and convey them to hospital. If in doubt the paramedic should not withhold resuscitation.

Drowning

Cardiac arrest in drowning may be primary (e.g. secondary to an acute myocardial infarction causing ventricular fibrillation while swimming) or secondary (hypoxia from the submersion causing cardiac arrest). Attempts to retrieve the casualty from water must ensure that the rescuer's personal safety is paramount.

There is a high incidence of spinal injury associated with drowning and appropriate steps to protect the spinal cord should be taken unless the history of the incident makes a spinal injury unlikely.

Treatment follows standard ALS protocols, but with increased emphasis on early ventilation and endotracheal intubation in order to correct hypoxia and protect the airway. Survival following prolonged immersion (>45 minutes) and resuscitation has been recorded and therefore attempts at resuscitation should not be abandoned in the prehospital environment.

Asthma

Cardiac arrest in asthma invariably arises due to hypoxia caused by severe bronchospasm and mucous plugging. Standard ALS algorithms should be followed with emphasis being placed on early intubation and ventilation.

Tension pneumothorax may be difficult to diagnose but should always be considered in the rapidly deteriorating asthmatic. The diagnosis is based on physical examination.

Pregnancy

Cardiac arrest during pregnancy is fortunately a rare event. Standard ALS protocols should be followed with the addition of manual displacement of the pregnant uterus to the left. Alternatively a wedge (pillows, blanket or rescuers' thighs) should be placed under the patient's right side in order to improve venous return.

The best chance for both the patient and the unborn baby is if an emergency caesarean section is undertaken within 5 minutes of the arrest, hence rapid transport to hospital is essential.

Anaphylaxis

Cardiac arrest due to anaphylaxis is usually caused by a combination of profound hypotension (secondary to vasodilation) and hypoxia due to acute airway obstruction and severe bronchospasm.

Resuscitation should aim to achieve early control of the airway and ventilation using a bag and mask followed by rapid intubation. Attempts at endotracheal intubation may fail due to upper airway swelling and if permitted, paramedics may need to consider an emergency needle cricothyroidotomy.

The circulation should be supported with a rapid infusion of intravenous fluids and adrenaline. Intravenous steroids and antihistamines may be given.

Trauma

Immediate cardiac arrest due to trauma is likely to be due to massive neurological or cardiac injury and is likely to be unsurvivable.

Cardiac arrest in the first few minutes may be due to a reversible cause such as hypovolaemia or tension pneumothorax. Massive external haemorrhage must be identified and stopped. Hypovolaemia is likely to result in PEA and may respond to fluid resuscitation.

> Do not forget to protect the cervical spine where indicated.

Additional support

Consider requesting further support to the scene. A first responder or a second crew may be available. If another crew cannot be obtained, an Immediate Care doctor or nurse can be extremely helpful.

Paramedics will on occasion encounter doctors and other healthcare professionals at the scene of a cardiac arrest who may or may not be helpful. It can take confidence, tact and experience to reason with doctors and nurses, some of whom will have less up-to-date training in resuscitation.

While the doctor at the scene of a cardiac arrest will carry overall responsibility for any actions or omissions in their care of the patient, it may be necessary for paramedics to remind doctors of local resuscitation protocols.

Post-resuscitation care

If a return of spontaneous circulation is achieved then post-resuscitation care should be instituted. Warn the receiving hospital of your arrival.

On Scene

The following actions should be completed before leaving the scene:

- Airway: a patent airway must be established and high-flow oxygen administered
- Breathing: adequate respiratory effort and symmetrical chest movement must be ensured and air entry to both lungs and tracheal position checked. An SpO_2 monitor must be attached and the patient ventilated if he is in

respiratory arrest. Titrate the inspired oxygen concentration to maintain between the range of 94–98%. Both hypo- and hyper-ventilation must be avoided. If available, an end-tidal CO_2 monitor is invaluable in confirming ET tube placement and to ensure normo-capnia.

En route to hospital

The following actions should be carried out *en route* to hospital:

- Circulation: cardiac monitoring must be continued and the blood pressure recorded. Intravenous access should be obtained if it is not already in place. Record a 12-lead ECG
- Disability: neurological status should be recorded using the AVPU score
- Environment: keep your patient warm and record a blood glucose level. Following ROSC, blood glucose should be maintained at ≤ 10 mmol L^{-1}. Hypoglycaemia and strict blood glucose control should be avoided.

Ethical matters

Withholding CPR

- The paramedic's safety is paramount in all resuscitation attempts. If it is not possible to make the scene safe then resuscitation should not be attempted until such time that additional help arrives and the scene is made safe
- There are a limited number of other occasions when it is considered inappropriate to commence resuscitation. These situations include those in which there is no possibility of survival such as when there is decapitation, rigor mortis, decomposition, incineration or massive cranial destruction
- Certain patients may have an active 'do not attempt resuscitation' (DNAR) order or have an Advance Directive drawn up about their wishes, as those with malignant or end-stage disease
- These directives must be written (not verbal), be in-date and the paramedic must be confident that the documentation is valid and relates to the patient being treated and the circumstances have not changed. If there is any doubt then advanced life support should be started and the matter referred to hospital
- With the exception of the examples stated above, resuscitation should generally be started in all other cases of cardiac arrest. Judgements about the present or future quality of life made at the time of cardiac arrest are frequently inaccurate.

Discontinuing resuscitation efforts

The paramedic may consider discontinuing resuscitation in the presence of persistent asystole (longer than 20 minutes) provided that no exclusion criteria are present (children and young adults, pregnant females, electrocution, drowning, trauma, suspected hypothermia and overdose). Paramedics should be guided by their own local protocols in this regard.

If patients fall into the exclusion groups listed above, then they should be rapidly transported to hospital with ongoing attempts at resuscitation while *en route*.

If a patient remains in asystole after full advanced life support for 20 minutes, resuscitation may be discontinued provided that there are no signs of life:

1. No heart or breath sounds
2. No palpable pulse over 30 seconds
3. No movement or response to pain
4. Fixed and dilated pupils.

In these circumstances, a 30-second rhythm strip should be recorded and attached to the patient's report form when confirming death.

Patient handover

- Advanced warning should be given to the receiving hospital that you will be arriving with a patient in cardiac arrest
- Consideration should be given to the essential information required by hospital staff. This includes:
  1. Approximate time from collapse to arrival at scene ('down-time')
  2. Administration and efficiency of any bystander CPR
  3. Paramedic interventions so far (e.g. cannulation, defibrillation, intubation)
  4. Any available medical history
  5. Likely cause and any complications that have arisen
  6. Response to resuscitative efforts.

For further information, see Ch. 14 in *Emergency Care: A Textbook for Paramedics*.

CHAPTER 15

Cardiovascular emergencies

Ischaemic heart disease is the most common cardiovascular problem in the UK. Approximately one in four men and one in five women die from the disease. Acute manifestations of ischaemic heart disease are dealt with together under the term Acute Coronary Syndrome (ACS). Myocardial infarction (where prolonged ischaemia is causing irreversible damage to the myocardium) should be identified because reperfusion can be achieved by thrombolysis or by primary angioplasty. The factors that contribute to the development of ischaemic heart disease include:

- Cigarette smoking
- High blood cholesterol levels
- Hypertension
- Diabetes
- Family history
- Obesity.

The association of two or more risk factors greatly increases the chance of developing ischaemic heart disease. Cardiovascular events may still occur in individuals without identifiable risk factors. Ischaemic heart disease occurs when the supply of oxygenated blood to the heart is insufficient for the demands of the myocardium.

Ischaemic cardiac pain

Angina pectoris

- The discomfort of angina is caused by reversible myocardial ischaemia and usually occurs during conditions of increased oxygen demand in the presence of a fixed supply, most typically during physical exertion or mental and emotional stress

- When the patient ceases the activity and rests, the discomfort passes off rapidly (within 2–3 minutes)
- Patients with angina often describe a feeling of tightness in the chest ('like a tight band') or liken the discomfort to a weight on the chest
- The pain is felt retrosternally (behind the sternum) and may radiate across the chest, spreading into the arms
- In some patients, the pain may also radiate into the throat or jaw.

Acute coronary syndrome (unstable angina)

- The term *unstable angina* is used to describe a rapidly progressive, deteriorating pattern of angina often occurring in patients whose angina has been previously stable
- The patient's exercise tolerance is reduced and ischaemic pain occurs more frequently
- The consumption of glyceryl trinitrate is often increased
- Ischaemic pain occurring at rest or on only minor exertion is a particularly worrying feature
- Unstable angina is a medical emergency and most patients are admitted to hospital for investigation and treatment, as there is a high instance of subsequent myocardial infarction.

Myocardial infarction

- The pain of myocardial infarction is similar in nature, site and distribution to that of angina, although it usually persists longer and is associated with more profound extra effects, such as profuse perspiration, dizziness and nausea and vomiting
- The intensity of the pain is not a reliable indicator of the immediate risk to the patient
- Only about half those with acute myocardial infarction will have a history of previous heart disease
- In elderly people and diabetics, pain may be absent (the 'silent' MI).

Myocardial infarction

The effects of an MI depend on the extent and location of the muscle loss, as well as on the pre-existing state of the myocardium.

The complications of myocardial infarction (see box 15.1) may be difficult to diagnose prehospital. Electrical effects are easier to diagnose using prehospital cardiac monitoring and indeed, are more commonly seen early in the course of the acute coronary event. Ischaemic and infarcted myocardial segments are electrically unstable and prone to ventricular fibrillation or tachycardia, both causes of cardiac arrest and sudden cardiac death. Atrial fibrillation also may occur which leads to a further reduction in cardiac output and an increase in

---

Box 15.1 **Major complications of myocardial infarction**

- Cardiogenic shock – systolic output is reduced so that major organs are underperfused
- Mitral regurgitation – papillary muscles rupture causing an incompetent valve
- Cardiac tamponade – the myocardium ruptures and blood enters the pericardium
- Ventricular septal defect – the myocardium ruptures between the ventricles.

---

risk of intracardiac thrombosis and peripheral embolisation. Interruption in the blood supply of the sinus node or atrioventricular node is a cause of bradycardia and degrees of heart block.

Diagnosis

- The diagnosis is made by combining the history and examination with the findings on ECG
- The patient will be anxious, pale, sweaty and may be complaining of severe chest pain, nausea and may be short of breath
- A tachycardia is likely, hypotension is an ominous sign
- Pulmonary oedema may have developed
- The 12-lead ECG may show ST segment elevation (an 'ST elevation MI'), which will give information about which area of the myocardium is affected.

Treatment

- Sit the patient up, give them high flow oxygen, put them on cardiac monitoring and establish intravenous access as a precaution in the first instance
- Record a 12-lead ECG at the earliest opportunity, if available
- Morphine should be given; as well as providing analgesia it will have the effect of reducing myocardial demand and improving coronary blood flow
- An antiemetic should be given, both to reduce the effects of the MI and the effects of the morphine (avoid cyclizine, which may produce vasoconstriction)
- Sublingual GTN may improve the patient's pain (only give if the systolic blood pressure is >90 mmHg). GTN reduces the workload of the heart as well as causing the coronary arteries to dilate. Sublingual administration of 0.4–0.8 mg is either by tablet or spray
- Unless contraindicated, all patients with acute coronary syndrome (ACS) or suspected myocardial infarction (MI) will benefit from 300 mg aspirin orally (contraindications include active peptic ulcer disease, bleeding disorders or allergy to aspirin)
- Consider thrombolysis dependent on local protocols.

Box 15.2 **Primary treatment of myocardial infarction**

- Oxygen
- Analgesia
- Antiemetic
- Glyceryl trinitrate
- Aspirin
- Thrombolysis.

- Address complications such as arrhythmias or pulmonary oedema
- Diuretics such as frusemide 40–120 mg IV may be used to address clinically significant heart failure and pulmonary oedema.

Thrombolytic therapy

- Thrombolytic agents activate the natural mechanism for producing clot breakdown (*lysis*)
- Dissolution of the obstructing thrombus occurs with reperfusion of ischaemic myocardium
- Treatment is most effective when given as soon as possible after the onset of symptoms. The most serious side-effect is intracerebral bleeding
- Generally thrombolysis is used when primary angioplasty is not available or transfer times are prolonged
- The diagnosis of MI and the administration of thrombolysis may be made autonomously by the paramedic or may be achieved via telemetry with the receiving hospital
- Tenecteplase and reteplase are the preferred thrombolytic agents for prehospital use, as each is administered in bolus doses rather than as an infusion. Tenecteplase is given in a single dose adjusted according to the patient's weight. Reteplase is given as two bolus doses that must be administered 30 minutes apart
- Concurrent treatment with heparin is usually required
- Adverse events following thrombolytic therapy include ventricular fibrillation, ventricular tachycardia and other arrhythmias. Hypotension and shock may also occur. These complications should be addressed as per normal protocols
- Rarely, anaphylaxis may occur, and is also treated according to standard protocols, ensuring that administration of the thrombolytic agent is discontinued immediately
- The incidence of haemorrhagic stroke (through disruption of an existing intracerebral clot) is 1 per 200 patients thrombolysed, and half of these cases will result in death

- In order to ensure that the benefit of prehospital thrombolysis outweighs the risk of adverse events, only patients meeting the criteria established by the Joint Royal Colleges Ambulance Liaison Committee (JRCALC) should be administered thrombolytic agents by paramedics.

Dissecting aortic aneurysm

A dissecting aortic aneurysm is one of the most serious cardiovascular emergencies. The condition is more common in men and hypertension is an important predisposing factor. The condition starts with a tear in the intima of the aorta, usually in the ascending part of the arch of the aorta and the dissection may involve one or more major branches of the aorta, including the coronary arteries. Rupture of the aorta into the pericardium or pleura may occur and is usually rapidly fatal.

The pain of dissecting aneurysm is similar to that of myocardial infarction, although perhaps a little more abrupt in onset. It is sometimes described as having a 'tearing' quality and often radiates into the back between the scapulae.

A dissection is sometimes manifest as a discrepancy in the pulses in the arms or a marked difference in blood pressure on the two sides. The same may occur with the carotid or femoral vessels: disturbance of consciousness occurs with interruption of cerebral blood supply. Myocardial infarction (from obstruction of the coronary arteries), stroke or paraplegia (from obstruction to spinal blood flow) may be seen. The administration of thrombolytic drugs for MI due to aortic dissection will seriously jeopardise the outcome.

Management

In many cases, the patient will be suspected to be suffering from myocardial infarction. ECG monitoring, oxygen therapy and analgesia are equally appropriate in both conditions, while sublingual nitrates will do no harm in dissection. Venous access will be established at an early stage and used to provide effective analgesia. Do not administer thrombolysis if an aortic dissection is suspected. Rapid transfer to hospital is mandatory.

Pulmonary embolism

Pulmonary embolism is commonly under-diagnosed. It occurs when a thrombus that has formed in a large vein in the leg or pelvis becomes dislodged and is carried through the venous system and right ventricle into the pulmonary circulation.

Conditions associated with a high risk of thromboembolism include pregnancy, recent operations (particularly orthopaedic and gynaecological procedures), chronic heart failure or pulmonary disease, fractures and other injuries of the legs, chronic venous insufficiency affecting the lower leg, prolonged immobility, including prolonged travel and the presence of carcinoma.

The immediate result of pulmonary thromboembolism is obstruction of all or part of the pulmonary arterial bed which, when severe, will lead to pulmonary hypertension with acute right ventricular dilation and failure, tachycardia and a decline in cardiac output. Pulmonary embolism can therefore present with collapse due to electromechanical dissociation.

Diagnosis

- In milder cases examination findings may be normal
- The chest pain in pulmonary embolism is often pleuritic in nature (made worse by breathing).

Box 15.3 **Clinical features of pulmonary embolism**

- Chest pain
- Central cyanosis
- Tachycardia
- Dyspnoea
- Remember to check for deep vein thrombosis.

Treatment

- Outside hospital, treatment will centre on emergency resuscitation where appropriate, the administration of oxygen, instituting cardiac monitoring and securing intravenous access
- Thrombolysis is not recommended prehospital.

Box 15.4 **Treatment of pulmonary embolism**

- Oxygen
- Cardiac monitoring
- Intravenous access
- Opiate analgesia.

Cardiac tamponade

Cardiac tamponade occurs when fluid collects in the pericardial cavity in quantities sufficient to interfere with cardiac filling and obstruct venous return. The most common cause is a penetrating injury to the anterior chest wall which penetrates the myocardium allowing blood to fill the pericardium. Other causes produce fluid which builds up more gradually.

Box 15.5 **Causes of cardiac tamponade**

- Trauma – blood
- Following myocardial infarction – blood or serous fluid
- Following surgery – blood or serous fluid
- Malignancy – serous fluid
- Infection – purulent fluid (pus).

Diagnosis

- The cardinal diagnostic feature of cardiac tamponade is a reduction in cardiac output associated with systemic venous congestion
- With rapidly developing effusions, as may occur with cardiac trauma, quiet heart sounds occur but the recognition of this sign is difficult
- Electromechanical dissociation may occur
- When tamponade develops slowly, the clinical features may resemble heart failure: dyspnoea, tachycardia, congestion of the neck veins, hepatic engorgement and peripheral oedema.

Treatment

Immediate treatment may be life-saving and in most cases, will be undertaken in hospital after confirmation of the diagnosis by echocardiography. Only very rarely is pericardial aspiration or open thoracotomy by medical staff performed before hospital admission. Treatment by the paramedic will be the provision of oxygen, establishment of intravenous access and cardiac monitoring.

Cardiac arrhythmias

The treatment of asystole, pulseless ventricular tachycardia, ventricular fibrillation and pulseless electrical activity follows Advanced Life Support guidelines.

All arrhythmia patients require oxygen.

In prehospital care, treatment of arrhythmias is relatively simple. The golden rule is to treat the patient and not the arrhythmia.

TREAT THE PATIENT, NOT THE ARRHYTHMIA.

Treatment of tachycardia

Prehospital treatment should only be undertaken if the arrhythmia presents a significant threat to the patient's cardiovascular status or life and wherever possible during ECG monitoring, with a paper record made of the initial tachycardia and any response to treatment.

Box 15.6 **Types of tachycardia**

Regular narrow complex

- Sinus tachycardia
- AV nodal tachycardia
- Macroreentrant AV tachycardia (in Wolff–Parkinson–White syndrome)
- Atrial tachycardia with fixed AV conduction
- Atrial flutter with fixed AV conduction.

Irregular narrow complex

- Atrial fibrillation
- Atrial flutter with variable AV conduction
- Atrial tachycardia with variable AV conduction.

Regular broad complex

- Ventricular tachycardia
- Any cause of regular narrow complex with coexistent bundle branch block.

Irregular broad complex

- Atrial fibrillation with coexistent bundle branch block.

Tachycardias may be classified as regular or irregular with narrow or broad (>120 ms) QRS complexes.

Sinus tachycardia

Treatment should be directed towards the cause of the tachycardia (e.g. hypovolaemia due to haemorrhage).

Atrial tachycardia and atrial flutter

Drug treatment may be considered during rapid transfer to hospital.

Carotid sinus massage or the Valsalva manoeuvre (*'Take a huge breath in and strain as if you were on the toilet'*) is unlikely to terminate the arrhythmia but may abolish ventricular activity long enough for the underlying atrial abnormality to be recognised and the correct diagnosis made. Both of these are 'vagal manoeuvres' and are more effective in the younger patient and when lying flat. Vagal stimulation with a Valsalva occurs on *release* of the manoeuvre.

Carotid sinus massage (massage over the carotid artery level with the upper border of the larynx) should not be performed for more than 5–10 seconds.

The patient with acute paroxysmal cardiovascular compromise is best treated by synchronised cardioversion after arrival in hospital.

Amiodarone (150 mg IV given over 10 minutes, repeated once) may be administered by paramedics.

Atrial fibrillation

Atrial fibrillation with a moderate ventricular response (pulse rate <120/min) usually responds to a course of oral digoxin.

In the patient with pronounced tachycardia, intravenous digoxin, verapamil or β-blocker may slow the ventricular rate.

Administration of more advanced drugs or synchronised defibrillation is best undertaken in hospital.

Junctional tachycardia

Junctional tachycardia (or AV nodal reentrant tachycardia – AVNRT) may be terminated by vagal manoeuvres (carotid sinus massage or the Valsalva manoeuvre).

If vagal manoeuvres fail, the first-line treatment is adenosine 6 mg by rapid IV injection, followed if unsuccessful after 1–2 minutes by 12 mg and followed again if unsuccessful by 12 mg.

Paramedics are not currently licensed to administer adenosine. Immediate evacuation for treatment in hospital is appropriate. Cardiac monitoring must be maintained during the treatment.

Amiodarone (150 mg IV given over 10 minutes repeated once) may be administered by paramedics.

> Remember to print a rhythm strip.

Ventricular tachycardia

If ventricular tachycardia is pulseless the resuscitation algorithm for ventricular fibrillation should be followed.

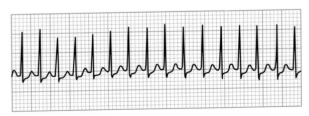

Figure 15.1 Junctional tachycardia (AVNRT).

If a pulse is present, oxygen should be given, followed by immediate rapid transfer to hospital.

Administration of intravenous amiodarone is indicated, subject to local protocol, followed if necessary after arrival in hospital by DC cardioversion.

Isolated ventricular complexes (ventricular premature beats) do not require treatment unless they occur in salvos in which case 150 mg of amiodarone should be given IV.

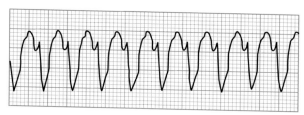

Figure 15.2 Ventricular tachycardia.

Treatment of bradycardia

First- and second-degree heart block rarely require treatment. Very occasionally, enough complexes fail to be transmitted in second-degree heart block to cause bradycardia with cardiovascular compromise (hypotension or chest pain). Atropine 0.5 mg (repeated if necessary to a maximum dose of 3 mg) should then be given.

If third-degree heart block ('complete heart block') is accompanied by an adequate cardiovascular status, it may be appropriate to delay treatment until arrival in hospital. Otherwise treatment is with intravenous atropine (0.5 mg, repeated if needed to a maximum dose of 3 mg). If this is unsuccessful, external pacing (if available) should be attempted.

In summary, bradycardia or heart block requires the following treatment.

1. First-degree block – none
2. Second-degree block – none or atropine
3. Third-degree block – none, external pacing or atropine
4. Sinus bradycardia – none or atropine.

For further information, see Ch.15 in *Emergency Care: A Textbook for Paramedics*.

CHAPTER 16

The unconscious patient

The unconscious patient is unable to ensure their own safety and in deeper levels of coma may be unable to protect their own airway.

Assessment of the unconscious patient

The first priority is to ensure safety before approaching the patient. Use the SAFE approach and evaluate the ABCs.

If there is any suspicion that the patient may have been a victim of trauma, the neck is immobilised in a rigid cervical collar while the airway is being assessed.

Give high-concentration oxygen, open the airway, check breathing and circulation status.

If there is no cardiac output, then immediately start CPR.

The next stage is to perform the rapid neurological checks – AVPU and assessment of pupillary responses.

> DEFG: Don't Ever Forget Glucose – a capillary glucose level (BM stix) MUST be checked in all unconscious patients.

Take a baseline set of observations and transfer the patient to hospital with monitoring on.

The assessment must be repeated regularly. A change in conscious level is the most important single sign in the assessment of the unconscious patient with a head injury.

AVPU

A – is the patient **A**lert?

V – is the patient responding to **V**erbal stimuli?

P – is the patient responding to **P**ainful stimuli?

U – is the patient **U**nresponsive?

A response by speech or movement scores 'V'. If there is no response, a painful stimulus is applied. The best stimulus to use is pressure over the supraorbital ridge, above one of the eyes: a response to this stimulus scores 'P', no response scores 'U'.

Signs to look for in the unconscious patient

- Any sign of head injury (protect the C-spine)
- 'Raccoon eyes' (base of skull fracture)
- A bitten tongue and urinary incontinence (epileptic fit)
- Pyrexia and rash (meningococcal septicaemia)
- Pinpoint pupils, needle marks and slow, shallow respiration (signs of an opiate overdose. Give naloxone (Narcan) and assess response)
- Empty medication packaging (possible overdose)
- Medi-alert bracelet
- Insulin, needles, glucose monitor (diabetic patient).

Bilateral pinpoint pupils virtually always indicate opiate overdosage (although a brainstem stroke can produce the same appearance). Bilateral dilated pupils are less helpful because there are many potential causes.

A dilated pupil on one side may indicate an expanding intracranial haematoma on the same side.

Further neurological examination

Two other useful neurological checks can be performed: a more detailed assessment of the conscious level of the patient using the Glasgow Coma Scale, and a brief neurological examination to determine if the patient has any areas of localized weakness or paralysis (focal neurological deficit).

Glasgow Coma Scale

The Glasgow Coma Scale uses three areas of patient response to determine a score that indicates coma level: these are *eye opening*, *speech* and *best motor response*.

The highest score (the alert patient) is 15 and the lowest (in deep coma or dead) is 3.

> 'Coma' is defined as a GCS score of 8 or less.

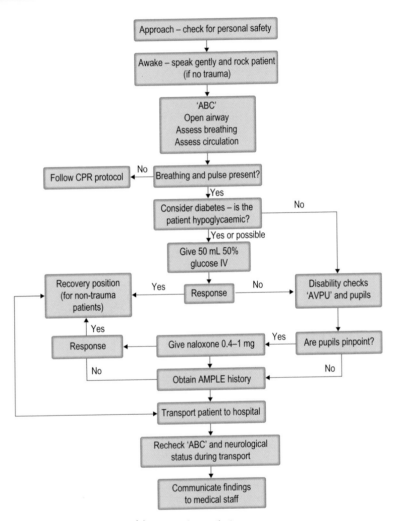

Figure 16.1 Management of the unconscious patient.

Table 16.1 Pupillary changes and possible diagnosis (adult)

Pupillary signs	Possible diagnosis
Bilaterally fixed and dilated	Death; hypovolaemic shock; drugs such as atropine, adrenaline and Ecstasy
Unilaterally fixed and dilated	Head injury; stroke
Bilateral pinpoint constriction	Opiate overdose
Bilateral constriction	Brainstem stroke
Irregular pupil	Trauma; previous eye operation

Table 16.2 The Glasgow Coma Scale

Component	Response	Score
Best motor response	Obeys commands	6
	Localises to pain[a]	5
	Withdraws from pain[b]	4
	Flexor response to pain[c]	3
	Extensor response to pain[d]	2
	No motor response to pain	1
Best verbal response (speech)	Oriented	5
	Confused conversation[e]	4
	Inappropriate speech[f]	3
	Incomprehensible speech[g]	2
	No speech	1
Eye opening	Spontaneous	4
	In response to speech	3
	In response to pain	2
	No eye opening	1

[a]Moves hand towards pain.
[b]Moves away from pain.
[c]Bends arm at elbow and wrist in response to a painful stimulus.
[d]Straightens at elbow and knee in response to a painful stimulus.
[e]Disorientated in time, person and place.
[f]Inappropriate response to question.
[g]Moans and groans.

Focal neurological deficit

On close examination of the face, note should be made of a drooping of the smile on one side, indicating a facial paralysis, common in patients who have had a cerebrovascular accident (stroke).

After a painful stimulus, movement of the patient's limbs should be observed and may reveal paralysis in one or more of the limbs. Weakness and paralysis are signs of focal neurological deficit and should be recorded and communicated to the receiving medical facility.

Common causes of altered conscious level

These may be remembered with the mnemonic CID CID F, see below.

CID CID F

C – Cerebral causes

I – Injury to the head

D – Diabetes and metabolic problems

C – Cardiac causes

I – Infection

D – Drugs, poisons and alcohol

F – Failure of organs and hypothermia

Cerebral causes

Common cerebral causes of unconsciousness are epilepsy, cerebrovascular accident (stroke) and subarachnoid haemorrhage.

Cerebrovascular accidents (CVAs) or strokes have two basic causes:

- *Haemorrhagic stroke* – from bleeding into the brain
- *Cerebral infarction* – a blood vessel becomes blocked.

If the features resolve completely over the space of several hours then the episode is known as a *transient ischaemic attack* (TIA).

Subarachnoid haemorrhage is usually caused by the sudden bursting of a small swelling (an aneurysm) of a cerebral vessel.

The characteristic history is of a patient who develops a sudden headache (often described as 'like being hit on the back of the head with a hammer') and who then collapses.

Epilepsy is a condition of abnormal brain activity, which presents with convulsions or 'fits'.

The most common type of epilepsy is 'grand mal' epilepsy, which has the following phases:

1. The patient collapses and the whole body contracts – the *tonic phase*; this usually lasts for a period of up to 30 seconds
2. Then follows a period of generalised contractions and relaxations, the *tonic-clonic phase* (the 'fit'), the duration of which can be very variable
3. The convulsion stops and consciousness slowly returns: this is the *postictal phase*. The patient may at first be confused before gradually returning to full awareness.

> If the tonic–clonic phase continues for more than 15 minutes, the patient is said to be in *status epilepticus* which is a medical emergency.

The patient who is immediately alert after an episode of collapse is unlikely to have had a grand mal fit.

Management of the fitting patient

- Ensure that the patient comes to no further harm
- Do not attempt to put anything in the patient's mouth
- Place an oxygen mask on or near the face of the patient
- If the convulsion shows no sign of ceasing give diazepam 10–20 mg IV or PR
- Transport the patient rapidly to the nearest available hospital with resuscitation facilities
- Ensure that the individual is protected from self-injury during the ambulance journey
- Check the patient's blood glucose level to exclude hypoglycaemia as the underlying cause.

Head injury

The diagnosis of head injury should not be overlooked, particularly in the drunk or intoxicated patient. Signs of trauma such as a head wound or palpable depressed fracture may be present.

Signs that indicate a base of skull fracture are:

- Bruising around both eyes ('raccoon eyes')
- Bruising over the mastoid process (Battle's sign, which usually takes a number of hours to develop)
- Blood or cerebrospinal fluid leaking from an ear.

Any episode of hypoxia or fall in blood pressure will significantly increase the head injured patient's morbidity and mortality.

Diabetes and metabolic problems

A low blood glucose level is one of the most common causes of coma found in the community. It is seen most often in diabetic patients who have taken too much insulin in relation to their food intake and activity level.

Chronic alcoholics have very low sugar stores and may develop acute hypoglycaemia after a bout of drinking.

The features of hypoglycaemia develop rapidly, usually over a period of a few minutes. Give glucose urgently, orally if possible, IV if absolutely necessary.

High blood sugars cause unconsciousness less commonly.

Clinical presentation of diabetic emergencies

Hypoglycaemia

- Dizziness and light-headedness
- Sweating (may be profuse)
- Confusion
- Aggression
- Weakness and loss of coordination
- Coldness and clamminess
- Fitting.

Hyperglycaemia

- Slow onset
- Thirst
- Weight loss
- Passing large amounts of urine
- Dehydration (dry skin, sunken eyes)
- Smell of ketones (not every one can smell these)
- Deep sighing breathing (Kussmaul's respiration).

Cardiac causes of unconsciousness

Cardiac arrhythmias

Major cardiac arrhythmias such as ventricular fibrillation result in collapse and should be treated using the cardiac arrest protocols.

Non-arrest arrhythmias may only cause transitory upset in cardiac output and result in a brief loss of consciousness.

A Stokes–Adams attack is when a patient (who is usually elderly) has a short run of a haemodynamically compromising arrhythmia. Patients have no warning symptoms of the collapse and recover quickly.

The patient should be transported to hospital with ECG monitoring.

Simple faint

Clinical features

- Sudden transient loss of consciousness.

Precipitating causes

- Emotional triggers include fright, sexual desire and the sight of blood

- Physical triggers such as pain
- Drugs (such as glyceryl trinitrate)
- Standing up too quickly or for prolonged periods (especially in hot weather)
- Anaemia (rarely).

Management

- The patient should be laid flat with the feet raised or in a head-down position
- If rapid recovery does not occur, consider an alternative diagnosis
- When the patient awakens, they should be asked about any possible precipitating causes of the faint
- If the patient does not fully recover or is unsafe at home, transfer to the ED.

Infection

Infection is a rare but serious cause of collapse. It is most commonly encountered in the young child or adolescent who develops meningococcal septicaemia.

These children or young people should be administered benzyl penicillin without delay and transported to hospital as rapidly as possible.

Other infections of the brain such as encephalitis and cerebral abscess can also cause collapse.

Overwhelming septicaemia, whatever the organism, may cause unconsciousness.

The diagnosis should be considered in an unconscious patient who is tachycardic with a low blood pressure and no signs of blood loss.

Intravenous fluids should be started and the patient transferred to hospital as soon as possible.

Drugs, poisons and alcohol

Alcohol

A drunk patient is not necessarily unconscious because of the alcohol; the cause may be a head injury, hypoglycaemia or an overdose.

Hypoglycaemia may be present and should be treated with intravenous glucose.

It is important to be wary of leaving an apparently drunk patient in police custody when other possible causes of decreased consciousness have not been excluded.

When a drunk patient is unconscious THINK:
- HEAD INJURY, HYPOGLYCAEMIA

Only then THINK:
- ALCOHOL

as the cause of the loss of consciousness.

Opiate poisoning

The features of opiate overdose are pinpoint pupils, respiratory depression and coma.

Assist respiration as necessary and consider using the opiate antagonist naloxone (Narcan).

Naloxone is given intravenously in a dose of 0.4–10 mg. Response to the drug is rapid, with wakening within 1 min, but the drug is short-acting, with a half-life of about 40 minutes.

If IV access is not possible, naloxone can be given intramuscularly (IM).

Other drugs that can cause coma

The next most common group of drugs causing coma is the antidepressants, particularly tricyclic antidepressants such as amitriptyline and mianserin.

Signs that may indicate tricyclic overdose include:

- Dilated pupils
- Convulsions
- Respiratory depression
- Cardiac arrhythmias.

The patient's cardiac rhythm must be monitored during transport to hospital.

Diazepam, temazepam and nitrazepam can cause drowsiness and coma when taken in overdose.

Carbon monoxide poisoning from faulty gas fires or attempted suicide from car exhaust fumes can cause coma. Be aware that carbon monoxide is odourless and invisible and may pose a threat to rescuers.

Drugs commonly causing coma:

- Alcohol
- Opiates
- Tricyclic antidepressants
- Benzodiazepines
- Carbon monoxide.

Hypothermia

A core body temperature of less than 35°C can be a cause of or a result of coma. The diagnosis should be suspected in the collapsed elderly patient or in anyone who has been exposed to the environment (such as the entrapped trauma victim).

For further information, see Ch. 16 in *Emergency Care: A Textbook for Paramedics.*

CHAPTER 17

The acute abdomen

Abdominal emergencies usually present with acute abdominal pain in association with other symptoms and signs. The causes range from life-threatening conditions that require immediate resuscitation and laparotomy to those that require more conservative management.

Diagnosis may be difficult, consequently the paramedic should concentrate instead on assessing the severity of the patient's condition and on managing it appropriately. In particular, it is important to detect patients who require immediate resuscitation and urgent transfer.

Pain is the major symptom of abdominal emergencies. It also has characteristics that can provide a clue to the underlying problem.

Irritation of the diaphragm, e.g. by blood, may produce pain referred to the shoulder-tip on the same side (due to shared innervations). A ruptured ectopic pregnancy may produce referred shoulder-tip pain.

Box 17.1 **Important aspects of the medical history and examination**

- History
- Pain
- Vomiting
- Bleeding (haematemesis or per rectum)
- Altered bowel habit
- Shock
- Abdominal distension.

Box 17.2 **Questions to ask the patient with abdominal pain**

- Where is the pain?
- What type of pain is it (i.e. inflammatory, colicky or ischaemic)?
- Does the pain move?
- What makes the pain better?
- What makes the pain worse?
- How long has the pain been present?
- How rapid was the onset of pain?
- Have you had this pain before? If so, what happened?

Box 17.3 **Signs and symptoms of peritonitis**

- Patient can localise the area of tenderness precisely (early)
- Coughing precipitates abdominal pain in the area of tenderness (early)
- There is rebound tenderness in the painful area (intermediate)
- Reluctance to move (aggravates the pain)
- No abdominal movement with expansion of the chest on inspiration (late)
- Generalised rigidity of the abdominal wall (very late)
- Pyrexia.

Table 17.1 Sites of referred pain from abdominal pathological conditions

Site of referred pain	Site of abdominal disease
Shoulder tip	Diaphragm
Retrosternal	Oesophagus and upper stomach
Epigastrium	Distal stomach to the second part of the duodenum
Periumbilical	Second part of the duodenum to the mid-transverse colon
Hypogastrium	Mid-transverse colon to the rectum
Left loin and back	Abdominal aortic aneurysm
Flank and genital pain	Ureter
Back	Pancreas

Vomiting and GI haemorrhage

- Vomiting may accompany severe pain or be directly caused by the abdominal disease. It is a common presentation in most acute abdominal conditions
- Intestinal obstruction is one of the causes of vomiting
- Vomiting blood indicates disease of the upper gastrointestinal tract Unaltered, bright red blood (haematemesis) suggests an oesophageal lesion, whereas altered blood, resembling 'coffee grounds,' due to partial digestion, indicates a gastric or duodenal site
- Upper gastrointestinal bleeding can also give rise to melaena, altered blood being lost as sticky, black, 'tarry' stools with a characteristic smell
- Bleeding from the lower gastrointestinal tract is seen as altered blood if the lesion is in the proximal part of the large bowel (e.g. caecal or small bowel carcinoma) or as bright red blood if it lies more distally (e.g. haemorrhoids or rectal carcinoma)
- Patients will need intravenous fluids to treat dehydration or replace blood loss.

Box 17.4 **Abdominal causes of hypovolaemic shock**

- Acute gastrointestinal bleeding
- Ruptured abdominal aortic aneurysm
- Trauma leading to abdominal vessels or organs being torn or ruptured
- Intestinal obstruction
- Mesenteric infarction
- Continuous vomiting or diarrhoea without fluid replacement
- Ectopic pregnancy (ruptured).

Common abdominal emergencies

Stomach and proximal duodenum

Diseases of the upper GI tract (e.g. gastritis and duodenitis, peptic ulcer disease) commonly present with:

- Epigastric or retrosternal inflammatory pain
- Mild epigastric tenderness
- Nausea
- Haematemesis (less common).

Gastroenteritis (most commonly due to 'food poisoning') presents with:

- Mild to severe, colicky abdominal pain (poorly localised)

- Vomiting, especially initially
- Diarrhoea
- Dehydration
- Raised temperature
- Diffuse, mild abdominal tenderness
- Guarding and rebound tenderness (rare).

Severe tenderness with localised signs of peritonitis (guarding and rigidity) suggests that the bowel may have perforated. If this is left untreated, the area of tenderness and pain increases as more of the gastric contents leak into the peritoneal cavity. Ultimately the patient will become shocked and critically ill and may die from overwhelming septic shock.

Biliary tract obstruction

Biliary tract obstruction (biliary colic) is caused by gallstones in the biliary tract. Epigastric colicky pain (may be provoked by eating fatty meals):

- Nausea
- Vomiting and belching
- Jaundice (rare).

Secondary infection is common in the stagnant bile trapped in the biliary tree proximal to the obstruction resulting in the symptoms and signs of acute cholecystitis (gall bladder inflammation).

Gall bladder inflammation (acute cholecystitis) can occur without stones in the biliary tract and presents with:

- Acute right upper quadrant pain (referred to the scapula) and tenderness
- Nausea
- Vomiting
- Anorexia
- Fever.

Intestines

Colic from small and large bowel obstruction is usually localised to the periumbilical and hypogastric regions, respectively.

The frequency of vomiting and dehydration as an early associated feature increases with the more proximal location of the intestinal obstruction.

Appendicitis

Appendicitis is usually associated with poor appetite, vomiting and a mild pyrexia. As with all inflammatory conditions, if it is left untreated the patient's condition will become more pyrexial and toxic as infection and necrosis develop.

Box 17.5 **Signs of acute appendicitis**

- Poorly localised abdominal pain shifting to right iliac fossa
- Anorexia
- Nausea and vomiting
- Diarrhoea or constipation
- Pyrexia (low).

Pancreas

Patients with pancreatitis have epigastric tenderness and severe inflammatory pain, which may radiate to the back. The most common causes are gallstones and alcohol abuse.

In order to gain some relief, the patients will either sit and lean forward or lie curled up on their side. Nausea and vomiting are common. Severe cases are associated with dehydration and a major metabolic disturbance.

Bruising of the flanks and abdomen indicates a more fulminant presentation with internal haemorrhage.

Begin IV fluid replacement and give opiate analgesia.

Kidneys and ureters

Obstruction in the kidneys or ureters from renal calculi presents as severe pain localised to the posterior aspect of the flank (renal angle). Pain may radiate to the groin ('loin to groin pain'). Severe pain is commonly associated with vomiting and may be associated with urinary symptoms.

Give analgesia and antiemetics as appropriate.

Blood vessels

Aortic aneurysm

Aortic aneurysms develop progressively with age and enlargement may be relatively painless until catastrophic haemorrhage occurs following rupture or dissection.

Ruptured aneurysms present with collapse, sweating and abdominal ischaemic pain which may radiate through to the back. An abdominal pulsatile mass may be palpable.

Ruptured aortic aneurysm

Resuscitate the patient with 250 mL boluses of crystalloid fluid, titrated to the radial pulse. Excess fluid administration may make the bleeding worse.

Box 17.6 **Symptoms and signs of ruptured aortic aneurysm**

- Collapse
- Sweating
- Abdominal pain: can be referred to the back or even the left flank
- Abdominal tenderness
- Abdominal pulsatile mass
- Respiratory and circulatory compromise
- Vomiting – RARE
- Haematemesis – RARE
- Lower limb pain and neurological deficit – VERY UNCOMMON.

Mesenteric artery embolus

Mesenteric artery embolism has a sudden onset. Initially there is colicky abdominal pain, which after about 1 hour becomes unrelenting and poorly localised.

With subsequent progression localised peritonitis and dehydration develop, the latter being due to impaired absorption, vomiting and fluid becoming trapped in the atonic bowel.

Later, when the bowel wall becomes gangrenous and necrotic, generalized peritonitis and septic shock occur.

Box 17.7 **Symptoms and signs of mesenteric artery embolism**

- Sudden onset colicky abdominal pain becoming unrelenting and poorly localised
- Nausea and vomiting
- Shock
- Localised peritonitis
- Dehydration
- Vomiting.

Genital tract

Pelvic inflammatory disease

This is a blanket term used to cover inflammation of the female upper genital tract and the adjacent peritoneum and bowel, usually from bacterial infection.

Usually there are also signs of infection such as pyrexia, tachycardia and occasionally rigors. The lower abdomen may be tender.

Ectopic pregnancy

Ectopic pregnancy occurs when a fertilised ovum becomes implanted outside the uterus. These patients require immediate resuscitation and urgent transfer to hospital so that haemostasis can be achieved surgically. This must not be delayed.

Box 17.8 **Symptoms and signs of ectopic pregnancy**

Before rupture

- Lower abdominal pain
- Tenderness and guarding
- Amenorrhoea 'fainting' feelings
- Irregular vaginal bleeding.

After rupture

- Bleeding
- Pain in the iliac fossa or hypogastrium
- Generalised tenderness and guarding
- Shoulder tip pain can occur (when there is much free intraperitoneal blood and the patient has been lying with her head down).

Ovarian cyst torsion

Ovarian cyst torsion presents as sudden onset of recurrent colicky pain in the ipsilateral iliac fossa. Nausea and vomiting are common associated features. In addition, the abdominal wall overlying the torsion is tender and may be rigid during the attacks.

Testicular torsion

Twisting of the testis on its cord causes intense ischaemic pain localised in the testis. Usually there is localised tenderness and vomiting (which may be the sole presenting feature), but no significant swelling. These patients require urgent surgery to salvage the testis and must be transferred immediately to hospital.

Hernias

HERNIA: a protrusion of an organ or tissue out of the body cavity in which it normally lies.

Box 17.9 **Types of hernia**

- Inguinal
- Femoral
- Hiatus
- Epigastric
- Lumbar
- Incisional.

Hernias may become incarcerated and may obstruct causing the signs and symptoms of acute intestinal obstruction.

For further information, see Ch. 17 in *Emergency Care: A Textbook for Paramedics*.

CHAPTER 18

Poisoning

Four crucial questions must be asked:

- What was taken?
- How much was taken?
- When was it taken?
- What was taken with the overdose (e.g. alcohol)?

If possible, the paramedic should take any medicine containers found at the scene to the hospital along with the patient.

> Always consider the possibility of alcohol consumption.

Box 18.1 **Poisoning in children**

Poisoning in children is common, but not commonly serious. A typical case of poisoning in childhood is the accidental ingestion of a mildly toxic substance by a child aged 1–3 years. Most incidents are minor.

In the UK, the majority of children ingest therapeutic agents: paracetamol, iron, benzodiazepines, tricyclic antidepressants and the contraceptive pill are the most common. The remainder are usually poisoned by a variety of household products. The accidental ingestion is usually noticed rapidly by the parents and the children often present very soon after ingestion.

As a general rule, most cases of poisoning require no treatment other than maintenance of the vital signs. If this is achieved, the majority of patients will have a favourable outcome.

Examples of alerting clinical syndromes include:

- Rapid pulse rate – tricyclic antidepressants, antihistamines, amphetamines or other arrhythmogenic agents
- Low blood pressure – anticholinergic medications or vasodilators such as alcohol
- Increased respiratory rate – substances that cause shock, also salicylate overdose
- Decreased respiratory rate – opiate ingestion
- Dilated pupils – tricyclic antidepressants, amphetamines ingestion
- Constricted pupils – opiate ingestion
- Nasal bleeding or perioral sores – solvent abuse.

Specific poisons

Medications

Almost any medication can be harmful if taken in excess.

Table 18.1 Treatment for over dosage of specific drugs

Drug	Effects	Treatment
Tricyclic antidepressants	Heart rate increased Blood pressure lowered Drowsiness Convulsions	ABC IV fluids Diazepam (for fits) Bicarbonate (in hospital)
β-blockers	Heart rate increased Blood pressure lowered Possible drowsiness	ABC IV fluids Atropine Glucagon May need external pacer
Opiates	Drowsiness Respiration reduced Pinpoint pupils Blood pressure lowered	ABC Naloxone
Insulin	Agitated Conscious level lowered Pale, clammy appearance Low blood glucose level	ABC Dextrose Glucagon

Benzodiazepines

Symptoms and signs

- Drowsiness
- Unconsciousness
- Respiratory depression (if taken with alcohol).

Management

- Clear and maintain the airway
- Support respiration (bag-mask ventilation if required)
- Monitor
- Transfer to hospital.

Antidotes

Although there is a specific antidote to benzodiazepines (flumazenil), there are dangers with its use. The patient may develop seizures as a result of benzodiazepine withdrawal or because other medications (e.g. tricyclic antidepressants) may also have been ingested. Should this happen, the seizures are extremely difficult to treat as the usual anticonvulsant in this situation – diazepam – will not work in the presence of the flumazenil. A further problem arises with the patient who revives following the administration of flumazenil, refuses further treatment and leaves the scene; because the effects of the flumazenil are short-lived, unlike the effects of the benzodiazepines, the patient may succumb again to the overdose, possibly when no witnesses are present to call for help.

Paracetamol

The most common over-the-counter medication taken in overdose is paracetamol. As noted previously, the great danger of this drug is that it is perceived as harmless.

Signs and symptoms

Early

- None
- Because there are often no immediately felt ill-effects after taking this drug, there may be a prolonged delay in seeking treatment and a reluctance to attend hospital.

> Drowsiness suggests the ingestion of other medication, commonly a compound analgesic.

Late

- Hepatic failure
- Death.

Management

Immediate transfer to hospital for assessment of blood paracetamol levels and management.

Antidote

N-Acetyl-cysteine is a specific and highly effective antidote to paracetamol.

Tricyclic antidepressants

Tricyclic antidepressants are commonly prescribed to the patients who are most at risk of attempted self-harm. It is unfortunate that this group of drugs are among the most toxic medications when taken in overdose.

Signs and symptoms

- Depressed consciousness
- Seizures
- Cardiac arrhythmias (sinus tachycardia to ventricular tachycardia)
- Hypotension
- Tachypnoea
- Impaired ventilation.

Management

The management of these patients can be very challenging; however, the ABC approach will provide sufficient prehospital care for most of them.

- Clear and protect the airway
- Give oxygen via a face mask
- Ventilate if necessary via a bag-valve-mask system (hyperventilating the patient will help correct both metabolic and respiratory acidosis)
- Treat hypotension with an intravenous fluid challenge
- Monitor ECG – only treat symptomatic arrhythmias
- Control seizures with diazepam.

Antidote

In hospital, sodium bicarbonate is effective in treating acidosis.

β-Blockers

Signs and symptoms

- Bradycardia
- Hypotension
- Depressed conscious level.

Management

- Secure the airway
- Assist breathing
- Treat hypotension with intravenous fluid
- Treat bradycardia with 0.5 mg atropine intravenously*
- Use of an external pacemaker may also be considered.

Antidote

Glucagon 0.5–1.0 mg given IM or IV (and repeated up to 5 mg) has been shown to be of benefit in severe β-blocker poisoning. In such cases, the patient may require insertion of an intravenous pacemaker, therefore there should be no delay in taking the patient to the nearest hospital.

> *Further doses (to a maximum of 3 mg) may be given if there is no effect or if the patient deteriorates after transient improvement.

Insulin

It is uncommon for insulin to be taken as a deliberate overdose, unless there is a genuine desire to die and steps are taken to avoid discovery, but accidental overdoses occur frequently.

Signs and symptoms

- Loss of consciousness
- Aggression
- Confusion
- Sweating.

Management

- Clear and maintain airway
- Obtain IV access
- IM glucagon

or

- Intravenous glucose.

Warm sweat drinks or Hypostop may be effective in aborting mild hypoglycaemia before it progresses.

> NEVER FORGET TO CHECK THE BLOOD SUGAR IN A PATIENT WITH AN ALTERED CONSCIOUS LEVEL
>
> Glucagon raises blood sugar by mobilising glucose from glycogen in the liver. In alcoholics or those with chronic liver disease, these stores will be depleted and glucagons will be ineffective.

Opiates

Opiates may be taken in overdose accidentally (in the case of the patient with chronic pain), intentionally, with a view to self-harm, or recreationally, by injecting drug abusers.

Signs and symptoms

- Depressed level of consciousness
- Depressed respiration (breathing tends to be slow and deep)
- Pinpoint pupils
- Hypotension
- Hypoxia
- Risk of aspiration of stomach contents
- Needle marks from IV drug abuse.

Management

- Secure the airway
- High flow oxygen
- Assist breathing
- Establish intravenous access
- Administer naloxone.

Naloxone dosage

IV boluses of 0.4 mg repeated to a maximum dose of 10 mg or until the patient begins to recover.

Failure to respond to a dose of 2 mg suggests that opiates are not responsible for the loss of consciousness.

The half-life, and therefore the effect, of naloxone is shorter than the effect of most commonly used opiates. The result of this is that the improvement in the patient's condition may be short-lived and coma may return. A patient who is allowed to leave the scene may well lapse into another coma, possibly with no witnesses to summon help. One method that may be used in such cases is to administer intramuscular naloxone (1 mg) to the poisoned patient before giving the intravenous dose. In this way, if the patient leaves the scene following recovery, naloxone will be slowly released into the circulation from the IM dose and may prevent a relapse.

Household substances

Most household products in current use are of low systemic toxicity if accidentally ingested. Commonly ingested substances include bleaches, turpentine substitute, paraffin and household cleaning products. The treatment of ingestion of these substances is to administer oral fluids (milk) and rapidly transfer the patient to hospital. There may be local irritation of the mouth or oesophagus, but systemic toxicity is unusual. The patient should not be encouraged to vomit, as this may lead to a potentially fatal pneumonitis.

Plants and fungi

It is unusual for adults to eat poisonous plants, although mistakes occur occasionally. Poisoning is more common in children.

The quantities involved are usually small because the plant material is sufficiently unpalatable to prevent consumption of more than very minimal amounts.

The most common plant poisoning in Britain is the ingestion of laburnum seeds ingestion of more than 10 seeds is considered dangerous.

The treatment of laburnum poisoning is the same as that for all plant ingestions: evaluation and support of the airway, breathing and circulation and transportation of the patient to hospital.

Many poisonous fungi can be mistaken for edible mushrooms, but serious poisoning is rare.

Usually, patients who have ingested fungi have a violent but self-limiting attack of abdominal pain, diarrhoea, nausea and vomiting about 2 hours after the ingestion.

There may be signs of excessive cholinergic stimulation (bronchospasm, bradycardia, constricted pupils and collapse). This can be treated with boluses of intravenous atropine, but this may exacerbate any agitation or hallucinations.

The patient and the fungi should be taken to the nearest hospital as soon as possible.

> Wherever possible, take a sample of the ingested plant to hospital for identification.

Effects of laburnum ingestion
- Burning mouth and throat
- Nausea
- Abdominal pain
- Vomiting
- Diarrhoea
- Drowsiness
- Incoordination
- Delirium
- Twitching
- Coma.

Inhalational agents

A number of substances are harmful if inhaled. The two main groups of inhalational 'poisons' are the recreational drugs and substances inhaled accidentally or for deliberate self-harm (carbon monoxide and other gases). The treatment of the first group is rapid assessment of the airway, breathing and circulation, supportive care, administration of naloxone in the case of opiate poisoning and rapid transport to hospital.

The second group is important because in these cases, there is a danger to the paramedic. Care should be taken that the paramedic does not become a secondary casualty by inhaling the toxic fumes. If it is possible to approach safely, the patient should be removed from the environment and given high-concentration oxygen.

Recreational drugs

The general effect of these drugs is to affect the central nervous system, producing depression (opiates and benzodiazepines) or stimulation (Ecstasy, amphetamines and cocaine). The treatment of poisoning by these substances is the assessment and support of airway, breathing and circulation, the administration of naloxone in opiate poisoning and rapid transport to hospital.

For further information, see Ch. 18 in *Emergency Care: A Textbook for Paramedics*.

CHAPTER 19

Microbiology and infection

Infection can be spread by a number of different routes, these include:

- Droplet spread – the common route of infection for respiratory disease
- Direct contact – hand to wound, mouth to mouth, biting, injection
- Faecal–oral – transmission on the hands from the lower GI tract to the mouth
- Indirect contact – contaminated material or equipment is brought into contact with another casualty.

Bacteria

Small, unicellular organisms that have evolved to live in very specialised environments.

Viruses

Much smaller organisms that cannot be seen with a normal light microscope.

Carrier

Someone harbouring a microorganism but not showing evidence of disease.

Source

Area in which a microorganism grows.

Reservoir

The vehicle of transport of infection (e.g. the hands in a faecal–oral transmitted infection).

Incubation period

The time during which the microorganism is multiplying in body tissue before the signs and symptoms of illness have developed.

Infectious period

The time during which the infection may be transmitted to other people.

Important infectious diseases in the UK

Bacterial Infections

Tuberculosis

Organism

- Bacteria of the mycobacterium species.

Symptoms and signs

- Shortness of breath
- Cough
- Discharging skin sinuses in lymph node involvement (rare).

Mode of spread

- Droplet
- Direct spread.

Incubation period

- 4–8 weeks.

Infectious period

- Until treated.

Prehospital precautions

If a patient with active tuberculosis has been transported, the ambulance must be thoroughly aired, linen laundered and contaminated respiratory equipment such as face masks and tubing destroyed. Concerns about staff contracting the disease should be discussed with occupational health.

Notes

The incidence has recently risen in the UK, possibly owing to the increasing number of immigrants, a decrease in the uptake of vaccination and poor living standards in inner cities.

Patients continue to be infectious until their illness has been treated. All paramedic staff should ensure that they are fully immunised against tuberculosis and have a Heaf test (intradermal tuberculin) every 3 years to check their immunity.

Meningitis

Meningitis is an infection of the membranes that surround the brain. When the infection is bacterial and organisms spread to the blood stream, septicaemia is present.

Organism

Bacteria or viruses. The most common bacteria are *Haemophilus influenzae, Neisseria meningitidis* and *Streptococcus pneumoniae.*

Symptoms and signs

- Headache
- Photophobia (light hurting the eyes)
- Neck stiffness
- Non-specific flu-like illness
- Bruising rash (non blanching) in associated septicaemia – especially *N. meningitidis*.

Mode of spread

Droplet.

Incubation period

Incubates for 2–3 days in meningococcal meningitis (due to the bacteria *N. meningitides*).

Infectious period

Infectious until treated.

Prehospital precautions

When transporting such a patient, a face mask should be worn and the ambulance and all equipment thoroughly cleaned afterwards. Hand washing is essential. If the final diagnosis is proved to be meningococcal meningitis, the occupational health department will consider giving a course of antibiotics to reduce any possible risk of acquiring the infection, although prophylactic antibiotics are *not* usually given to paramedic or medical staff unless they have been 'kissing' contacts (mouth-to-mouth ventilation).

Notes

The child with meningococcal disease may deteriorate very rapidly and must be administered benzyl penicillin and transported to hospital as soon as possible.

Whooping cough

Organism

Bordetella pertussis (bacterium).

Symptoms and signs

- Severe cough, with characteristic inspiratory whooping sound between bouts
- Vomiting
- Weight loss
- Pneumonia.

Mode of spread

Droplet.

Incubation period

Incubates for 7–10 days.

Infectious period

From 7 days after exposure until 21 days after first symptoms.

Prehospital precautions

Whooping cough does not represent a great risk to paramedic staff, but an ambulance should be thoroughly cleaned and aired if a child with the illness has been transported.

Notes

Whooping cough mainly affects children and is most severe in those under 6 months of age. The disease often lasts several months.

Viral infections
Hepatitis A – infectious hepatitis

Organism

Hepatitis A virus.

Symptoms and signs
- General malaise
- Jaundice
- Nausea and vomiting.

Mode of spread
Faecal–oral.

Incubation period
Incubates for 15–40 days.

Prehospital precautions
Universal precautions. Care when handling sharps. Report personal contamination immediately.

Notes
Common in conditions of poor sanitation and tends to occur in outbreaks, for instance in prisons or mental health institutions. The disease tends to run a benign course and usually resolves over a period of 1–2 months.

Hepatitis B – serum hepatitis

Organism
Hepatitis B virus.

Symptoms and signs
- General malaise
- Jaundice
- Nausea and vomiting
- Liver failure.

Mode of spread
- Intravenous (including dirty needles)
- Sexual contact.

Incubation period
Incubates for 40–160 days.

Infectious period
Variable – beware chronic carriers.

Prehospital precautions

Universal precautions. Care when using sharp instruments or needles. Significant contamination with infected or potentially infected blood or body fluids (e.g. needlestick injury) must be reported immediately. The name of the index patient should be recorded for subsequent serological blood testing subject to the patient's consent. Expert advice should be sought at the earliest opportunity.

Note

An effective vaccine is available for immunisation against hepatitis B. All ambulance staff should ensure that they are vaccinated and have their antibody levels checked every 3 years.

Hepatitis C

Organism

Hepatitis C virus.

Symptoms and signs

- General malaise
- Jaundice
- Nausea and vomiting.

Mode of spread

- Intravenous (including dirty needles)
- Sexual contact.

Incubation period

Incubates for 40–160 days.

Infectious period

Variable – beware chronic carriers.

Prehospital precautions

Care when using sharp instruments or needles. Significant contamination with infected or potentially infected blood or body fluids (e.g. needlestick injury) must be reported immediately. The name of the index patient should be recorded for subsequent serological blood testing subject to the patient's consent. Expert advice should be sought at the earliest opportunity.

HIV infection and AIDS

Organism

Human immunodeficiency virus 1 or 2 (HIV1 or HIV2).

Symptoms and signs
- Usually secondary to increased susceptibility to infection
- Certain characteristic rashes.

Mode of spread
- Sexual contact
- Intravenous (including dirty needles).

The risk of becoming infected from a needlestick injury is 10 times lower for HIV than for hepatitis B virus, taking equivalent inoculating doses of the virus.

Incubation period

Months to years.

Infectious period

Unknown.

Prehospital precautions

Universal precautions will minimise the infection risk. The ambulance should be thoroughly cleaned and disinfected after use and all disposable items placed in labelled double bags and sent for incineration.

Notes

The chances of acquiring HIV while at work are very small, but disease transmission has occurred in medical and nursing staff through needlestick injury and there are occasional instances of contamination through non-intact skin.

If an accident occurs which puts health service personnel at risk of contracting HIV infection, it is essential that medical advice is sought *immediately*. Post-exposure prophylactic drug therapy (PEP) is effective in reducing the serum conversion rate from HIV and must be started as soon as possible, ideally within 1 hour.

Herpes virus infections

The herpes viruses cause a variety of different blistering eruptions.

Symptoms and signs
- Herpes simplex type I – cold sores on the mouth, 'whitlows' on the fingers
- Herpes simplex type 2 – blistering painful lesions on the genitalia
- Chickenpox virus – diffuse blistering rash, common in children.

Mode of spread
- Sexual contact
- Direct contact.

Incubation period
- Usually 2–10 days
- Chickenpox 14–21 days, remains infectious until the vesicles are dry.

Infectious period

From 2 weeks before rash until vesicles are dry.

Prehospital precautions

Spread of the infection can be prevented by wearing gloves when dealing with such patients and regularly washing the hands.

Chickenpox can affect adults more seriously, so it is best to avoid carrying an infected patient if any member of the crew has not had the illness as a child. Even so, repeat infection can occur.

After carrying such a patient, the ambulance should be cleaned thoroughly to avoid the possibility of spreading the infection to other casualties.

Notes

Chickenpox virus remains dormant in nerve endings and may reactivate at a later date, resulting in 'shingles.' This is characterised by vesicles erupting in small areas corresponding to the spinal nerves that supply the skin (dermatomes). It commonly occurs in the elderly, precipitated by stress or underlying disease, and can be very painful.

Pregnant women should not be allowed in contact with chickenpox cases.

It is possible in the non-immune to contract chicken pox from active shingles.

Influenza

Organism

Influenza RNA viruses (multiple serotypes).

Symptoms and signs
- Pyrexia
- Aches and pains
- Cough.

Mode of spread
- Air-borne droplet spread
- Contact with contaminated surfaces.

Incubation period
Incubates for 2–4 days.

Infectious period
Infectious for 4–5 days following onset of symptoms.

Prehospital precautions
Simple precautions required: use gloves and masks and wash hands after treating suspected cases. Front-line care workers should receive annual vaccination against seasonal influenza strains.

Notes
Unusual serotypes such as H1N1 'swine-flu' have the potential to cause serious epidemics in non-immune populations.

Other childhood infectious diseases
Measles
Organism
Measles virus.

Symptoms and signs
- Rash
- Fever
- Cough
- Conjunctivitis.

Mode of spread
Droplet.

Incubation period
Incubates for 10 days.

Infectious period
From beginning of symptoms until 4 days after appearance of rash.

Prehospital precautions
Patients with measles do not present any particular risk to paramedic staff, but the ambulance and equipment should be thoroughly cleaned after use to prevent transmission of infection to others.

Notes
Measles is infectious from the beginning of symptoms until 4 days after the appearance of the rash. The illness is not always benign and can result in deafness and brain damage.

German measles (rubella)

Organism
Rubella virus.

Symptoms and signs
- Transient rash
- Lymphadenopathy.

Mode of spread
Droplet.

Incubation period
Incubates for 14–21 days.

Infectious period
From 7 days before until 4 days after the rash.

Prehospital precautions
All female ambulance staff should ensure that they are immunised against the disease and if pregnant, should not transport patients who are suspected of having the disease.

Notes

The most important aspect of rubella infection is the potential fetal damage, which can result when mothers are exposed to the virus in the early months of their pregnancy. For this reason, all British girls are immunised against rubella prior to leaving school.

Mumps

Organism

Mumps virus.

Symptoms and signs
- Swelling of the parotid glands
- General malaise
- Orchitis (testicular inflammation) and sterility after infection in adulthood.

Mode of spread

Droplet.

Incubation period
- 14–21 days
- The patient is infectious for several days before the parotid gland swells and for the subsequent 5 days.

Infectious period

From 2 days before parotid swelling until 5 days after.

Prehospital precautions

Adult males who have not had mumps should avoid transporting children who are suspected of having the illness.

Notes

Inflammation of the ovaries (oophoritis), thyroid (thyroiditis), brain (encephalitis) and pancreas (pancreatitis) can all result from mumps infection.

Minimising the spread of infectious diseases

The risk of catching an infectious disease is small and can be minimised further by the observation of some simple precautions.

Immunisation

Paramedical staff should ensure that their immunisation schedules are up-to-date.

General hygiene

- Hands should be thoroughly washed after each patient
- Nails must be kept clean and regularly trimmed otherwise they may act as a reservoir for bacteria
- Hair should be kept short or tied back so that it cannot contaminate a wound
- A paramedic with any large wound or open weeping areas should not work until the injury has healed. Small lacerations should be cleaned and dressed with a waterproof dressing to decrease the risk of infection.

Equipment

Whenever possible, disposable equipment should be used and then replaced.

Disposable sharps should be kept in puncture-resistant containers.

Other disposables should be placed in plastic bags and clearly marked before being sent to be destroyed.

The ambulance should be aired regularly and the interior cleaned thoroughly at least once a day.

All non-disposable equipment should be scrubbed with an antiseptic solution after each patient and linen should be changed and sent for cleaning to the laundry.

Immunisation requirements for ambulance service staff

- Tetanus – a booster should be given every 10 years
- Tuberculosis – a Heaf test is necessary every 3 years to check on immunity
- Hepatitis B – a full course of three injections should be given and then antibody levels checked. If levels are low a further booster dose may be necessary. Antibody levels should be checked every 3 years
- Rubella – antibody titres should be checked and immunisation offered to female personnel who are not immune.

Measures to avoid the spread of infectious disease

- Ensuring that one is fully immunised
- Observing good general hygiene
- Using disposable equipment when possible
- Having a regular cleaning schedule for equipment and the ambulance
- Using 'universal precautions' (see below)
- Taking extreme care when using sharps.

Universal precautions

- Ensure that protective equipment is always available in the ambulance
- Observe blood and body fluid precautions with ALL casualties

- Wear gloves whenever exposed to blood or other body fluids
- Protect eyes, face and trunk if blood is likely to be splashed
- Wash immediately if blood or body fluid is splashed onto skin.

Sharps Safety

- Extreme care should be taken when using needles, blades and other sharps
- Sharps should be disposed of immediately in a puncture-resistant container
- Needles should never be re-sheathed or broken because of the risk of needlestick injury
- Sharps should not be handed from one person to another
- Beware of sharp items such as broken glass or edges of metal.

High-risk situations

There are several situations in which ambulance staff may be subjected to a higher risk of exposure to an infectious disease. In these situations further precautionary measures may be necessary.

Cardiopulmonary resuscitation

There have been no case reports of HIV or hepatitis B infection caused by transmission of the virus during mouth-to-mouth ventilation. However, both viruses are present in saliva so a small risk may be present. In addition, there have been isolated cases of transmission of herpes virus, tuberculosis and meningitis. For these reasons mouth-to-mouth ventilation should be avoided if at all possible. Instead, ventilation should be performed using a Laerdal pocket mask with a one-way valve or a self-inflating bag with mask.

Transport of high-risk patients

On some occasions an ambulance may be called upon to transport a patient with a known infectious disease. In this case some anticipatory measures can be taken. A crew with known immunity to the disease should be selected where possible (e.g. mumps). Disposable linen should be used in the ambulance, and gowns and masks should be worn by the crew whenever they examine the patient. After the transfer of the patient all disposables should be placed in plastic bags and sent for incineration.

Action to take in case of exposure to infectious disease

Crew members who have been exposed to an infectious disease and are worried that they may have contracted the infection should contact their occupational health department.

Needlestick injury

- After a needlestick injury, immediately wash the area of the injury in running water
- Ask the patient if he is known to have an infectious disease
- If the patient gives consent take a blood sample to assess hepatitis and HIV status (*the patient will need counselling before having these investigations*)
- Attend the occupational health unit or local Emergency Department without delay
- Ensure blood is taken for checking hepatitis serology and to ensure immunity.

Any treatment will be based on a risk assessment depending on one's own (or likely) hepatitis status and that of the patient. The occupational health department may offer HIV counselling.

Infections transmitted from paramedic staff to patient

All paramedic personnel have a duty to ensure that they are healthy and are not harbouring any potentially infectious diseases. Any concerns about illness should be discussed with the occupational health department. Paramedics should not work if they have large open wounds and must ensure that any small cuts or abrasions are covered with waterproof dressings.

For further information, see Ch. 19 in *Emergency Care: A Textbook for Paramedics*.

CHAPTER 20

Trauma

The trauma patient requires rapid assessment and management prior to transport to hospital for definitive care. This early evaluation and resuscitation must be structured and methodical and must identify time-critical cases where patients have life-threatening injuries. These patients need the urgent services of a major receiving hospital, trauma team and trauma surgeons. The medical history of the patient and the mechanism of the injury are the two essential requirements of the trauma history and must be obtained at a speed appropriate to the clinical state of the patient.

Taking a history from a trauma patient

- History-taking must not delay immediate resuscitation within the primary survey where this is clearly required
- After an appropriate introduction, the patient should be asked about what has happened
- A positive and appropriate response will also provide the information that the patient is conscious, has a patent airway, sufficient tidal volume to speak and sufficient cardiac output to provide an adequate cerebral circulation
- The major complaints and location of pain must be sought next, followed by accompanying symptoms such as breathing difficulty and nausea
- Any episode of altered level of consciousness and any events or symptoms preceding the accident, such as chest pain, must be established
- The mnemonic AMPLE is a helpful aide-mémoire for the components of the trauma history when under pressure
- Knowledge of medications such as beta-blockers or warfarin will alter the management of the patient

- The past medical history is important in that patients who have previous significant illnesses (particularly cardiac or respiratory) have a relatively poor prognosis following injury
- It is always wise to assume that an injured patient has a full stomach and that there is a constant risk of vomiting and aspiration
- Some environmental factors to consider are the temperature, the presence of toxic substances (chemicals and radiation) and material which may contaminate a wound
- Identification of a chemical contaminant is the responsibility of the fire service.

The mechanism of injury

The hospital trauma team has little or no perception of the clues at the scene that relate to the nature, direction and force of injury. Therefore, ambulance personnel are the 'eyes and ears' of the emergency department and they are privileged to know far more about the mechanism of injury – this understanding should be conveyed in the handover.

> Consider taking Polaroid photographs of the scene for the Emergency Department.

Road traffic collisions

- Certain mechanisms of injury, such as side-impact collisions, can be used to predict the pattern of injury found in an individual patient
- The paramedic should therefore assess the pattern of damage to the vehicles – a process known as 'reading the wreckage'
- Ejection from the vehicle in a road traffic collision increases the likelihood that the patient has sustained spinal cord and other serious injuries and is associated with a threefold increase in mortality rate
- Death of another occupant of the vehicle implies that the live patient has been subject to a high-energy collision and is therefore at risk of major injury even if injuries are not immediately apparent
- Entrapment for over 15 minutes is associated with an increased magnitude of injury severity
- Rollover incidents tend to be associated with an increase in cervical spine injuries. This is consistent with the forceful lateral bending and flexion–extension forces involved and the increased likelihood of axial loading of the spine.

Falls from a height

- Falls from a height inevitably involve sudden deceleration on impact. The distance of the fall, type of surface contacted and anatomical points of impact will determine the injury pattern

- Most adult falls involve lower limb fractures, often including the calcaneum, femur and, by transmitted force, the pelvis
- Lower limb injury is commonly bilateral although the patient may only complain of pain in one limb
- The spine, in particular the lumbar and thoracic areas, is frequently affected, often with multiple crush fractures of the vertebral bodies
- Any complaint of back pain should raise the suspicion of vertebral fractures
- Even trivial falls may cause serious injury in the elderly, particularly where disease has rendered the patient vulnerable to injury
- The elderly man who falls down two or three stairs and strikes his forehead on the ground may hyperextend his relatively rigid cervical spine enough to produce a fracture.

Penetrating trauma

Knife wounds

- Knife wounds cause direct injury in the direction of blade penetration. The damage depends on the length of the blade and the degree of penetration hence a description of the weapon will be of use to the surgeons
- Knife wounds to the neck and chest may be particularly dangerous owing to the presence of important blood vessels and organs
- Chest wounds may involve abdominal structures and vice versa
- A wound in the epigastrium may penetrate the diaphragm, causing ventricular puncture and pericardial tamponade.

Bullet wounds

- Civilian bullet wounds in the main tend to be from either a handgun or a shotgun
- Lethal damage from these injuries depends largely on the anatomical area of injury and the type of projectile; e.g. if a projectile breaks up during the first few centimetres of penetration it will cause increased tissue injury
- The energy transferred from the missile along its wounding path will depend on the density and elasticity of the tissue. High-energy transfer is likely if the missile strikes bone.

Blast injuries

Six patterns of injury are commonly associated with explosions:

1. Primary blast injury: the shock wave

    Primary injury commonly causes damage to cavities within the body: the ears, lungs and gastrointestinal tract. The injuries to the lung range from pinpoint haemorrhages to massive intrapulmonary haemorrhage ('blast lung')

2. Secondary blast injury: injuries from flying debris

    Secondary blast injuries are directly related to the types of flying debris and the sites of penetration

3. Tertiary blast injury: injuries due to the blast wind such as amputations
4. Crush injury
5. Flash burns
   Flash burns tend to affect those nearest to the site of the explosion and will burn exposed areas of skin (often hands and face)
6. Psychological trauma.

For further information, see Ch. 20 in *Emergency Care: A Textbook for Paramedics*.

CHAPTER 21

The primary and secondary survey

The initial assessment of the trauma patient requires a methodology which can be applied consistently and in priority order.

Primary survey

> Primary Survey = Assessment + Management of life-threatening injuries.

A primary survey may be completed rapidly if there are no life-threatening injuries. The ability to converse normally with a patient demonstrates a normal airway, adequate breathing and circulation to the brain and an alert conscious level.

The primary survey follows the sequence:

- Catastrophic haemorrhage control (<C>)
- Airway with cervical spine control (A)
- Breathing with ventilation (B)
- Circulation (C)
- Disability and neurological assessment (D)
- Exposure and environment (E).

Patients with significant trauma require immediate evacuation to hospital. Highly organised on-site care is essential. The aim is to prepare the patient for departure from the scene in no more than *10 minutes* from the ambulance's arrival.

'Scoop and run'

Survival rate is increased if the time taken to reach definitive care in hospital is short. This is reflected in the modern 'scoop and run' method which incorporates:

- Control of exsanguinating external haemorrhage
- Airway and cervical spine protection
- Breathing assessment and support
- Arrest of major external haemorrhage
- Immobilisation on a long spinal board (where appropriate)
- Rapid evacuation to an appropriate hospital
- Cannulation *en route*.

Performing the primary survey

The primary survey and resuscitation permit identification of life-threatening conditions and their simultaneous treatment.

Catastrophic haemorrhage

The management of severe, life-threatening, external haemorrhage can take precedence over the rest of the primary survey. This situation is likely to be rare, e.g. a traumatic amputation, and is likely to be obvious when encountered.

Management

Direct pressure on a bleeding wound followed by pressure dressings and elevation should deal with most bleeding peripheries.

Rarely, pressure will need to be applied to pressure points (where an artery can be compressed) such as the brachial or femoral arteries. Improvised tourniquets should not be employed, as they cause venous distension without stopping arterial flow.

Specifically designed tourniquets such as the Combat Application Tourniquet (CAT) can be used to temporarily get control of bleeding from a limb but in the civilian environment should be loosened after 15 minutes to see if control can then be gained by conventional means.

Bleeding from large wounds to the torso will be more difficult to manage and will require packing and constant, direct pressure. If available, novel haemostatic agents may be used. These include Hemcon®, Quikclot® and Celox®.

Airway and cervical spine

Assessment

Any injury severe enough to compromise the airway may also damage the cervical spine. Always assume that the cervical spine is injured and thus it must be protected from movement during airway interventions and transport.

Causes of airway obstruction include:

- Tongue prolapse
- Foreign bodies

- Vomit
- Major facial injury.

Obstruction may occur at any level from the mouth and nose to the trachea.
   Complete obstruction of the airway will manifest as an absence of breathing.

Management

If complete or partial airway obstruction is identified it must be rectified as rapidly as possible without endangering the cervical spine. This involves a series of stepped airway interventions of increasing complexity until obstruction is relieved.

Box 21.1 **Stepped airway care**

1. Airway clearance – manual and aspiration
2. Manual airway opening manoeuvres
3. Jaw thrust
4. Oropharyngeal airway
5. Nasopharyngeal airway
6. Orotracheal intubation
7. Cricothyroid transtracheal jet insufflation
8. Definitive surgical airway.

Box 21.2 **Actions in the patient with a clenched jaw**

- Insert a nasal airway
- Administer high-flow oxygen
- Consider needle cricothyroidotomy
- Transfer urgently to hospital for induction of anaesthesia and intubation.

Cervical spine immobilisation

Once the airway is secure, neck immobilisation must continue with the application of a correctly sized semi-rigid cervical collar and head immobilisation device.
   The patient must subsequently be fully immobilised on a long spinal board with at least four body straps.
   Restless patients should only be fitted with a semi-rigid collar, since full immobilisation may only exacerbate movement in the cervical spine if the rest of the body is flailing.
   If the history conclusively excludes the possibility of a spinal injury, immobilisation is not necessary.

DO NOT immobilise the neck if the patient is restless and thrashing about.

Breathing

Assessment

The following signs should be sought in the neck:

- Swelling
- Surgical emphysema
- Tracheal deviation
- Neck vein distension
- Bruising
- Lacerations.

Breathing must be assessed for:

- Rate
- Adequacy
- Equal bilateral ventilation.

The chest must be inspected to assess:

- Movement
- Instability
- Flail segment
- Wounds.

The chest wall must be felt to detect:

- Surgical emphysema
- Tenderness
- Paradoxical movement.

Percussion bilaterally may reveal one-sided hyper-resonance over a large pneumothorax. Finally, auscultation for the presence of breath sounds bilaterally must be performed.

Distress, confusion and abnormally rapid or slow respiratory rate are alarming signs and the patient may require assisted ventilation.

Clearing the airway does not assure adequate ventilation

Management

The spontaneously breathing patient with significant trauma requires the provision of supplemental oxygen, with a non-rebreathing reservoir mask and an oxygen flow rate of 10–15 L/min.

In adults, a respiratory rate of <10/min or >30/min suggests significant ventilatory inadequacy. Inadequate ventilation demands assisted ventilation. This is most easily performed using a bag-valve-mask and reservoir device.

Formal intermittent positive pressure ventilation with bag and mask or endotracheal tube may be necessary in the event of respiratory arrest. A mechanical ventilator may also be useful, especially for longer transfers.

Displacement of an endotracheal tube in transit, or development of tension pneumothorax secondary to positive pressure ventilation, may occur at any time.

The use of pulse oximetry and end-tidal CO_2 monitors can assist greatly in transit but repeated auscultation is essential.

Immediately life-threatening conditions

Box 21.3 **Life-threatening breathing problems (ATOMIC)**

A – **A**irway obstruction (intrathoracic)
T – **T**ension pneumothorax
O – **O**pen chest injury
M – **M**assive haemothorax
i – Fla**i**l chest
C – **C**ardiac tamponade

Airway obstruction

Intrathoracic airway obstruction is fortunately rare. It is usually untreatable in the prehospital environment. If there is a history of foreign body aspiration, a chest thrust or Heimlich manoeuvre may be beneficial. Otherwise apply high flow oxygen and evacuate immediately.

Tension pneumothorax

Tension pneumothorax may be present during initial assessment or appear secondary to positive pressure ventilation, where a simple, undetected pneumothorax is expanded by the pressure of the ventilating gases. The features of tension pneumothorax are given in the table.

Immediate decompression using needle thoracocentesis is required (see p. 133).

Open chest injury

Open chest wounds must be covered with an Asherman® or Bolin® seal or occlusive dressing sealed on three sides.

Massive haemothorax

Massive haemothorax requires a chest drain, best inserted in hospital. Intravenous access can be achieved en route. Needle thoracocentesis is not indicated in haemothorax.

Flail chest

Patients with significant flail chest may require ventilatory support; apart from this, simple support to the flail segment is the only treatment necessary pending arrival in hospital.

Cardiac tamponade

Unless there is a penetrating wound in the appropriate area, cardiac tamponade is extremely difficult to diagnose prehospital. Unless a doctor is present (who may perform an emergency thoracotomy), the patient's only hope is rapid evacuation to hospital.

Circulation

Pale, cool skin, tachycardia, delayed capillary return and altered mental state indicate significant shock. Hypotension frequently is not apparent until at least 30% of the blood volume has been lost.

> Shock is a disorder of the circulation characterised by reduced organ perfusion and tissue oxygenation

Management

Any external blood loss should be arrested by the application of direct pressure. Pelvic and long-bone fractures should be rapidly immobilised. Unless the patient is trapped or the transfer time is likely to be very long, intravenous access should be obtained in transit.

In general, a policy of hypotensive resuscitation should be followed:

- If the patient has a palpable radial pulse, *fluid should not be given*
- Access should be obtained during transit (unless the transit time is very short)

Box 21.4 **Clinical features of tension pneumothorax**

- Rapidly increasing breathlessness
- Unilaterally absent breath sounds
- Hyper-resonance on percussion of the affected hemithorax
- Raised and congested neck veins
- Hypotension
- Cyanosis
- Tracheal shift away from the affected side (late)
- Resistance to ventilation in the ventilated patient.

- *If the radial pulse is not palpable*, small aliquots of 250 mL of warm normal saline (or a similar crystalloid) should be given until a palpable pulse returns and repeated to maintain it
- Under no circumstances, however, should any of these actions delay transfer to hospital since patients who are actively bleeding require urgent life-saving surgical intervention
- Elevation of the blood pressure above the level of 90 mmHg may precipitate rebleeding as well as diluting clotting factors and result in a worse prognosis.

Assessment of the circulation

- Skin colour
- Skin temperature
- Pulse rate and volume
- Capillary refill time (normal less than 2 seconds)
- Mental state
- Assess the thorax, abdomen, pelvis and femurs for evidence of injury and consequent concealed haemorrhage (think 'blood on the floor and four more').

Disability

Quickly assess responsive pupil size and reactions. The AVPU mnemonic should be used or GCS recorded to establish a baseline level of consciousness.

An AVPU response of P or U is an indication for serious concern due to the likelihood of significant intracranial injury. The blood sugar should be estimated.

Expose and environment

Complete exposure of the patient is impractical in the prehospital environment and will potentially render the patient hypothermic. The chest and neck area are exposed as part of the primary survey.

The patient's temperature and blood sugar should be checked at this stage.

If during the primary survey the patient deteriorates restart the primary survey from the beginning.

The secondary survey

The secondary survey is the more detailed head-to-toe examination to identify every injury the patient has sustained and is generally performed in hospital.

In prolonged transfers a secondary survey may occasionally be appropriate.

Performing the secondary survey

There will rarely be time to complete a secondary survey in the prehospital environment. It may occasionally be possible, for example, in an entrapment. In the majority of cases, evacuation to the hospital for the management of life threatening (1° survey) injuries is paramount.

Assessment of the head

Look for:

- Lacerations
- Bruising
- Blood and/or cerebrospinal fluid from ears or nose (suggesting basal skull fracture)
- Check pupil size and response
- Battle's sign and 'raccoon' or panda eyes
- Pallor and sweating
- Cyanosis.

Feel for:

- Scalp haematomas
- Depressed skull fractures
- Facial tenderness and fractures.

Listen for:

- Airway 'noise' suggesting obstruction
- Breathing adequacy and rate.

Assessment of the neck

To assess the neck, the collar may need to be removed while a colleague maintains in-line immobilisation of the neck.
  Look and feel for:

- Lacerations
- Swelling
- Surgical emphysema – skin 'crackling'
- Distension of neck veins
- Spinal deformity, tenderness or haematoma
- Tracheal deviation
- Laryngeal crepitus.

Assessment of the chest

Look for:

- Wounds and evidence of penetrating injury
- Deformity and abnormal movements
- Breathing distress and pain on inspiration
- Patterning from clothing or seatbelts.

Feel for:

- Tenderness
- Instability and 'clunking' of flail segment
- Surgical emphysema.

Listen for:

- Percussion revealing increased resonance over a pneumothorax or stony dullness over a haemothorax
- Presence of equal breath sounds
- Unilateral absence or reduction of breath sounds suggestive of pneumothorax
- Unilateral, usually basal reduction of breath sounds associated with haemothorax (only if the patient is sitting up).

Assessment of the abdomen

Look for:

- Penetrating wounds and contusions
- Seatbelt contusions and clothing imprints
- Distension.

Feel for:

- Tenderness – either localised or generalised
- Guarding – involuntary muscle spasm on gentle palpation
- Rigidity.

Assessment of the pelvis

The need for pelvic splintage should be determined based on the mechanisms of injury and symptomatology.

Assessment of lower and upper extremities

Look for:

- Obvious wounds and contusions
- Deformity and swelling associated with fractures
- Voluntary movement.

Feel for:

- Tenderness and deformity
- Distal pulses
- Intact nerve supply – sensation to touch and pain, motor function
- Normal movement in joints.

On completion of the secondary survey, any injuries which are found should be stabilised and any wounds covered.

Assessment of the totality of the patient's injuries comprises the secondary survey.

For further information, see Ch. 21 in *Emergency Care: A Textbook for Paramedics.*

CHAPTER 22

Shock

Shock is a clinical syndrome which is defined as 'inadequate tissue perfusion resulting in hypoxia and ultimately in cell death'. Shock can be classified according to the mechanism by which it occurs:

Types of shock

- *Hypovolaemic or haemorrhagic shock* due to loss of circulating volume. Causes include: blood loss, burns and diarrhoea and vomiting
- *Cardiogenic shock* due to loss of normal cardiac function ('pump failure'). Causes include: myocardial ischaemia, infarction, contusion, cardiac tamponade, massive pulmonary embolism
- *Septic shock* due to dilation of blood vessels by substances released in overwhelming infection. Causes include: bacterial viral or fungal infection
- *Neurogenic shock* due to dilation of blood vessels caused by spinal injury
- *Anaphylactic shock* due to dilation of blood vessels as part of a severe allergic reaction.

Hypovolaemic shock

The most common cause of shock in the prehospital environment is hypovolaemia (inadequate blood volume), usually related to blood or plasma loss from trauma, ruptured aortic aneurysm, ectopic pregnancy or gastrointestinal haemorrhage.

The priorities in the management of shock are:

- Identification of the patient at risk of significant bleeding
- Identification of shock
- Control of compressible haemorrhage
- Urgent transfer to hospital for surgical intervention.

Box 22.1 **Clinical features of shock**

- Tachycardia (arrhythmias may develop)
- Change in blood pressure (initially reduced pulse pressure, later lowered systolic and diastolic pressures)
- Altered mental state
- Tachypnoea
- Cool, clammy skin
- Cyanosis
- Oliguria

Compensatory mechanisms in hypovolaemic shock

- Tachycardia
- Peripheral vasoconstriction (with diversion of blood to vital organs)
- Increase in frequency and depth of respiration
- Diversion of blood within the lungs to areas of maximal gas exchange
- Increased release of oxygen from haemoglobin
- Reduced urine output.

Classification of haemorrhagic shock

Hypovolaemic shock can be divided into four grades depending on the extent of circulating volume lost.

Exact estimation of blood loss will almost never be possible and is usually over-estimated. However, the following factors should be taken into consideration:

- Age (the elderly are less able to compensate for volume loss and have signs associated with a higher grade of shock but with lower blood loss)
- Fitness (athletes and fit individuals may compensate and hence have few signs or symptoms even with major losses): eventual decompensation may be very rapid
- Medications (drugs such as β-blockers, antihypertensives and antianginals may mask normal responses such as tachycardia)
- Pre-existing disease (patients with underlying conditions such as ischaemic heart disease, cerebrovascular disease and pregnancy are less able to cope with the effects of shock).

A pulse of 95 bpm may be normal in an elderly patient, but can represent severe vascular compromise in a marathon runner whose resting pulse is 40 bpm.

All grades of shock will progress if the bleeding is not stopped, the only end-point of uncontrolled bleeding is death.

Table 22.1 Classification of hypovolaemic shock (adult)

Grade	Blood loss	Symptoms
Grade I	Up to 750 mL, 15%	Minimal blood pressure unchanged Occasionally tachycardia occurs
Grade II	750–1500 mL 15–30%	Pallor, tachycardia 100/min, decreased pulse pressure Subtle changes in mood may be seen, e.g. anxiety, aggression or fright
Grade III	1500–2000 mL 30–40%. This is the minimum volume loss that results in a decrease in blood pressure	Classic signs of inadequate perfusion are usually noticed: pallor, sweating, altered mental state (anxiety, confusion, aggression), tachycardia >120/min, tachypnoea, hypotension
Grade IV	Over 2000 mL life-threatening and catastrophic	Pulse is weak and thready. Tachycardia may deteriorate to bradycardia. Systolic blood pressure drops markedly with a very narrow pulse pressure or unobtainable diastolic pressure. Drowsiness, lethargy or unconsciousness

Treatment principles
- The delivery of the patient to hospital must never be delayed by interventions such as intravenous access or volume replacement
- Catastrophic external haemorrhage should be addressed immediately
- The primary objective in the management of shock is to restore tissue perfusion, with the delivery of adequate oxygen and other metabolites. Only the start of this process will occur before the patient reaches hospital
- All shocked patients require the highest possible concentration of inspired oxygen delivered to the lungs
- Clearance and maintenance of a patent upper and lower airway are mandatory. This may require the patient to be intubated and positive pressure ventilation commenced
- Factors impeding ventilation, such as pneumothorax, haemothorax or gastric dilation, will require specific correction

- Identification of the patient who is at risk of injury likely to cause shock is the key first stage of the assessment of C
- Circulatory assessment includes a general assessment of the patient for:
  - Coldness
  - Clammy skin
  - Sweating
  - Mental state
  - Pulse (rate and quality, presence or absence of a radial pulse)
- Once external bleeding has been identified and controlled, a brief attempt should be made to identify sites of *significant* internal bleeding. Potential sites of bleeding are:
  - Chest
  - Abdomen (and retroperitoneum)
  - Pelvis
  - Long bones (usually from fractured femurs)
  - External
- This is often referred to as *'blood on the floor and four more'*.

Intravenous fluid therapy

- Aggressive administration of intravenous fluids is discouraged due to:
  - Displacement of blood clot
  - Dilution of clotting factors
  - Promotion of hypothermia and secondary metabolic derangement
  - Delay in reaching surgery whilst attempts to gain intravenous access are made
- If the patient is trapped or transfer times are likely to be prolonged, vascular access should be obtained.

Vascular access is often difficult because of the combination of hypovolaemia with collapsed veins and an adverse environment. If two attempts at venous access are unsuccessful then consideration should be given to the use of intraosseous access.

Once intravascular access has been achieved, crystalloid should be administered in aliquots of 250 mL to maintain the presence of a radial pulse. If the presence of a radial pulse cannot be achieved, in the circumstances of prolonged transfer or entrapment, survival is unlikely and vigorous fluid administration pending extrication and transfer to definitive care is the only option available.

Choice of fluid

- It is standard practice in the UK to start intravenous volume replacement with isotonic crystalloid solutions such as 0.9% (normal) saline or sodium lactate (Hartmann's or Ringer lactate) solution
- Colloid solutions are significantly more expensive than crystalloids and have a small but recognised risk of anaphylactic reaction

- In the restoration of hypovolaemic shock, colloids are relatively more efficient volume for volume than crystalloid solutions. Colloid solutions may have a role in fluid therapy during prolonged transfers or in entrapment.

All fluid given should be warmed to 37°C to prevent the adverse effects of rapid infusion of cold fluid into a shocked patient.

Cardiogenic shock

Cardiogenic shock is inadequate tissue perfusion: caused by failure of the pump mechanism (the heart). It may be caused by failure of the heart muscle owing to ischaemia of the myocardium, myocardial infarction or contusion secondary to trauma. Rupture of the heart following ischaemia or penetrating trauma will also result in cardiogenic shock, exacerbated by compression of the heart caused by blood within the pericardium (*cardiac tamponade*).

Massive pulmonary embolism prevents normal cardiac function and will also produce cardiogenic shock but the most common cause of cardiogenic shock is myocardial infarction producing cardiac muscle or valve rupture. This results in a mortality rate greater than 90%.

Cardiogenic shock due to tamponade may occur as a result of blunt or penetrating trauma. In blunt trauma the outlook is extremely poor however cardiac tamponade due to penetrating trauma may respond to aspiration of blood from the pericardium or thoracotomy, when the chest is opened and the hole in the heart is closed, either by the insertion of a finger, a catheter (with the balloon inflated) or a stitch.

The possibility of tamponade should be considered with any penetrating injury to the upper torso. Thoracotomy or pericardiocentesis must be performed by an experienced doctor and is best undertaken in the Emergency Department.

Other causes of cardiogenic shock require oxygen therapy, management of the underlying cause and immediate evacuation.

Causes of cardiogenic shock

Heart muscle (myocardial) dysfunction:

- Ischaemia
- Infarction
- Contusion (blunt trauma).

Cardiac tamponade:

- Trauma
- Post infarction

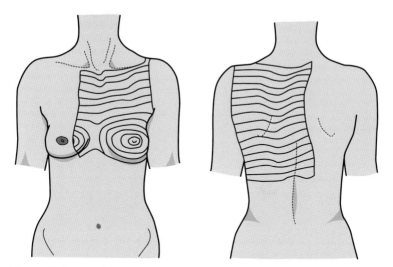

Figure 22.1 Areas where a penetrating injury may be associated with cardiac tamponade.

- Pulmonary embolism
- If the penetrating object is still in situ it must be left there and carefully protected from dislodgement or movement during a rapid transfer to hospital.

Septic shock

Septic shock results from the action of substances (mediators) released from cells as a consequence of severe infection (usually bacterial). Dilation of blood vessels, leakiness of tissue capillaries and a defect of oxygen utilisation by the tissues produce shock. The appropriate treatment for a patient with septic shock is investigation of the source of infection, intravenous antibiotics and intensive supportive care.

Septic shock usually takes some time to develop following the onset of infection. An exception is shock following suspected meningococcal infection when the patient may progress from health to death within a few hours. In this situation benzylpenicillin should be given intravenously or intramuscularly as soon as the diagnosis is made.

- All cases of septicaemic shock require oxygen and IV fluids should be started if the transfer is likely to be delayed.

Neurogenic shock

Neurogenic shock results from injury to the spinal cord, there is interruption of the nervous mechanism maintaining blood vessel wall tension; as a consequence vessels dilate, blood pressure falls and shock ensues. Neurogenic shock is therefore not associated with cold peripheries, which are instead warm and well perfused. In addition, the neurological interruption prevents a compensating tachycardia. Neurogenic shock is most commonly seen with lesions at the level of T6 and above.

> The hallmarks of neurogenic shock are hypotension, warm peripheries and bradycardia.

Shock due to spinal injury is rare. Therefore shock in the trauma patient is far more likely to be due to unrecognised haemorrhage. Protect the spine, start IV fluids and transfer the patient for hospital assessment of their spinal injury.

> Isolated head injury is not a cause of shock.

Clinical features of septic shock
- Low blood pressure
- Tachycardia
- Warm peripheries.

Anaphylactic shock

Anaphylactic shock results from an allergic reaction to a foreign protein such as nuts, bee stings or drugs.

The reaction is mediated by immunoglobulins and histamine and results in vasodilation and drop in blood pressure with a compensatory tachycardia.

For further information, see Ch. 22 in *Emergency Care: A Textbook for Paramedics.*

CHAPTER 23

Head injuries

The central nervous system has no stores of oxygen or glucose; if the blood supply is interrupted, depriving the brain of oxygen, consciousness is lost within 15–20 seconds. The brain cells will then die within 3–4 minutes.

Because the skull is a rigid box, tissue swelling or bleeding within it will lead to an increase in pressure. As the pressure rises, the brain is pushed down, impacting on rigid structures such as the tentorium and the foramen magnum. This leads to reduced consciousness and eventually causes death by coning, the compression of cardiorespiratory centres within the brainstem.

Any head injury should raise the suspicion of associated c-spine injury.
Risk factors for head injury include:

- Alcohol abuse
- Drug abuse
- Anticoagulants
- Blood clotting disorders
- Other drugs including tranquillisers
- The elderly especially with dementia.

> The key to the optimal management of head-injured patients is the prevention of secondary brain damage by appropriate attention to the airway, breathing and circulation.

Primary and secondary brain injury

> Definitions: The brain injury sustained at the time of the accident is known as the primary injury and cannot be reduced once it has occurred
>
> Secondary brain injury is a combination of factors that lead to additional brain injury and cell death following the primary injury

Any episode of hypoxia or hypotension will significantly worsen the patient's outcome from head injury. As hypoxia affects the brain as a whole there is generalised swelling – cerebral oedema – which results in raised intracranial pressure (ICP). When the intracranial pressure approaches the arterial pressure, blood cannot flow through the brain and so cells will die.

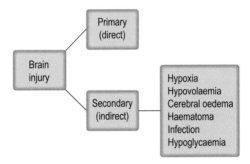

Figure 23.1 Primary and secondary brain injury.

The important blood pressure for the brain is not the mean arterial pressure (MAP) alone, but the perfusion pressure (PP). The cerebral perfusion pressure is the mean arterial pressure minus the mean intracranial pressure (MICP): $PP = MAP - MICP$.

Both a fall in mean arterial pressure and a rise in intracranial pressure may therefore reduce cerebral perfusion pressure and produce secondary brain injury.

Treatment should aim to maintain the cerebral perfusion pressure and keep the patient's arterial pressure near normal limits and above 100 mmHg in the adult. Raised central venous pressure also leads to increased ICP. Anything that increases central venous pressure, for example a tension pneumothorax, must also be treated.

Signs of raised intracranial pressure:

- Decreasing level of consciousness
- Increasing blood pressure (late)
- Falling pulse rate (late)
- Decreasing respiratory rate (late)
- Pupillary dilation (late).

Generalised brain injury

Generalised or diffuse injuries represent a spectrum of injury from mild concussion with rapid and complete recovery to diffuse axonal injury (DAI) which is the principal cause of long-standing coma following head injury. Coma may last days or weeks or may be permanent.

Localised or focal brain injuries consist of:

- Cerebral contusion
- Intracranial haemorrhages
- Lacerations and penetrating injuries.

Intracranial haemorrhage

Intracranial haemorrhage may be:

- Extradural bleeding: <1% of injuries, may be fatal but complete recovery is possible if treated within 2 hours
- Subdural bleeding: 30% of injuries, good recovery if treated within 2 hours but some residual disability is common
- Intracerebral bleeding: this is within the brain tissue itself
- Subarachnoid bleeding: within the subarachnoid space, produces headache and decreasing consciousness.

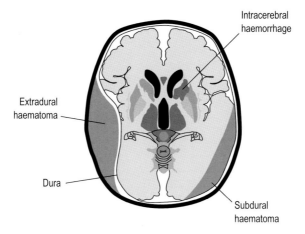

Figure 23.2 Anatomy of intracranial bleeding.

Extradural haematoma – a history of rising intracranial pressure

An extradural haematoma is bleeding within the skull. Although the initial injury to the brain is liable to have caused concussion, the patient often recovers temporarily (a lucid interval) before deteriorating. As the size of the haematoma increases, intracranial pressure increases and the conscious level deteriorates.

As the pressure increases on one side of the brain, part of the temporal lobe herniates into the small space between the brain stem and the tentorium cerebelli. In this space is the third cranial nerve and as this is compressed, the pupil on the same side dilates.

As intracranial pressure continues to rise the herniating temporal lobe forces the brainstem against the opposite fold of tentorium, causing the opposite pupil to dilate and paralysis of the arm and leg of the opposite side of the body to the haematoma. This is a pre-terminal sign.

An alternative site of herniation is the foramen magnum. This is known as coning and results in the late development of bradycardia, hypertension and hypoventilation.

Classical clinical features of extradural haematoma:

- Loss of consciousness (initial concussion), followed by recovery
- Then increasing headache
- Then declining conscious level
- Weakness on the opposite side of the body to the head injury
- Dilated and fixed pupil on the same side as the injury.

Diagnosis can be difficult. The definitive investigation is a computed tomography (CT) scan. Patients with a significant period of unconsciousness (2–3 minutes or more) should be taken to a hospital that has 24-hour CT scanning facilities.

Penetrating injury

Brain haemorrhage can also be caused by penetrating trauma, inflicted by a low-velocity implement such as a knife, or by impalement in an industrial or traffic accident. The severity of the injury and any long-term disability is determined by the area of the brain which is injured. If the patient is unconscious after the penetrating injury the prognosis is exceedingly poor. Patients who are conscious and talking after such an injury can survive.

Skull fractures

Damage to the brain is demonstrated by an altered conscious level.

The clinical significance of a skull fracture is its potential relation to intracranial bleeding. The combination of a fracture of the skull and alteration of consciousness increases the chance of intracranial bleeding from 1 in 5000 to 1 in 4.

Linear skull fractures require no specific treatment. The emphasis is on the underlying brain injury, but when the skull fracture is depressed, and pressing on the brain tissue, urgent neurosurgical intervention is required.

Signs of a base of skull fracture may not appear until several hours after the injury and rarely develop before the patient arrives in hospital. Signs of basal skull fracture include:

- CSF leakage from nose (rhinorrhoea)
- CSF leakage from ear (otorrhoea)
- Panda (raccoon) eyes
- Battle's sign
- Bleeding from the ears.

Very severe open injuries may expose the brain. Moist non-adherent dressings are needed to cover the area and to stop the brain tissue drying out. Scalp wounds should not be probed with a finger in the prehospital environment. They should be covered and left alone.

Patient assessment

The priorities in management are to protect the airway and ensure the delivery of oxygen to the brain

To achieve this there must be:

- an adequate airway (A)
- uncompromised breathing (B)
- adequate cerebral perfusion (C).

Assessment of the head-injured patient assumes the primary survey has been carried out, with appropriate management for the airway and protection of the cervical spine in every patient who is concussed or who has an altered conscious level. The level of consciousness should be assessed using the AVPU scale or the GCS.

Loss of consciousness and amnesia

Many patients cannot tell you whether they have been knocked out and certainly cannot reliably judge the period of unconsciousness.

> Patients cannot remember the duration of coma.

Patients will say they lack memory of an event. This lack of memory is known as amnesia which can be post-traumatic or retrograde. Post-traumatic or anterograde amnesia is common. The duration of amnesia should be recorded. Retrograde amnesia (with memory loss of events prior to the head injury) is usually a sign of more significant injury.

'Minor' head injuries, where the patient has been knocked out for 1–2 seconds but then makes a full recovery, are extremely common, large numbers of these patients are admitted to hospital for head injury observation.

> Symptoms attributed to head injury are known as concussion.

Any patient who has undergone loss of consciousness should be taken to hospital. Patients who have prolonged post-traumatic amnesia of 5 minutes or more should also be assessed in hospital.

Always exclude head injury in:

- Epilepsy (post-ictal state)
- Alcohol abuse
- Drugs
- Dementia.

The above should never be simply accepted as the cause of an altered conscious level.

Lateralising signs

Assessment of upper and lower limb movement and sensation should be carried out. Loss of movement on one side of the body suggests an intracranial bleed – these are known as lateralising signs.

Pupils

Assessment of pupil function, documenting the size of the pupils and their response to light is an essential part of the primary survey.

Vital signs

The patient's vital signs are of great significance, as they provide direct assessments of brain function. These signs include pulse rate, blood pressure, respiratory rate and temperature.

Blood glucose

Hypoglycaemia contributes to secondary brain injury and must be corrected. Recording of blood glucose levels by paramedics should be routine not only in diabetic patients but also in patients with major head injury.

Management

Effective and rapid management of the airway, breathing and circulation will effectively manage disability and head injury. There are additional details which can improve the management of the head injured patient.

Airway

- If the patient is irritable, aggressive and has a gag reflex, adequate airway maintenance can be one of the most difficult prehospital problems
- Use stepped airway management to establish a patent airway
- Insert an OP or nasal airway if tolerated, apply oxygen if tolerated. Otherwise evacuate immediately

- Patients with a GCS score of 8 or less (AVPU rating P or U) will require formal intubation to protect their airway
- Intubating without the use of paralysing drugs will likely increase the patient's ICP. A careful 'neuroprotective' anaesthetic will be needed. This can only be carried out by a team trained in anaesthesia
- If the patient is trapped or cannot be transported to hospital within 15 minutes, the paramedic must consider calling medical help to the scene.

Breathing

- A normal respiratory rate is 10–18 breaths per minute in an adult, any respiratory rate above 18 breaths per minute should be assumed to be a sign of hypoxia, indicating that the patient requires oxygen
- Slow respiratory rates may be caused by drugs or by significant head injury
- A major aggravating factor in head injury is a tension pneumothorax As the pressure builds up in the chest cavity there is an increase of central venous pressure, resulting in a further increase in the intracranial pressure and precipitating further cerebral oedema. Relief of a tension pneumothorax as soon as possible by needle thoracocentesis can have a dramatic effect in reducing high cerebral pressures as well as improving ventilation.

Circulation

- Head injuries themselves do not cause low blood pressure, however, infants may lose a significant percentage of their blood volume into a scalp haematoma. This is less of a problem in adults although scalp lacerations can bleed heavily
- In the multiply injured patient the policy of maintaining a palpable radial pulse is appropriate
- This is less than ideal physiologically for the brain, as it may reduce cerebral perfusion, and a higher blood pressure endpoint is acceptable if there is definite isolated head injury.

Disability

- If possible, the patient should be transported at a slight 'head-up' angle of about 15°. This is only possible with some designs of stretcher trolley. This helps to maintain correct intracranial pressure.

Environment and exposure

- The unconscious patient will lose heat rapidly so keep them warm
- Blood glucose (BM Stix) should be checked and hypoglycaemia treated as low blood sugar will also lead to secondary brain injury.

Transfer to hospital

Ideally the assessment of a patient should be completed within 5 minutes, as longer on-scene times will be detrimental. Once the airway and cervical spine and breathing are stabilised, the patient should be rapidly transported to the nearest appropriate hospital. Obtaining IV access is best attempted in transit. At this stage a GCS score can be accurately assessed and can be continually monitored during the journey.

An appropriate hospital is one that has a 24-hour accident and emergency department and access to an available and working CT scanner. It is best to transfer the patients with serious head injuries to a hospital that has trained trauma teams and rapidly available neurosurgeons.

It is not efficient to treat patients by transferring them to the nearest hospital where they may be assessed over a period of 1–2 hours and then require a secondary transfer to a neurosurgical unit. The critical time for surgery may have passed, leading to increased mortality and morbidity rates.

For further information, see Ch. 23 in *Emergency Care: A Textbook for Paramedics.*

CHAPTER 24

Facial injuries

Most facial injuries will be managed as part of the secondary survey. Severe facial injuries may however compromise the airway through anatomical disruption or by bleeding.

Airway problems

Airway problems arise from:

- Inhalation of foreign bodies
- Posterior impaction of the fractured maxilla
- Loss of tongue control in a fractured mandible
- Intraoral tissue swelling
- Direct trauma to the larynx
- Haemorrhage.

Severe facial injury may necessitate advanced airway procedures such as cricothyroidotomy.

Circulatory problems

Haemorrhage from facial fractures may produce:

- airway obstruction
- hypovolaemic shock.

Two percent of facial injuries have associated cervical injuries and the patient's cervical spine should be protected using a semi-rigid collar, spine board and head blocks until injury can be excluded.

Soft tissue injuries

Soft tissue injuries may be divided into superficial cuts and grazes, lacerations and penetrating wounds. There may be loss of tissue or degloving injuries, as seen for example in the lower labial sulcus (groove behind the lower lip) when the skin over the chin is forcibly pushed downwards and backwards.

Treatment

- Profuse haemorrhage from cuts and lacerations should be stopped during the primary survey. Pressure applied over the wound with a gauze swab held firmly in place may be all that is required
- Penetrating injuries should not be explored. It is dangerous to explore neck wounds, which should be covered and managed in hospital
- Foreign bodies should be left in place, including those piercing the cheek or penetrating the other intraoral tissues, unless they are causing airway obstruction
- A cheek wound may sever the parotid duct, resulting in an escape of saliva onto the cheek
- During the secondary survey a thorough examination of the scalp and face will be carried out in order to identify all the soft tissue injuries.

Eye injuries

The most common superficial injury is a corneal abrasion in which the superficial layers of the cornea are removed. The resulting injury is exactly analogous to an abrasion of the skin and is very painful.

Blunt injury to the globe of the eye can produce a variety of injuries including haemorrhage into the anterior or posterior chambers and injury to the individual structures of the eye.

As well as a late sign of intracranial haemorrhage a unilateral dilated pupil may be caused by severe concussion to the globe (traumatic mydriasis). Similarly a unilateral constricted pupil may result from blunt trauma to the eyeball (traumatic miosis).

Penetrating injuries may be immediately apparent, especially given knowledge of the mechanism of injury. Foreign bodies on the surface of the eye are remarkably irritant and painful. Chemical injuries to the eye are extremely common, occurring in both domestic and industrial settings and can be eyesight-threatening.

Treatment

- No immediate treatment is usually required for corneal abrasions, although some patients may gain relief from covering the eye with a pad
- Patients with penetrating injuries should be transported to hospital urgently in the supine position. Both eyes should be covered to prevent eye movements but any protruding foreign body must not be forced further into the globe
- Small superficial foreign bodies will require removal in hospital although irrigation with clean water may be helpful in removing general debris if the injury has occurred in a dirty or contaminated environment
- Chemical injuries must be irrigated with copious saline
- Under no circumstances should any attempt be made to 'neutralise' an acid with an alkali or vice versa

- Eye injuries from alkalis have a worse prognosis than those from acids
- All such injuries require urgent assessment in the Emergency Department.

Injuries to teeth

Teeth may be loosened, partially extruded or completely avulsed (extracted). They may be fractured at the level of the crown or lower down on the root. Fractures involving segments of tooth-bearing bone may occur and are known as dentoalveolar fractures. Loose and avulsed teeth (and dentures) may be inhaled and are a cause of airway obstruction. Assessment of the patient's airway and inspection of the mouth are mandatory. Well-fitting dentures may be left in place.

In a patient without a head injury, a completely avulsed tooth (usually a front tooth in a child) can be immediately reinserted. The patient should be asked to hold the tooth in position and the advice of a dentist or maxillofacial surgeon sought. Alternatively, the tooth may be placed in a container of milk and transferred with the patient to hospital. Patients with an associated head injury are at particular risk from inhaling foreign bodies and should not be asked to hold their tooth in the inside of the cheek. If the tooth is fractured, where possible, the pieces should be found and taken with the patient to hospital. A chest radiograph may be necessary if there is any suspicion that a tooth or fragment may have been inhaled.

Fractures of the facial skeleton

Fractures of the mandible

A patient with a fractured mandible will give a history of recent trauma to the jaw. A blow to the right side of the jaw may lead to a fracture through the right angle and/or a fracture of the left condylar neck. An injury to the chin may produce a midline fracture together with bilateral condylar neck fractures.

The patient will complain of pain and swelling over the site of the injury and be unable to open the mouth fully. A number of teeth may have been lost or displaced and the patient may notice that their teeth no longer fit together properly (malocclusion).

Examination may reveal a step deformity along the line of the lower jaw. Intraoral inspection may show lacerated and bleeding gums and loose teeth. Bruising underneath the tongue (sublingual haematoma) usually occurs adjacent to the fracture line.

Loss of tongue control in a fractured mandible

The fractured mandible may become an immediate airway management problem when there are bilateral symphysial fractures or there is extensive bone loss resulting in loss of tongue support.

The musculature of the tongue is attached to the genial tubercles in the midline and if this fragment becomes detached, the tongue may fall backwards to obstruct the oropharynx. Patients at particular risk from this complication are those with a depressed conscious level who are unable to control their tongue.

Immediate management involves pulling the tongue forward and holding it in an unobstructed position. This may be achieved manually or a doctor may use a large suture (0 gauge black silk) placed transversely through the dorsum of the tongue (a large safety pin may even be used) and the suture taped to the side of the face. A transverse stitch is less likely to cut through the tongue when traction is applied.

Fractures of the maxilla

A patient with a fractured upper jaw is likely to have sustained high-impact trauma to the face. Gentle manipulation of the maxilla will reveal mobility of the upper jaw and the patient may have a 'dish-face' deformity.

Marked swelling is a feature of the Le Fort II and Le Fort III fractures and may be accompanied by bruising around the eyes. The patient may complain that the teeth do not meet properly.

Posterior impaction of a fractured maxilla

A fractured maxilla may cause obstruction of the nasopharynx by backward and downward displacement along the slope of the base of the skull.

Disimpaction of the maxilla can relieve the obstruction and is performed by placing the gloved middle and index fingers behind the soft palate and pulling forwards.

Management of haemorrhage

Profuse haemorrhage can result from a fractured maxilla after damage to the terminal branches of the maxillary and ethmoidal arteries. Nasal Epistats® should be inserted – the distal balloon is inflated first, traction applied and then the proximal balloon inflated.

This may further displace a fractured maxilla downwards in which case bite-blocks (such as rolled up gauze) should be placed between the teeth to splint the upper jaw.

Orbital and zygomaticomaxillary complex fractures

Fractures in this region potentially involve the eye. Trauma to the cheek can produce marked periorbital swelling and bruising. A step deformity may be felt along the zygoma and there may be flattening of the cheek.

Swelling of the eyelids may make examination of the eye more difficult but it is important that any globe injuries are not missed. Examination of the pupils should be undertaken to assess size and reactivity.

The patient may also complain of double vision (diplopia).

A blow to the eye may cause a fracture to the weak orbital floor, tethering the globe and restricting eye movement when looking up (orbital blow-out fracture).

Nasal complex fractures

Nasal fractures can be accompanied by profuse haemorrhage. The patient should bend forward (c-spine injuries permitting) to prevent blood filling the posterior oropharynx.

If simple compression of the anterior part of the nose (Little's area) does not stop the bleeding then it can be controlled by inserting expanding foam packs (Merocel® packs). The packs should be lubricated, inserted into the nostril and activated by injecting some normal saline with a syringe. The strings should be taped to the patient's face to prevent the pack displacing into the airway.

For further information, see Ch. 24 in *Emergency Care: A Textbook for Paramedics*.

CHAPTER 25

Chest injuries

Deaths following injuries to the thorax usually result from a lack of oxygen (hypoxia) or lack of circulating blood volume (hypovolaemia). Injuries may be blunt or penetrating. In blunt trauma the force can be spread over a wide area. After low-energy impacts, damage is usually localised to the superficial structures. In contrast, following high-energy impacts considerable tissue disruption can be produced with severe injuries that may be difficult to manage. The significance of the local damage following penetrating trauma is dependent on both the site and the depth of penetration. In gunshot wounds the degree of injury is also determined by the amount of energy transferred to surrounding tissues.

Blast injuries cause particular injury to the lungs. The shockwave transmits through the tissues and causes injury to the alveoli within the lung tissues. This syndrome is known as blast lung and may lead to hypoxia. High blast pressures can also lead to air emboli which may precipitate sudden death if they obstruct the coronary or cerebral arteries.

Primary survey and resuscitation

The aim of the primary survey is to detect and correct any immediately life-threatening condition. In chest trauma there are six immediately life threatening conditions which can be treated.

These may be remembered using the mnemonic ATOMIC:

A – **A**irway obstruction

T – **T**ension pneumothorax

O – **O**pen chest wound

M – **M**assive haemothorax

I – Flail chest

C – Cardiac tamponade.

All trauma patients require high flow oxygen

Examination

To be confident that these conditions have been found or excluded, it is important that the chest and neck are examined.

Ideally, all the clothing covering the thorax should be removed so that a full inspection can be carried out.

The neck should be examined for the following:

- Swelling
- Surgical emphysema with crepitus
- Tracheal deviation
- Neck vein distension
- Bruising
- Lacerations.

Lacerations should only be inspected and *never* probed with metal instruments or fingers because catastrophic haemorrhage can be precipitated.

The chest can then be examined. This involves the following stages:

- Inspection of the chest
- Palpation of the trachea and ribs
- Auscultation of both axillae, top and bottom
- Percussion of both axillae, top and bottom
- Examination of the back: inspection, palpation, auscultation and percussion.

Inspection

The respiratory rate, depth and effort of respiration should be checked at frequent intervals. Rapid, shallow breathing and intercostal or supraclavicular indrawing are all sensitive indicators of underlying lung pathology. Both sides of the chest should be inspected and compared for symmetry of movement, bruising, abrasions and penetrating wounds. Paradoxical movement (movement of part of the chest wall in the opposite direction to the rest, inwards on inspiration and outwards on expiration) may be seen and is a sign of a flail segment.

Palpation

Starting at the top, the clavicles should be carefully palpated for deformity (which may be visible) and the chest wall should be gently felt for tenderness. Instability or crepitus may be noted. Feel down the sides of the chest and look on your gloves for any blood.

Auscultation

A stethoscope should be used to listen in both axillae in the upper and lower half of the chest to determine if the air entry is equal. Listening over the anterior chest detects air movement in the large airways which can drown out sounds of pulmonary ventilation, particularly if any secretions are present.

Percussion

If there is a difference in auscultation, the findings on percussion of both sides of the chest should be compared. The most likely findings are either hyperresonance (pneumothorax) or dullness (fluid or contusion) on one side compared with the other.

Check the back

It is important to assess the back quickly to determine if there is any evidence of a penetrating injury. If there is time, the examination should include palpation, auscultation and percussion of the posterior aspect of the chest.

Life-threatening conditions

*Airway obstruction (**A**TOMIC)*

Obstruction of a major airway can occur within the thorax. In many cases, there is little that can be done about this although cardiopulmonary resuscitation or the Heimlich manoeuvre may dislodge the obstruction.

*Tension pneumothorax (A**T**OMIC)*

- If there is a breach in either the lung or chest wall, then air can be sucked into the vacuum of the pleural space and a pneumothorax created
- It is important to remember that the pleural cavity and apex of the lung project above the clavicle. Consequently this can occur following penetrating injuries to the lower neck
- Following trauma, a one-way flap valve may be produced on the lung surface. This allows air to be sucked into the pleural cavity during inspiration, but obstructs its escape during expiration
- With subsequent breaths, the volume and pressure of air in the pleural cavity increase. This causes the underlying lung to collapse and profound hypoxia to develop
- In the later stages, the mediastinum is displaced towards the opposite hemithorax, impeding venous return and diminishing cardiac output. This is a *tension pneumothorax* and is fatal if not rapidly relieved
- It is important to remember that this condition can develop rapidly at any stage of the resuscitation. Consequently a high index of suspicion is always required

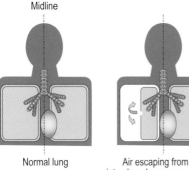
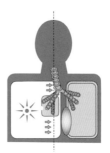

| Normal lung | Air escaping from lung into pleural space cannot return due to the hole acting as a 'one-way valve' | High air pressure in the pleural space (tension) forces structures across midline compressing great vessels and lung |

Figure 25.1 Development of a tension pneumothorax.

- Positive pressure ventilation may convert a simple pneumothorax into a tension pneumothorax
- If the patient deteriorates after artificial ventilation and ventilation becomes progressively more difficult, think: tension pneumothorax.

Signs of a tension pneumothorax

- Rapid respiratory rate
- Decreased air entry to the hemithorax
- Hyper-resonant hemithorax
- Rapid, weak pulse
- Decreasing level of consciousness
- Deviated trachea – away from the affected side
- Raised jugular venous pulse (if no accompanying hypovolaemia)
- Cyanosis (very late).

Management

- As an emergency measure, a 14-gauge cannula connected to a 10 ml syringe should be inserted into the second intercostal space in the midclavicular line on the affected side aspirating continuously
- The aim is to decompress the chest by equalising the pressures on either side of the chest wall. A rapid release of air confirms the diagnosis, following which the cannula is slid over the needle into the pleural cavity and the syringe and needle removed
- The cannula usually lasts no more than about 15 minutes before becoming kinked thus requiring a repeat needle decompression
- Insertion of a chest drain will be required when the patient reaches hospital.

Open chest wound (ATOMIC)

- An open chest wound will automatically produce an open pneumothorax on the same side
- If the wound is greater than two-thirds the diameter of the trachea then air preferentially enters the chest through this hole during inspiration ('sucking' chest wound)
- This causes failure of ventilation of the lung which eventually collapses
- If the wound or an inadequate dressing acts as a one-way valve then a tension pneumothorax will develop
- The immediate management of an open chest wound is to apply an Asherman® or Bolin® chest seal. Air can then escape during expiration, but cannot enter through the wound during inspiration because the valve is sucked closed
- The primary survey can then be completed and the patient transferred to hospital where a chest drain is inserted via a freshly created incision
- If an Asherman® or Bolin® seal is not available, a dressing sealed on three sides only can be used.

Massive haemothorax (ATOMIC)

- A massive haemothorax is defined as the presence of more than 1.5 litres of blood in the chest cavity; it usually results from laceration of either an intercostal vessel or the internal mammary artery
- Intravascular access must be achieved and fluid resuscitation following standard protocols should be followed
- The remainder of the primary survey should be completed and the patient rapidly transferred to hospital.

Signs of a massive haemothorax

- Decreased air entry on the affected side
- Dull percussion note over the affected side
- Shock, grade II, III or IV
- Jugular venous pressure usually low.

Flail chest (ATOMIC)

- Flail chest occurs when two or more ribs are fractured in two or more places or when the clavicle and first rib are fractured
- Normally the chest moves out during inspiration and in with expiration. When a rib is fractured in two places the middle section can move independently from the relatively fixed ends and tends to be drawn in during inspiration and pushed out in expiration. This is known as *paradoxical movement*
- Shortly after trauma, this type of movement will only be evident if there is either a large flail chest (over five ribs) or a central flail (multiple bilateral costochondral fractures with a flail sternum)

- More commonly, the spasm of the chest wall musculature is sufficient to splint the flail segment and mask paradoxical movement for a short time
- A flail segment can be a life-threatening condition, mainly because of the underlying pulmonary contusion which adds greatly to the hypoxia already produced as a result of the impaired breathing
- Manual stabilization of the flail segment may be considered.

Management

- Hypoxia must be corrected. Give high-flow, warm, humidified oxygen
- The patient may benefit from lying on the injured side
- Strapping the flail segment with adhesive tape may improve ventilation
- The definitive management is positive pressure ventilation so the patient should be transferred urgently to the Emergency Department
- The patient must be carefully monitored for signs indicating either the development of a tension pneumothorax or that immediate intubation and ventilation are required to prevent further deterioration
- The warning signs include:
  - Exhaustion
  - Respiratory rate greater than 30/minute
  - Significant associated injuries of the abdomen and head
  - Pulse oximeter reading of 85% or less on air
  - Pulse oximeter reading of 90% or less with supplemental oxygen.

Cardiac tamponade (*ATOMIC*)

- A small collection of blood within the pericardium will constrict the heart, compromising ventricular filling and hence cardiac output
- This condition is known as *cardiac tamponade* and usually follows penetrating chest wound within the anatomical area indicated in Figure 22.1
- Cardiac tamponade may be temporarily relieved by pericardiocentesis. Aspiration of even a few millilitres of blood may be life-saving
- In all cases an urgent thoracotomy is necessary if the patient is to survive: rapid transfer to hospital is essential
- Cardiac arrest warrants immediate ('*crash*') thoracotomy to expose the heart and decompress the pericardium if sufficient medical expertise is available.

Secondary survey

The secondary survey involves a detailed head-to-toe examination but is seldom performed in the prehospital environment. There are eight potentially life-threatening conditions which may be identified during a more detailed assessment of the patient:

1. Pulmonary contusion
2. Cardiac contusion

3. Ruptured diaphragm
4. Dissecting aorta
5. Oesophageal rupture
6. Simple pneumothorax
7. Haemothorax
8. Ruptured bronchi.

Most of these conditions are only ever identified on CT scan.

Monitoring the patient

The patient will require a baseline set of observations including pulse rate, blood pressure, respiratory rate, oxygen saturation, capillary refill time, temperature and if time permits a blood glucose measurement. He/she should be transferred on full monitoring including ECG leads, blood pressure and oxygen saturation probe and should not be left unattended.

Analgesia in chest injuries

Nitrous oxide and oxygen inhalation (Entonox) is contraindicated in chest injuries not only because it will reduce the inspired oxygen to 50% but also, and most importantly, because nitrous oxide will diffuse rapidly into a simple or potential pneumothorax to produce a life-threatening tension pneumothorax. The analgesia of choice is therefore intravenous opiates titrated to effect.

For further information, see Ch. 25 in *Emergency Care: A Textbook for Paramedics.*

CHAPTER 26

Abdominal and genitourinary trauma

A high index of suspicion is mandatory in potential abdominal trauma as signs and symptoms may be subtle or evolve slowly.

Mechanisms of injury

Three mechanisms of injury exist – blunt, penetrating and blast. In the majority of instances, injury results from blunt impact following a road traffic accident, sporting accident, fall or industrial accident. Blast injuries are fortunately rare.

Blunt injuries

Blunt impact results in definable injury patterns:

Bursting

Sudden, violent compression of the abdominal wall may dramatically raise intra-abdominal pressure leading to rupture of a bowel loop. An incorrectly fitted seatbelt is a common factor in these injuries.

Crush

Direct crush injuries occur when a viscus is injured by directly applied pressure. A common event is rupture of the retroperitoneal portion of the duodenum in bicycle accidents – the duodenum is compressed between a handlebar and the lumbar spine. The pancreas, liver and spleen are also readily injured in this way.

Shear

Shear force injuries occur when force is applied tangentially across vascular pedicles; structures at risk include the spleen, liver and small bowel mesentery. These injuries are commonly associated with sudden deceleration.

Collision

Collision injuries result typically from impact of a motor vehicle on a pedestrian. The pattern of injury will depend on the size of the victim – bumper (fender) impact on an adult usually involves the limbs and abdominal injury is relatively uncommon, but in a child the torso takes the brunt of the force and abdominal and chest injury should be assumed in the prehospital setting.

Ejection

Ejection from a vehicle can result in multiple injuries, including damage to the cervical spine, depending on how the casualty lands – the torso is a large target and the likelihood of abdominal injury under these circumstances is high.

> Injury to the chest + injury to the pelvis = injury to the abdomen until proven otherwise

Penetrating injuries

Intra-abdominal penetration may be obvious however penetrating objects, bullets, fragments, knives or damaged vehicle parts can reach the abdomen from the lower chest, the back, flanks, buttocks and perineum. In the case of bullets and missile fragments, the entry site may be anywhere, as they may travel unpredictable distances and readily deflect from their original line of flight.

Recognition of injury

As many as 20% of patients with significant intraabdominal bleeding reveal little or nothing in the way of physical signs.

Event history

The event history may be provided by the patient, other victims or bystanders. It is frequently unavailable.

Initial clinical assessment

In the primary survey, the first indication of abdominal trauma typically arises during assessment of circulation. Another clue may be when the extent of shock is out of proportion to the observed injuries. If shock is not a particular feature and the patient is readily stabilised, the secondary survey may reveal tenderness, rebound tenderness or even rigidity.

In particular, the paramedic should:

- Expose the abdomen as far as possible
- Inspect or look at the abdomen, including flanks, lower chest, back and pelvic region
- Palpate the abdomen, including the flanks and as much of the back as possible
- Wounds, bruises or abrasions should raise the level of suspicion.

The history in abdominal injury

Details of the following should be established:

- History of event
- Pain
- Location
- Radiation: is pain present in the shoulders or back
- Wounds
- Wounding instrument
- Loss of consciousness
- Presence of drugs or alcohol
- Obvious distracting injuries elsewhere.

> Establishing a specific diagnosis is not necessary: assess the likelihood of injury being present and arrange expeditious transport to hospital

Genitourinary trauma

Genitourinary trauma and abdominal trauma are normally considered together.

Because the kidneys and ureters lie in the retroperitoneal space, injury is often silent and easily missed. Haematuria is not a constant feature.

However, blood at the external urinary meatus or an inability to pass urine are clear signs of injury.

The lower urinary tract is also vulnerable to injury following pelvic trauma. There is little to be done in the prehospital setting apart from injury recognition, understanding the implications and transporting the patient to hospital as a priority.

Pelvic fractures

Pelvic fractures are common components in multisystem injury and they should be particularly looked for.

The more severe pelvic fractures are usually associated with high-speed impact and should therefore be suspected from the history and mechanism of injury.

- These are critical injuries to recognise. Unstable, complex pelvic injuries are associated with a very high mortality rate, principally due to uncontrolled haemorrhage
- Physical examination and extrication should be handled with great care
- Consider the application of a specialised pelvic splint. More simple techniques include the application of a pelvic binder or drawsheet
- In the absence of palpable radial pulses, initial management may require repeated 250 mL aliquots of crystalloid. This should be started *en route* to hospital if the patient is not trapped. Rapid transportation to hospital is of paramount importance. Large volumes of whole blood are typically needed and some patients will continue to haemorrhage until the pelvis is stabilised by operative fixation.

Abdominal trauma in pregnancy

The pregnant uterus remains inside the protection of the bony pelvis until the 12th week of gestation and pregnancy therefore may not be obvious, particularly in an unconscious patient.

After 12 weeks, the uterus rises above the pelvic brim and is palpable. The possibility of pregnancy should always be considered in a woman of childbearing age and should be actively sought.

The best possible care for the fetus is optimal care for the mother and this must be the aim.

Trauma to the abdomen in later pregnancy when the uterus is thin-walled may result in uterine rupture or placental abruption associated with significant blood loss.

Shock management must be prompt and vigorous and the patient quickly transported to hospital. Remember the problem of postural hypotension due to compression of the inferior vena cava by the gravid uterus, which may require manual displacement of the uterus to the left, elevation of the right hip or, if a spine board is available, tipping the spine board and patient towards the left side at a 30° angle during transportation.

Treating the mother well is the best treatment for the foetus

---

For further information, see Ch. 26 in *Emergency Care: A Textbook for Paramedics.*

CHAPTER 27

Bone and joint injuries

Bone and joint injuries range from the relatively trivial to the life-threatening. The <C>ABC system must be followed. Only when life-threatening injuries have been excluded or treated should limb injuries be assessed.

Mechanism of injury

Fractures

Fractures may be classified in several ways. Injuries may be:

- Closed (simple), if the skin and soft tissues overlying the injury are intact, or
- Open (compound) if bacteria could have entered the wound through damaged skin.

When fractures are treated, wherever possible the normal anatomical alignment should be re-established. This reduces pain and bleeding and helps to prevent damage to adjacent structures. It is perfectly acceptable to reduce a bony fragment back into a wound in order to achieve this.

Fracture anatomy

After a bone has been fractured, the fragments may remain in their normal anatomical relationship to one another (undisplaced) or their relative positions may change (displaced).

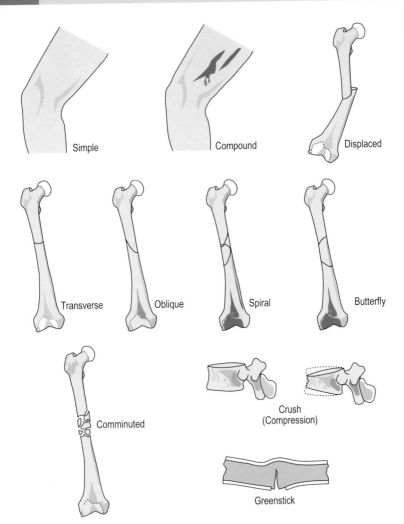

Figure 27.1 A classification of fractures.

Fractures in children

Even although fracture patterns may differ in children, potential injuries should be assessed and managed in the same way as adults.

Dislocations

Dislocations may occur when similar forces are placed on joints, but the soft tissue structures fail before the surrounding bone fractures.

There are some injuries where fracture and dislocation occur at the same time; e.g. posterior dislocation of the hip with a fracture of the posterior lip of the acetabulum (hip socket). In this case, the acetabulum is fractured by the femur as it passes posteriorly, striking the lip.

General examination

The majority of fractures and dislocations are not immediately life-threatening, but exceptions include fractures of the pelvis, multiple closed fractures or compound fractures of long bones, where serious haemorrhage may occur.

Fractures of the skull and face may lead to airway obstruction or be associated with life-threatening neurological injuries. Fractures may co-exist with injuries to the vital thoracic or abdominal organs.

Limb-threatening injuries are much more likely. Many fractures and dislocations can lead to lifelong disability and thus are very important for the individual patient.

The multiply injured patient may require immediate transfer to hospital without full assessment or treatment of such injuries.

Examination of bones and joint must be systematic if injuries are to be identified (see box below).

Look – The part should be inspected for swelling, deformity and overlying wounds. Are there any pre-existing scars? The joint should be compared with the normal side

Feel – Is the injured part painful and if so, where? Is there any protective muscle spasm? Are the pulses distal to the injury intact?

Move – Can the patient move the injured part?

If there is a fracture then the sensation of grating of the bone ends may be experienced ('crepitus'). This is extremely painful for the patient and deliberate attempts to elicit crepitus should be avoided.

Assess the limb for vascular injury. The palpation of a distal pulse alone is not sufficient. It is important to assess capillary refill in order to assess tissue perfusion.

The nail bed is compressed for 5 seconds. The pressure is released and the time taken for the return of the normal pink colour is measured. If this is greater than 2 seconds, then tissue perfusion is abnormal. The capillary refill test is best performed in good light and a warm environment.

A neurological assessment of sensation and muscle power should be made in order to determine whether there is a possibility of any nerve damage.

General treatment considerations

All patients who have sustained a long-bone injury should be given oxygen via a Hudson mask with a non-rebreathe valve and a reservoir bag at a rate of 15 L/min.

Analgesia

Entonox is excellent for fractures and dislocations sustained as sports injuries. Intravenous opiate analgesia will be required for significant fractures.

Compound fractures and serious wounds

Infection of a fracture is a disaster for the patient. Osteomyelitis can be controlled, but rarely cured. Good wound care starting at the scene of an accident will help reduce the incidence of this complication.

The fracture must be stabilised to avoid further damage to the soft tissues. Some form of immobilisation or splinting is required. Traction splinting will reduce blood loss, but must not be applied excessively if traction injuries to the nerves are to be avoided.

The wound should be covered in a sterile dressing, soaked in 0.9% saline or aqueous iodine solution. Life-threatening bleeding should be controlled by direct pressure.

> Splinting a fracture or dislocation to prevent movement of the injured part is one of the best and simplest forms of pain relief

Simple splintage

Simple splintage of the lower limb may be achieved by securely fastening the injured part to the opposite uninjured leg using triangular bandages or a purpose-built splint.

The limb may be placed in a box splint which should be well padded and should be of the appropriate size for the injured limb.

Vacuum splints are even more effective.

> Immobilise the joints above and below the fracture

Traction splintage

Traction splintage is generally employed for femoral shaft fractures. Modern traction splints work on the principle of traction at the ankle and countertraction via a ring at the ischial tuberosity, except for the Sager® splint (a padded T-bar that fits between the legs) which exerts countertraction on the symphysis pubis.

The principle is to reduce the fracture and overcome the deforming force of the surrounding muscles which are in spasm. The restoration of the normal length and shape of the limb also has the advantage of reducing blood loss by up to 20–30%.

Splints that apply traction to one (e.g. the Hare®, Donway® or Trac-Ill® splints) or both lower limbs (e.g. the Sager® splint) are effective.

Adequate splintage of a fractured limb will result in:

- Pain relief
- Reduction of blood loss
- Prevention of further soft tissue damage
- A reduced incidence of fat embolism.

Bone and joint injuries in specific regions

Skull, facial skeleton and cervical spine

Patients who have sustained a fracture to the skull or facial bones have sustained a serious head injury. The airway may be compromised, either directly owing to instability of the facial skeleton (e.g. an unstable fracture of the mandible) or owing to secondary factors such as swelling, bleeding or loss of consciousness. All patients with a head injury should be assessed for injury to the cervical spine.

> There is a 5% chance of significant cervical spine injury in the unconscious patient

The airway must take priority, but all reasonable precautions to prevent cervical spine movement must be taken. Neck collars which are combined with immobilisation on a spinal board effect the most secure immobilisation when properly applied.

Pressure necrosis of the skin and soft tissues can be caused by even short periods on a spinal board.

Scoop stretchers can be used when transferring patients from the floor to a stretcher or bed.

The patient's clothing must be checked for sharp or lumpy objects such as coins or wallets as these will quickly lead to the development of pressure sores in the immobilised patient. This is particularly important in the unconscious patient.

The upper limb

Fractured clavicle

Cause

Fall on the outstretched hand (FOOSH), when the forces transmitted up the upper limb may indirectly result in a fracture, or from a direct blow.

Signs and symptoms

Pain occurs at the site of the fracture whenever the upper limb is moved. The patient often supports the injured arm at the elbow in an attempt to reduce movement of the limb. There is usually swelling at the site of the fracture, which typically occurs at the junction of the outer (lateral) third and inner (medial) two-thirds of the bone.

Treatment

The upper limb should be immobilised in a broad arm sling. A collar and cuff should not be used, as this will act to separate the bony ends of the fracture due to the weight of the arm.

Potential problems

This is usually a straightforward injury to treat. The sling will often control the pain as it prevents movement at the fracture site. As with all limb injuries, there is a chance of damage to important vascular and neurological structures close to the fracture site. The subclavian artery and vein are in close proximity to the clavicle and although injury to them is rare, it can be serious. Similarly, the nerves that supply the upper limb may be injured, particularly when the fracture has been caused by direct rather than indirect force. Direct injury to this region may also result in chest injury and the assessment must not be confined to the clavicle.

> Always check distal neurovascular function

Fractured scapula

Cause

Usually due to a direct blow, most commonly after a fall from a motorcycle, from a blunt weapon during an assault or accidentally during a sporting event with a stick or bat (e.g., a hockey stick). The scapula is surrounded by muscle and this is an unusual injury, considerable force being required.

Signs and symptoms

Pain occurs over the site of the fracture and may be made worse with movement of the upper limb.

Treatment

Immobilisation of the upper limb in a broad arm sling will reduce the discomfort.

Potential problems

There may be associated injuries to the thoracic cage and ribs and these need careful examination.

Dislocation of the sternoclavicular joint

Cause

Fall on the outstretched hand (FOOSH) or by direct injury to the anterior aspect of the shoulder, levering the medial end of the clavicle away from its usual articulation with the manubrium of the sternum.

Signs and symptoms

There is pain localised at the medial end of the clavicle, made worse by movement of the upper limb. There may be swelling and deformity over the sternoclavicular joint.

Treatment

The vast majority of these injuries are subluxations or partial dislocations. They are best treated in a broad arm sling.

Potential problems

Occasionally there is severe displacement. If the medial end of the clavicle has been dislocated posteriorly, then the major vessels are in danger of injury. The patient should be examined for signs of chest injury and shock. If there is evidence of shock, they should be considered to have a severe, potentially life-threatening injury and evacuated to hospital immediately. Intravenous access can be achieved in transit and any delay in reaching hospital should be avoided. Occasionally posterior dislocation of the sternoclavicular joint may produce airway obstruction: the clavicle should be pulled forwards, as a matter of urgency.

Dislocation of the acromioclavicular joint

Cause

Usually a fall onto the point of the shoulder. It is a common injury in rugby football. This injury results from partial or complete disruption of ligaments between the clavicle and the acromion and in severe cases also the ligaments between the clavicle and the underlying coracoid process of the scapula.

Signs and symptoms

Pain at the lateral end of the clavicle, made worse by attempting to carry any weight with the affected arm. There will be a variable amount of local swelling and usually a step is visible between the lateral end of the clavicle and the acromion (this is the expanded anterolateral process of the scapula which forms a bony roof over the shoulder joint and muscles and normally articulates with the clavicle).

Treatment

The upper limb should be immobilised in a broad arm sling.

Potential problems

The mechanism of injury should lead to a high level of suspicion of associated injuries to the cervical spine and nerves in the brachial plexus.

Anterior dislocation of the shoulder

Cause

Usually caused by forced external rotation of the glenohumeral joint (the joint between the humerus and the glenoid process of the scapula). Typically, this results from a fall or a mistimed rugby tackle. If the shoulder has previously been dislocated, then less force is required to produce a recurrent injury.

Symptoms and signs

The patient will be supporting the forearm with the elbow flexed. The shoulder will look abnormal (square contour) compared with the other side, with a loss of the usual rounded contour of the upper arm. The lateral edge of the scapula may well appear prominent. It is important to assess the sensory portion of the axillary nerve which provides sensation to the 'regimental badge' area of skin on the lateral aspect of the proximal arm.

Treatment

Treatment should be directed at immobilising the upper limb during transfer to hospital for relocation of the joint. An acceptable method is to allow the patient to sit upright and support the arm, perhaps resting it on a pillow. The sooner the joint is relocated the better.

Potential problems

The longer the joint is dislocated, the more permanent damage is done to the articular surface of the bone and to the soft tissues. All the nerves of the upper limb can be at risk. Damage to the major blood vessels may occur and proper examination and reexamination of the distal limb circulation is essential. Severe fractures and fracture-dislocations of the surgical neck of the humerus may mimic simple anterior dislocation.

Posterior dislocation of the shoulder

Cause

Often a fall on the outstretched hand with the arm internally rotated or a direct blow to the anterior aspect of the shoulder. An electric shock, epileptic fit or chronic muscle spasticity such as is seen in cerebral palsy can also cause posterior dislocation.

Symptoms and signs

These are similar to those of anterior dislocation, with pain, swelling and local deformity.

Treatment

The arm should be immobilised and the patient transported to hospital.

Potential problems

The nerves in the brachial plexus are particularly susceptible to damage due to pressure from the humeral head. Recognition and early relocation are essential. The X-ray changes are very subtle and this injury can be easily missed in hospital.

Inferior dislocation of the shoulder

Cause

Inferior dislocation is extremely rare but can follow a violent convulsion or an electric shock.

Symptoms and signs

The arm is held extended above the head and the injury is extremely painful. The condition is often bilateral.

Treatment

Analgesia and support during the transfer to the hospital are all that is required.

Potential problems

Fitting the patient onto the stretcher may be difficult.

Fracture of the proximal humerus

Cause

Usually either a fall onto the outstretched hand (FOOSH) or a direct fall onto the upper arm, particularly in elderly patients and those with osteoporosis. The fracture can occur in younger patients following direct violence.

Symptoms and signs

There is pain at the upper end of the arm. The patient will usually be supporting the arm at the elbow with the other hand. There may be obvious deformity. Swelling is almost immediate, but the severe bruising which accompanies this injury may not be apparent for several days and can track distally down the lateral aspect of the arm.

Treatment

The arm is supported in a broad arm sling initially. Once the diagnosis has been confirmed in the accident and emergency department, the sling should be changed to a 'collar and cuff.' This allows the weight of the arm to apply traction to the fracture and tends to reduce the fractured bone into its normal anatomical position.

Potential problems

As with all fractures, the surrounding nerves and blood vessels can be injured directly at the time of the fracture.

Fracture of the shaft of the humerus

Cause

The shaft of the humerus may be fractured through direct injury such as a fall onto the arm or a blow from a blunt weapon. Indirect force can cause these fractures, although the fracture pattern may be different.

Symptoms and signs

The arm is painful and may be supported at the elbow by the other hand. There may be obvious angular deformity, but rotational malalignment is not always obvious. There may be significant swelling and bruising. It is essential to examine the distal portions of the limb to exclude vascular and neurological injury.

Treatment

The arm should be supported in a broad arm sling.

Potential problems

The radial nerve runs in a groove, closely applied to the humeral shaft posteriorly. It may be damaged directly or secondarily due to swelling (compartment syndrome). Loss of radial nerve function may lead to weakness of the muscles that extend the wrist and as a result the patient will demonstrate 'wrist drop' (inability to extend the wrist). The arterial blood supply to the upper limb is via just one vessel at this point, the brachial artery. This artery may suffer direct injury or may be constricted owing to a compartment syndrome.

Supracondylar fracture of the humerus

Cause

Supracondylar fractures of the distal portion of the humerus just proximal to the elbow joint are common in childhood. They are typically caused by a fall onto the outstretched hand. The fractures can range from an undisplaced crack to a completely displaced injury with vascular and neurological damage.

Symptoms and signs

There is pain at the elbow after a fall. The child will support the elbow with the other hand. There may be obvious swelling and deformity and serious interference with the blood supply to the distal part of the limb.

Treatment

The arm should be immobilised in a broad arm sling in slight extension. Constant evaluation of the distal circulation is essential. If the circulation is compromised the elbow should be extended (straightened).

Potential problems

The brachial artery can be kinked over the bone ends, trapped between the bone ends or directly damaged by the fracture. If the circulation to the distal forearm is not restored then there is real danger of Volkmann's ischaemic contracture (the death of all the muscle in the forearm), leaving a contracted, painful, useless arm. This can also be the result of compartment syndrome caused by swelling after this injury. Volkmann's contracture is a serious injury which often leads to long-term disability.

Fracture of the radial head

Cause

Fall on the outstretched hand (FOOSH).

Symptoms and signs

There is pain over the lateral aspect of the forearm just distal to the elbow joint. There is often pain on rotation of the forearm (pronation and supination) and the elbow cannot be fully extended.

Treatment

The arm should be placed in a broad arm sling. Once the diagnosis has been confirmed at the accident and emergency department this may be replaced by a collar and cuff.

Potential problems

The distal circulation should be assessed, but this injury rarely leads to complications.

Fracture of the olecranon

Cause

Fall directly onto the elbow or from violent contraction of the triceps muscle in an attempt to extend the elbow against resistance.

Symptoms and signs

The elbow is very painful and there is considerable swelling. If the triceps tendon is still attached to the distal part of the ulna then it will still be possible to actively extend the elbow, although this will be very painful. If the attachment has been pulled off or is solely to the proximal fragment, then there can be no active extension of the elbow.

Treatment

The arm is immobilised in a broad arm sling. The distal neurological and vascular status is monitored.

Potential problems

The swelling may cause vascular insufficiency and compartment syndrome. There is a potential for damage to the nerves that cross the elbow joint. This is particularly true for the ulnar nerve which is closely applied to the medial side of the joint in the ulnar groove. Damage may lead to altered or lost sensation of the palmar surface of the small and ring fingers of the hand. It may also lead to loss of function of the small muscles of the hand with the exception of those that move the thumb.

Dislocation of the elbow

Cause

Fall on the outstretched hand. This injury may be associated with fractures of the distal humerus and/or the proximal radius and ulna.

Symptoms and signs

There is obvious deformity and gross swelling and the injury is usually very painful. Little movement is possible and attempts to do so are exquisitely painful. There is significant risk of vascular compromise due to swelling and neurological damage due to the stretching of the nerves at the elbow.

Treatment

The elbow should be immobilised in a well-padded splint. The distal circulation and neurological status require constant assessment.

Potential problems

The potential for vascular and neurological complications is high and the patient is best served by rapid transfer to hospital to enable early reduction of the dislocation.

Fractures of the shafts of radius and ulna

Cause

Falling on an outstretched hand may cause a fracture of both forearm bones, the radius and ulna. Direct injury such as a fall onto the forearm or a direct blow may also fracture both bones, but it is possible to fracture one or other in isolation. If one bone is fractured there is often an associated dislocation of the proximal or distal joint between the radius and ulna. Children may fracture the radius and ulna in the midshaft region or they may sustain a fracture involving the growth plate of the bones (epiphyseal injuries, see below).

Signs and symptoms

The forearm is painful and is supported by the other hand. There may be an obvious angular deformity.

Treatment

The arm requires immobilisation, which is best achieved using some form of splintage. However, if this is difficult to apply because of angulation or discomfort, then a broad arm sling may be appropriate. It is important that the sling prevents movement at the fracture site but that it does not compromise the circulation because it is too tight. It is almost impossible to apply a splint single-handed and attempts to do so may cause the patient unnecessary discomfort and even increase the soft tissue damage at the fracture site.

Potential problems

There is the ever-present possibility of circulatory compromise with these fractures and the distal portion of the limb must be regularly assessed. The skin and soft tissues directly overlying the fracture may be placed under tension if there is significant angulation. This may cause local skin ischaemia and necrosis. There is a real danger that closed fractures may become open if the forearm is not immobilised.

Fractures of the distal radius

Cause

Fracture of the distal radius is caused by a fall on the outstretched hand. This is particularly common in the elderly with osteoporotic bone resulting in Colles' fracture with displacement of the distal fragment away from the palm (dorsally). Younger age groups can also sustain fractures of the distal radius. With children the injury is usually through the soft cartilage of the growth plate of the bone or epiphysis.

If the patient falls onto the back of the wrist with the forearm supinated then the distal fragment of the fracture may be displaced towards the palmar (volar or ventral) surface. This is known as a Smith's fracture.

Symptoms and signs

There is pain and swelling at the wrist. If the distal fragment has been displaced dorsally there is said to be a 'dinner fork' deformity. If there is volar displacement of the fragment, there is said to be a 'garden spade' deformity. There may be symptoms of nerve injury in the palm of the hand. The median nerve is situated in the midline of the wrist and enters the hand via the carpal tunnel. It supplies sensation to the palmar surfaces of the thumb, index and middle fingers and supplies the motor branches to the small muscles of the thumb. It may sustain direct damage at the time of fracture or it may be compressed within the carpal tunnel owing to swelling or displacement of the fragments of the bone. The ulnar nerve may also be affected in fractures of the distal radius, but less frequently than the median nerve. The ulnar nerve supplies sensation to the little and ring fingers and motor branches to the remainder of the small muscles of the hand.

Treatment

The distal radius must be immobilised. A broad arm sling may be sufficient in some cases, a short box splint or vacuum splint may be used as alternatives. The sensation and circulation to the hand and fingers must be monitored.

Potential problems

The nerve injuries outlined above may cause symptoms. The hand must be examined to exclude vascular damage. If there is massive swelling then the hand and wrist should be elevated after the fracture has been immobilised.

Fractures of the carpal bones

Cause

Fractures of the carpal bones are caused by a fall on the outstretched hand. Scaphoid fractures (the most common) are caused when the wrist is forced into hyperextension.

Symptoms and signs

The wrist is painful with reduced movements. There may be no significant swelling.

Treatment

The arm should be placed in a broad arm sling.

Potential problems

If fractures of these bones are missed and not immobilised in plaster, the fracture may fail to unite and the patient will be left with a stiff wrist.

Fractures of the metacarpals and fingers

Cause

Injuries to the metacarpals and fingers are usually caused by direct falls or blows.

Symptoms and signs

The injured bone will be painful. There may be considerable swelling on the dorsum (back) of the hand. The palmar skin is firmly attached to the bony skeleton of the hand to allow good grip but the dorsal skin is loose and thus bruising and swelling track dorsally. There may be obvious bony deformity. The fifth metacarpal is most commonly broken, often as a result of a punch.

Treatment

The hand should be elevated in a high arm sling.

Potential problems

The blood supply to the digits may be compromised, either directly as a result of the injury or secondary to swelling. Rings should always be removed from an injured hand. If it is not possible to remove them prehospital then their presence must be communicated to the staff in the accident and emergency department so that arrangements can be made to cut the rings off. Failure to remove rings may lead to swelling, circulatory compromise and even loss of the digit. This applies to rings on uninjured digits because they will subsequently swell in any hand injury.

Dislocation of the fingers

Cause

Finger dislocation is usually caused by direct injury, for instance by a blow from a cricket ball.

Symptoms and signs

There is obvious deformity of the joint, which is painful.

Treatment

It is often said that these dislocations should be reduced quickly, without anaesthesia. This is not appropriate. Relocation of these joints is not always straightforward and there may be a fracture associated with the dislocation. It is better to transport the patient to the accident and emergency department where a fracture can be excluded by X-ray and reduction can performed painlessly under a ring block or other regional anaesthesia.

The thoracic skeleton

Fractures of the ribs and flail chest

Cause

Rib fractures are usually a result of direct trauma. They may be multiple.

Symptoms and signs

The fractured rib is painful. Clearly it is not possible to stop moving the injured rib without stopping breathing. Thus, pain is experienced with each inspiratory and expiratory movement. If there have been fractures of more than one rib in more than one place, then a segment of the thoracic cage may move independently of the main chest wall. This is referred to as a flail segment (flail chest). A flail segment will exhibit paradoxical movement; that is, it will move in the opposite direction to the rest of the chest wall. This has significant consequences for the ventilation of the underlying lung. Patients with significant chest injuries will have an abnormal respiratory rate (usually high).

A fractured rib may result in blood loss of up to 150 mL. Multiple rib fractures may therefore be a significant contributory factor in hypovolaemic shock.

Treatment

The patient must be given high-flow oxygen (15 L/min) through a mask with reservoir bag. Large flail segments may be treated by lying the patient on the injured side (remembering the cervical spine precautions) or by strapping the chest. If the patient is shocked then an intravenous infusion should be started, but this must not delay transfer to hospital.

Record the respiratory rate and monitor changes

Fractures of the sternum

Cause

Fractures of the sternum are characteristically caused when the chest strikes the steering wheel in a decelerating vehicle. The correct use of seatbelts, and more recently, the deployment of air bags during an accident, has prevented many of these injuries.

Symptoms and signs

There is pain in the anterior aspect of the chest. There may also be symptoms and signs of other significant chest injury.

Treatment

It should be assumed that there is also myocardial contusion. The patient should receive oxygen by face mask (15 L/min through mask with reservoir bag). Monitoring of the pulse, blood pressure, respiratory rate, ECG and oxygen saturation are mandatory. Intravenous access should be obtained following normal protocols. Urgent transfer to hospital is essential.

Potential problems

The main problem with these fractures is not the bony injury but contusion or bruising of the heart which lies just posterior to the sternum. This injury requires careful cardiac monitoring and observation in hospital. If cardiac arrhythmias occur they require urgent treatment.

The pelvis

Minor pelvic fractures
Fractures of the pubic ramus

Cause

The cause of a fracture of the pubic ramus is usually a fall, particularly in an elderly patient.

Symptoms and signs

The patient will complain of pain in the hip. Careful elucidation of the site of the pain will reveal that it is in fact groin pain. There is no external rotation or shortening of the leg. The patient is usually unable to walk. The injury is frequently confused with fracture of the femoral neck and correct differentiation of the two may only be possible on X-ray.

Treatment

The patient requires supportive treatment and transfer to hospital.

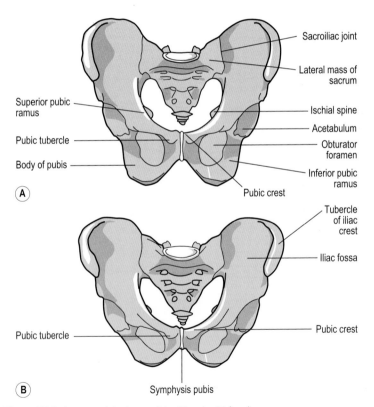

Figure 27.2 Anatomy of the bony pelvis. (A) male; (B) female.

Avulsion fracture of the pelvis

Cause

Many powerful muscles have attachment to the pelvis (for example, the hamstring muscles). Strong contraction of these, perhaps during sporting activity, may lead to an avulsion fracture (where the muscle inserts onto bone, a small fragment of bone is pulled off).

Symptoms and signs

The patient experiences acute pain after a muscular effort and may be unable to stand or walk. The symptoms are similar to those of a severe pulled muscle.

Treatment

The patient will need analgesia and should be transferred to hospital for assessment.

Major pelvic fractures

Cause

Major pelvic fractures are usually caused by severe violence. Falls directly onto the pelvis or force transmitted down the femoral shaft are common causes; direct injury by a heavy weight falling on the pelvis can also be responsible. The pelvis can be considered as a ring and usually fails in at least two places. The fracture pattern is dependent on the mechanism of injury.

Symptoms and signs

The patient will be in pain. There may be a leg length discrepancy in pelvic fractures with a vertical shear fracture. Major blood vessels lie on the inner pelvic surface anterior to the sacroiliac joint and pelvic fractures can be complicated by life-threatening haemorrhage. The patient must be examined and assessed for signs of hypovolaemia. The pelvic organs are also at risk of severe injury. The male patient may have blood at the tip of his penis and swelling of the scrotum as a result of rupture of the urethra. The pregnant woman will be susceptible to uterine rupture or detachment of the placenta (abruptio placentae). She will also mask the signs of hypovolaemia because she has a proportionately greater blood volume in pregnancy.

Treatment

The diagnosis of a major pelvic fracture may be made when instability is found on pelvic assessment during 'C' of the primary survey. The absence of obvious instability does not exclude the diagnosis which may be suspected from the mechanism of injury or in a shocked patient where no other obvious source of bleeding is identified. Avoid attempts to 'spring' the pelvis, as this may precipitate or exacerbate haemorrhage. The patient should receive high-flow oxygen (15 L/min through a mask with reservoir). Haemorrhage can be fatal and an external fixator may need to be applied as an emergency at hospital. Any delay will be detrimental to the patient, who must be transported to hospital quickly. Intravenous access should therefore be obtained during transit or, for short transit times, after arrival in hospital. If it is possible the pelvis should be stabilised during transfer. Pelvic 'wrap-around' splints (e.g. the SAM splint) have been proven to improve alignment and reduce bleeding in complex pelvic fractures.

Potential problems

Severe hypovolaemic shock may lead to pulseless electrical activity dissociation and death. The patient may also have sustained other life-threatening injuries which must be identified and treated.

Types of major pelvic fracture
Femoral acetabular fractures

Cause

Fractures usually occur when force is transmitted indirectly from the femoral shaft. This is a high-violence injury and usually follows a road traffic accident or a fall from a height. The exact injury will depend on the position of the femur. If the hip is flexed or extended then it will usually dislocate, perhaps fracturing the rim of the acetabulum. However, if the hip is in neutral then the force is transmitted directly to the acetabulum which will fracture.

Symptoms and signs

The patient will be in pain which is made worse by any attempt to move the leg. The leg may be short, adducted and internally rotated (see Dislocated hip, below). There may be extensive haemorrhage and thus the patient may show signs of shock.

Treatment

The patient should be given high-flow oxygen. An intravenous infusion should be started if this does not delay transporting the patient to hospital. The injured leg should be supported by splinting it to the other leg.

Potential problems

The patient may have sustained other life-threatening injuries which must be identified and treated. If there has been displacement of the femoral head into the pelvis then there may be severe haemorrhage and damage to other pelvic organs.

The lower limb

Fractured neck of the femur

Cause

Fracture of the neck of the femur occurs in the elderly population. A fall or twisting injury may result in this injury. Some children (often overweight adolescents) have a condition where the upper femoral growth plate slips. Minor trauma in these children may precipitate a complete slipped epiphysis which has similar signs and symptoms to fractured neck of femur.

Symptoms and signs

The hip is painful. There may also be referred pain to the knee of the same side. The leg may be shorter than the normal side and may lie in external rotation. All movements of the hip joint cause pain. It is often the case with the elderly person who lives alone that the patient has been lying on the floor for some time since the injury. This increases the possibility of chest infection, pressure necrosis to the skin and hypothermia. The elderly patient may have had some medical event to cause the fall in the first instance (e.g. a myocardial infarction).

Treatment

The leg should be immobilised during transfer to hospital. This is best achieved by using some form of strap or bandage to tie the injured leg to the normal one.

Potential problems

The patient may have been on the floor for some time. Underlying medical problems may require urgent treatment. Egress from the patient's home may be difficult. Analgesia will be required but must be used judiciously in the frail, elderly patient. Fluids can usually wait until hospital.

Dislocation of the hip

Cause

Hip dislocation is caused by a high-energy injury. Typically, the knee is struck when the hip is flexed, for example on the dashboard of a car in a high-speed road traffic collision. Posterior dislocation is most common and there is often an associated fracture of the lip of the acetabulum (see above). If the hip is in the extended position at the time of injury anterior dislocation may occur. Hip prostheses are particularly vulnerable to dislocation.

Symptoms and signs

The hip is painful. There may be referred pain down the thigh and in the knee joint. The hip is held flexed and adducted and the leg is internally rotated. There may be associated sciatica. Other life-threatening injuries are extremely likely and examination should identify these urgently.

Treatment

The patient should be given oxygen. It is not possible to place the femur in the normal position until reduction is performed under anaesthesia. Attempts to reduce the dislocation without anaesthesia will be fruitless, extremely painful and delay the patient at the scene. The injured leg should be immobilised by securing it to the uninjured side and the patient transported to hospital as soon as possible. The distal circulation should be monitored. Analgesia will certainly be required. If the patient is trapped then medical assistance should be requested. If the patient is responsive intravenous opiates will probably be required in addition to Entonox.

Potential problems

The mechanism of injury is such that the patient may have multiple injuries. There is considerable disruption to the muscles and soft tissues around the hip joint, leading to haemorrhage. The patient must be monitored and treated for hypovolaemic shock where appropriate but this should not delay transfer to hospital. Good analgesia is essential. The head of the femur will compress the sciatic nerve as it leaves the pelvis which may lead to temporary or permanent damage. If the displacement of the joint is significant then the femoral vessels may become kinked and the distal circulation threatened. It can be difficult to extricate a patient with this injury, even if the vehicle damage is minimal, and good liaison with the fire and rescue services will be essential.

Fracture of the shaft of femur

Fracture of the shaft of the femur is always a major injury.

Cause

Fractures of the femoral shaft are usually the result of high-energy injury, such as a road traffic collision or a fall from a height.

Symptoms and signs

The exact symptoms and signs will depend on the level of the fracture. There will be pain and usually swelling at the site of the injury. There is often some degree of deformity, which may be rotational or angular. The leg may be short. The distal circulation may be compromised. Other coexistent life-threatening injuries should be identified and treated.

Treatment

The patient should receive high-flow oxygen (15 L/min through a mask with reservoir). An intravenous infusion should be started particularly if there is a delay before the patient can be transferred to hospital; otherwise it may be commenced en route. Intravenous opiate analgesia will be required. A regional nerve block (femoral nerve block) may be administered by an immediate-care doctor. Some form of splintage is required: the best splintage will be afforded by a traction splint, but if this is not easily applied or unavailable then a long leg splint (box splint, lollipop splint) or splinting to the other leg will suffice.

Potential problems

Hypoxia must be avoided. Other major injuries must be identified and treated. A femoral fracture may lose up to 1500 mL blood. This may be doubled in a compound injury. The patient should be monitored for the signs of shock and treated with fluids or urgent evacuation. It should be remembered that the infusion volumes achievable in hospital are far greater than those at the roadside. Minimal delay is essential. It may not be possible to immobilise a badly displaced fracture without manipulation.

Fractures of the patella

Cause

Fracture of the patella (kneecap) may be sustained in a number of ways. The knee may strike the dashboard in a road traffic accident or it may strike the floor in a fall. Alternatively, a heavy object falling on the knee may cause a patella fracture, as may violent contraction of the quadriceps tendon.

Signs and symptoms

The knee is painful and swollen. There may be a laceration or abrasion over the patella. If the fracture is displaced, it may be possible to feel the gap between the ends of the patella. The extensor mechanism of the knee consists of the quadriceps tendon superiorly, the patella and the patella tendon inferiorly. The latter attaches to the tibia at the tibial tubercle which can be felt 4–5 cm below the patella. If any of these soft tissue or bony structures are disrupted then the knee cannot be extended.

Treatment

The leg should be placed in a well-padded, long leg splint.

Potential problems

A careful history will ensure that potentially serious associated injuries can be identified and treated.

Dislocation of the patella

Cause

The patella may dislocate with minor trauma. The patient will often have experienced this injury previously. The patient typically complains of a dislocated knee secondary to relatively minor trauma.

Symptoms and signs

The patella almost always dislocates laterally. The acute injury is usually painful. The knee appears abnormal with the patella located over the lateral femoral condyle. There may be swelling (effusion) inside the joint. The patient will not be able to move the joint.

Treatment

Analgesia with Entonox may be sufficient to allow relocation of the patella. The important manoeuvre is to extend (straighten) the knee while pressing the knee-cap medially. It will be very difficult to reduce while the knee is flexed (bent). If one attempt fails then the leg is placed in a long leg splint and the patient transported to hospital. If the patella is successfully relocated, hospital consultation is still required as the patient will need orthopaedic follow-up.

Potential problems

This condition can be extremely painful and the patient may not tolerate a splint.

Dislocation of the knee

Cause

Dislocation of the knee is a rare and serious injury which inevitably means that the majority of the ligaments of the knee have been disrupted. The vessels and nerves to the distal portion of the limb are frequently compromised. A great degree of force is required.

Symptoms and signs

The knee will be painful and swollen. There may be significant angular deformity of the joint, although elastic recoil may have returned it to an anatomical position. The disruption of the ligaments and capsule renders the joint unstable. There is a serious possibility of vascular and neurological deficit to all structures below the knee.

Treatment

The vascular status must be assessed and monitored. The leg should be placed in a long leg splint.

Potential problems

The joint is unstable and may have few ligamentous and capsular attachments remaining. Redislocation of the joint may further damage the vascular and neurological structures. When placing the leg in the splint, the limb must be supported above and below the knee.

Soft tissue and ligament injuries to the knee joint

Cause

Injuries to the ligaments of the knee joint are common and are frequently sustained during sporting activities such as football, rugby and skiing. Damage to the menisci of the knee (commonly known as 'cartilages') can occur in isolation or in concert with such ligament injuries. A common mechanism of injury is a twisting injury to the knee when the foot is fixed.

Symptoms and signs

The knee will be painful. It may swell immediately (if there is bleeding into the joint, a haemarthrosis), or over the next 12–24 hours (an effusion). It is important to ascertain the exact mechanism of injury as this will help the medical staff make the diagnosis.

Treatment

The leg should be immobilised in a long leg splint until a fracture has been excluded in hospital. The distal circulation should be assessed and monitored.

Potential problems

The joint may be potentially unstable when severe ligament disruption has occurred.

Fractures of the tibial plateau

Cause

Fracture of the tibial plateau is caused by a large valgus force (the lower tibia is forced away from the midline) or varus force (the lower tibia is forced towards the midline).

Symptoms and signs

There is pain at the knee and often a haemarthrosis (bleeding into the joint). The patient is unable to walk.

Treatment

The limb is immobilised in a well-padded splint.

Potential problems

The patient should be examined for other major injuries and the distal circulation monitored.

Fractures of the tibial shaft and fibula

Cause

Fractures of the tibial shaft and fibula may be caused by direct injury, such as in road traffic accidents and sporting injuries. In some cases of direct injury either the tibia or fibula may be fractured in isolation. Longitudinal compression as a result of a fall may lead to these fractures and they may also result from indirect torsional forces caused by rotation transmitted from the foot or from the upper body if the foot is fixed. Finally, the tibia may fracture as a result of completion of a preexisting stress fracture.

Symptoms and signs

There is localised pain and swelling. There may be angular or rotational deformity. The distal circulation may be compromised.

Treatment

Oxygen should be given (15 L/min). Hypoxia is common after tibial fractures and must be avoided. Similarly, there may be considerable haemorrhage. The patient must be examined for circulatory shock and monitored. An intravenous infusion should be started without causing undue delay in transferring the patient to hospital. The injured limb should be immobilised in a long leg splint.

It may be necessary to reduce the fracture before immobilisation is possible and therefore opiate analgesia is required. Only then should the limb be subjected to gentle longitudinal traction to reverse any shortening caused by muscle spasm and overlap of bone. Once limb length, rotation and angular deformity are corrected, the fracture will be in a near reduced position. Excessive traction must be avoided as this may lead to secondary injury to the vessels and nerves. Accurate fracture reduction will reduce the amount of haemorrhage at the fracture site and from the soft tissues.

Potential problems

The tibia is a subcutaneous bone. It is easy to convert a simple fracture to a compound fracture by careless handling of the limb. The vascular supply of the lower parts of the limb may become compromised.

There is a significant risk of compartment syndrome following fracture of the tibia. The muscles of the lower legs are enclosed in tough fibrous sheaths. If bleeding occurs into these compartments or if there is significant swelling following a soft tissue injury, then the pressure within the compartment will rise. The risk is highest when there is a closed fracture or a soft tissue injury such as a muscle haematoma following a kick. As the pressure rises, perfusion of the tissues and cells decreases and they are starved of oxygen. The pressure in the arteries may be high enough to allow continued flow into the compartment, making the situation worse. The presence of a palpable distal pulse does not guarantee that the tissues are adequately perfused. The capillary refill test must be performed to allow a more complete assessment of the vascular status of the tissues.

Fractures and dislocations of the ankle

Cause

The exact pattern of fracture depends on the mechanism of injury, but the pre-hospital treatment is identical regardless of the fracture type. The typical history is of 'going over' on or 'twisting' the ankle, which may be combined with a fall down a kerbstone or step. These injuries are usually referred to as inversion or eversion injuries. Injuries of this kind are also common on the sports field. The ankle may be trapped by the foot pedals in a motor vehicle or a fall may lead to a fracture or dislocation of the ankle.

Symptoms and signs

The ankle is extremely tender over the fracture site and swelling occurs rapidly. In general, eversion injuries are associated with fractures of the medial malleolus and inversion injuries with fractures of the lateral malleolus. In severe injuries, both may fracture. Any attempt at walking is painful. There may be associated deformity. Distal nerve or vessel injury may occur.

Treatment

The ankle should be immobilised in a well-padded splint – this will probably require analgesia. The neurological and vascular status of the foot must be carefully monitored. Dislocation of the ankle may occur with obvious deformity. This is a limb-threatening emergency requiring rapid reduction. Urgent transfer to hospital (or reduction on scene by a doctor in remote areas) is essential. With an unstable injury, the act of splinting the joint may lead to reduction. However, reduction often requires sedation and intravenous analgesia.

Potential problems

If there is significant deformity following this fracture then the skin overlying the joint can become tightly stretched over the bony fragments. This will quickly lead to pressure necrosis and death of that skin. Penetration of the skin converting a closed to an open injury must be avoided.

At times it can be difficult to distinguish between a fracture and a sprain of the ankle. Typically the pain and swelling of a sprain to the anterior talofibular ligament are distal and anteromedial to the lateral malleolus. If there is any doubt about the diagnosis it is best to treat these injuries as fractures until they have been assessed at hospital.

Fractures of the talus and calcaneum (os calcis)

Cause

The talus is situated between the lower tibia (and forms part of the ankle joint) and the calcaneum or os calcis (heel bone). Both these bones are vulnerable to fracture as a result of falls from a height. They can also fracture when struck or trapped by foot pedals in a motor vehicle.

Symptoms and signs

There is pain on attempts to walk or on direct palpation. There may be significant deformity if these fractures are associated with dislocation of either the ankle or the midfoot joints.

Treatment

The ankle and foot should be placed in a well-padded splint and elevated. The circulation to the foot should be monitored and the neurological state assessed.

Potential problems

The mechanism of injury usually causes associated injuries. A fall from a height may produce fractures of the calcaneum, talus, femoral neck, acetabulum and vertebrae and a thorough secondary survey is mandatory, although this will usually be deferred until the patient arrives in hospital.

Dislocations of the midfoot

Cause

Midfoot dislocations result from a fall from a height, landing on the foot with the toes pointing downwards.

Symptoms and signs

The deformity is usually obvious, although it may be obscured by the footwear, and swelling will occur quickly. There may be associated vascular injury, either directly or indirectly, because of a compartment syndrome.

Treatment

The paramedic should not attempt to relocate the dislocation at the scene. The foot should be placed in a well-padded splint and elevated and the patient evacuated to hospital. The circulation to the distal part of the foot must be assessed and recorded.

Potential problems

The possibility of other associated serious injuries should not be forgotten.

Fractures of the metatarsals and toes

Cause

Fractures of the metatarsals and toes can be caused by direct blows, falls and even by overuse (e.g. the 'march fracture' of the second metatarsal seen in army recruits unused to marching in boots). Overuse injuries will rarely present to the ambulance service as an emergency.

Symptoms and signs

There is pain over the fracture which is made worse when attempting to walk. The foot swells dorsally (the top surface), an analogous situation with hand injuries.

Treatment

The foot should be elevated. A splint is not always required, but when used it should be well padded.

Potential problems

The main problem is swelling which may compromise the circulation, particularly of the digits.

Traumatic amputation

Traumatic amputation can range from a relatively minor fingertip injury to a life-threatening avulsion of a limb. Recent improvements in microsurgical techniques have increased the likelihood of successful reimplantation of the amputated part.

In order to minimise the damage to the amputated part and thus improve the chances of successful surgery, the following steps should be performed.

- The time of amputation should be recorded
- The amputated part should not be placed in water or directly in ice, as this can cause further cellular damage
- The amputated part should be securely wrapped up in a sealed plastic bag, which should be placed in a second bag, and the double-wrapped part kept cool. It is safe to place the part in an ice-water mixture after wrapping it in this way as direct contact is avoided
- If the patient is still trapped then the part should be clearly labelled and sent to the receiving hospital after discussion with the medical staff who will be receiving and treating the patient.

However damaged the amputated part is, it should always be transported to hospital with the patient. Even if reimplantation is not possible, use of the skin for grafting may be considered.

Complications of fractures

The complications of any injury can be divided into immediate, early and late.

Immediate complications

- Haemorrhage
- Vascular injury
- Nerve injury.

Early complications

- Compartment syndrome
- Infection
- Fat embolism.

Late complications

- Reflex sympathetic dystrophy
- Osteomyelitis
- Non-union
- Malunion
- Arthritis.

For further information, see Ch. 27 in *Emergency Care: A Textbook for Paramedics.*

CHAPTER 28

Spinal injuries

Spinal cord injury may be either complete (i.e. with no motor or sensory function below the level of injury) or incomplete (with partial preservation of sensory or motor function, or both). In 50% of cases of spinal injury there are associated injuries which also may require their own urgent management. As with head injuries the aim is to avoid exacerbating the primary injury.

Three elements contribute to spinal cord injury:

- Biomechanical movement
- Hypoxia due to A or B problems
- Underperfusion – C problems.

Causes of spinal cord injury

The principal causes of spinal cord injury are:

- Motor vehicle collisions
- Falls
- Sports:
  Gymnastics and trampolining
  Rugby football
  Horse riding and hunting (female to male 5:1)
  Skiing
  Hang gliding
- Aquatic injuries, e.g. diving into shallow water
- Weight falling on the back.

Diagnosis

Signs and symptoms of spinal injury include:

- Pain (highly suggestive of bony injury)
- Tenderness

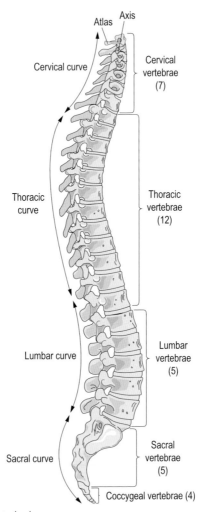

Figure 28.1 The spinal column.

Atlas

Axis

Cervical curve

Cervical vertebrae (7)

Thoracic curve

Thoracic vertebrae (12)

Lumbar curve

Lumbar vertebrae (5)

Sacral curve

Sacral vertebrae (5)

Coccygeal vertebrae (4)

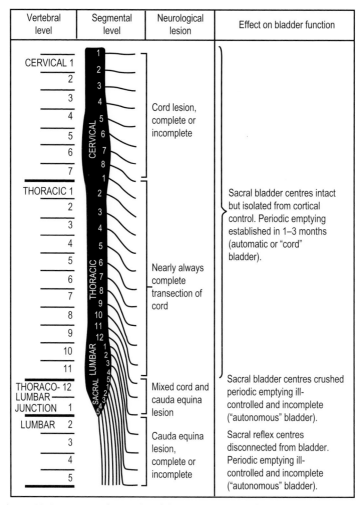

Figure 28.2 Damage to the spinal cord due to displaced bony fragments.

- Swelling
- Bruising (rare and usually late)
- Irregularity in the spine on palpation (a 'step') – occurs in only 10% of cases.

Sensory disturbances from spinal cord injury are even wider in their spectrum:

- 'Pins and needles' (paraesthesia)
- Electric shock-like pain at the moment of impact with no other indicator that injury has taken place
- Disturbances of proprioception, where the patient feels he or she is still in the same position as at the moment of impact, despite clearly now lying in another
- Burning pains through both arms or both lower limbs.

Burning pains in the upper limb are seen in motor vehicle deceleration accidents. In the lower limbs, burning pains are associated with 'hyperpathia' (touch registers as pain), seen most frequently in conus injuries.

Minor degrees of sensory or motor loss are frequently described by patients either in terms of 'clumsiness', 'stiffness' or 'heaviness' and such complaints must always be treated seriously.

Patients who have congenitally abnormal spines or diseases such as ankylosing spondylitis or rheumatoid arthritis do not require the same degree of force to produce a cord injury as those with a normal spine.

Assessment

- Any patient who is unconscious as a result of a head injury (or who could have had a head injury in association with unconsciousness) and any victim of trauma who is unable to give an account of the accident (e.g. through intoxication) must be regarded as having a spinal cord injury until proved otherwise
- It is essential to have a high index of suspicion. If the situation suggests that there could be a spinal cord injury the patient must be treated as if there is
- When a history is available and clearly excludes the possibility of a spinal injury or when it is apparent from the injury mechanism that a spinal injury has not occurred, immobilisation of the spine is not necessary.

Neurological examination at the accident site should not be detailed. In motor terms, attendants should be looking at voluntary power, e.g. bending large joints normally. It is important to observe whether the chest wall moves during breathing or whether it is the diaphragm alone which is responsible for respiratory effort (diaphragmatic breathing, see below).

- Do not let the patient get up
- Do not allow others to get the patient up
- Do not get the patient up yourself. Think spinal cord injury!

Sensory levels

- Root of the neck is C4
- The nipple line (in the male) is T4
- The umbilicus is T10
- Foot (sole) is S1.

Immediate management

Because of the risk of anoxic damage and damage from underperfusion, catastrophic haemorrhage <C>, airway (A), breathing (B) and circulation (C) must take priority over a cord injury or a potential cord injury.

The problems found in a primary survey are not only life-threatening but will inevitably make any spinal injury worse. Careful horizontal movement (e.g. a properly applied 'log roll'), will prevent further permanent damage.

The patient should be moved as little as possible.

Causes of deteriroration in established or suspected spinal injury

- Hypoxia from underventilation, airway obstruction or lung damage either as a result of associated injuries or from aspiration of vomit
- Underperfusion from reduced cord blood flow which may be due to positioning (e.g. sitting up) or to shock
- Mechanical displacement of vertebrae
- Displacement of vertebral fragments.

Reasons for missing a spinal injury

- Stress leading to endorphin release distracting injuries elsewhere or between release and distracting injuries
- Central nervous depression from brain injury
- Intoxication from alcohol or drugs
- Uncooperative or aggressive behaviour.

Emergency extrication

Emergency extrication, that is, without the availability of appropriate extrication devices or the assistance of relevant emergency services, is justifiable only when there is an immediate threat to life.

Airway

Airway obstruction leads to hypoxia and inevitably to cord deterioration. Airway clearance is therefore vital. The technique of jaw thrust (or chin lift if necessary) should be used, while the head and neck are simultaneously moved into a neutral position and manual in-line stabilisation is applied.

Breathing

Ventilation is often impeded in a thoracic or cervical cord injury. This may be because the patient is breathing using only the diaphragm (the intercostal and abdominal muscles being paralysed) or because of chest injuries and associated pain. It should be remembered that pain from chest injuries may mask the pain from the back injury. If ventilation is inadequate ventilatory assistance will be necessary.

Always administer high concentration oxygen

Intubation in potential cord injury

There are benefits in intubating the apnoeic and/or unconscious patient in terms of improved airway control, prevention of subsequent bronchial soiling, ease of bronchial toilet and ease of mechanical ventilation.

The hazards include:

- Neck injury may be associated with laryngeal damage
- Intubation may precipitate vagal asystolic arrest
- Endobronchial suction may precipitate vagal asystolic arrest
- Intubation may precipitate vomiting
- Neck movement may exacerbate a spinal cord injury.

In the majority of cases intubation will not be possible without the administration of anaesthetic drugs since the patient will be conscious.

Indications for intubation include

- Absence of spontaneous ventilation which is not restarted by airway opening
- Absent or inadequate spontaneous ventilation with evidence of vomiting, reflux or aspiration
- Adequate supine spontaneous ventilation which is associated with problems in airway control
- Adequate supine spontaneous ventilation associated with increasing ventilatory difficulty in association with thoracic or abdominal injury
- The unconscious spinal cord injury patient with isolated head and neck injuries

Spinal cord injury and disordered circulation

Spinal cord injury can be associated with disorders of central circulation, which may cause either cardiac arrest or a fatal arrhythmia.

After spinal cord injury, due to loss of function of the sympathetic nervous system, the parasympathetic nervous system can be unopposed.

This produces generalised vasodilation. Thus, even if the circulating blood volume is unchanged there will effectively be underperfusion. This produces neurogenic shock.

In an isolated cervical or thoracic cord injury, the 'normal' systolic arterial blood pressure will be found to be around 90 mmHg. At this level, because the vessels are vasodilated, perfusion should be adequate so long as the patient is kept flat. The heart rate may be either slow or normal.

A combination of bradycardia and hypotension should always raise the suspicion of spinal cord injury.

> Where a patient has a normal pulse and apparent hypotension, both spinal cord injury and covert trauma should be suspected. Shock in the patient with multiple trauma must never be assumed to be solely due to spinal cord injury.

In a patient with multiple injuries of which the cord injury is one element, the indications for infusion are the same as for any other polytrauma victim.

With the isolated cord injury, as may occur in a gymnastic or rugby accident, if given at all, the infusion must be given with extreme care.

So long as the patient is kept flat, perfusion should be adequate to maintain a radial pulse.

Where the radial pulse is lost, an infusion will be necessary to ensure that a palpable radial pulse returns. Only 500 ml of intravenous fluid should be given pre-hospital. This volume is sufficient to compensate for the increased vascular space.

While a head-down tilt can be used temporarily to clear vomit from the airway, continued use of this position on circulatory grounds may cause the abdominal contents to splint the diaphragm and reduce the vital capacity and so should be avoided.

Neurogenic shock is a cardiovascular condition resulting from loss of vascular tone as a result of loss of sympathetic activity and is manifested by a low blood pressure in a well-perfused individual with no evidence of tachycardia.

Spinal shock is a neurological condition manifested by flaccidity and loss of reflexes.

If the heart rate is below 45 bpm, a bolus dose of atropine (500 µg) should be given before any of the above interventions are attempted and should be given in any case if the heart rate falls as low as 40 bpm.

Unconsciousness

If the patient is alive when the first rescuer arrives, the incidence of a grossly unstable biomechanical cervical injury is of the order of 1 in 300.

Two maxims derive from this:

- In the presence of a significant head injury, a spinal cord injury should always be suspected and movement minimised accordingly
- Because of the relative incidences, any movement which is necessary to save life must take priority and must be carried out in accordance with the priorities of primary survey using the greatest care and best endeavours available.

The major risk of unconsciousness is that of aspiration pneumonia induced by inhalation of vomit or refluxed gastric contents.

Unconsciousness takes priority: the airway must be maintained and bronchial soiling avoided. The mortality of isolated spinal cord injury is under 1%, but this rises to 40% if aspiration pneumonitis supervenes.

The patient with neurogenic shock will appear warm, pink and well perfused, with a low or normal pulse despite a low blood pressure.

Indicators of possible spinal cord injury in the unconscious patient

- Different level of responsiveness above and below the level of possible cord injury
- Diaphragmatic ventilation (during inspiration the abdominal wall, instead of appearing to recede, balloons out)
- Bradycardia with hypotension and a head injury
- Priapism (sustained erection).

Basic management summary

- Always have a high index of suspicion for spinal cord injury
- Remember the history and mechanism of injury
- The patient must not stand or sit up
- Massive haemorrhage, airway, breathing, circulation and unconsciousness require immediate action
- Slow, careful movement is safe
- Careful movement in the horizontal axis preserves life and will also preserve residual cord function.

From this list it can be seen that the basic rules are as follows:

- Consider safety
- Consider the need for resuscitation (primary survey)
- Consider the possibility of a spinal cord injury
- Control the head and neck position while allowing optimal support of the airway, breathing and circulation
- Organise the team before embarking on complicated extrication and management procedures.

The use of equipment will always require assistance beyond the standard two-person ambulance crew. It may involve summoning ambulance colleagues, making use of fellow emergency service professionals or even seeking help from the general public. Assistants must always be adequately briefed before a task is undertaken.

Spinal immobilisation and patient handling

Control of the head and neck

Control of the head and neck must be undertaken as soon as possible. Control is secured by immobilising the base of the skull without exerting a positive traction force. In the unrecognised spinal injury, traction may induce a secondary distraction injury.

Collars

A semi-rigid collar must be used rather than a soft collar, improvised collar or rehabilitation collar.

The collar should restrict flexion, extension, lateral flexion and rotation of the neck and the resting position of the neck must be in neutral alignment.

The instructions for application should be rigorously followed. Another person must always control the head and neck while the collar is applied.

Lastly, any collar is only a restraint and must be supplemented by manual head control or the use of headblocks and tape.

A tight collar may interfere with venous return from the cerebral circulation and accordingly raise the intracranial pressure in patients whose cerebral perfusion is already compromised.

Movement at the accident site

Movement at the scene is usually:

- From prone to supine to maximise ventilation with a conscious patient and place the head in neutral alignment
- From supine to side to protect an otherwise unprotected airway or to assist the clearance of vomit
- From side to supine once vomit has been cleared or to intubate or otherwise maintain ventilation of someone whose ventilation is inadequate on their side.

Movement is effected by a 'log roll'. The log roll requires ideally six people and at least five people if it is to be carried out without moving the full length of the spine. Log rolling using three people has been described but this produces a movement of the dorsal and/or lumbar spine. Equally, in hospital, four people can be used but this works only where: (a) the conditions are ideal and the patient is at the right height and (b) where the team is highly experienced at the manoeuvre.

Orthopaedic ('scoop') stretcher

For retrieving casualties from the ground, the scoop stretcher is preferable to the long spinal board which requires a log roll procedure.

It is almost exclusively a transfer stretcher, although it can be used to remove people from difficult locations, after which they can be transferred to a conventional stretcher or an evacuation mattress.

Once the patient is on the ambulance trolley cot or the evacuation mattress, the scoop stretcher should be removed unless the transfer time to hospital is short.

Evacuation (vacuum) mattresses

The mattress should be tested before the ambulance goes on duty to make sure that there are no leaks.

When laid out it needs to be smoothed flat. Once the patient is positioned on it manual contouring is required between the legs and around the head, neck and shoulders.

The scoop stretcher can be placed underneath it with safety and will add to overall rigidity.

Extrication devices

The designs that are easiest to use have a leading edge which can be applied from either side (and which can be cleared of straps, buckles and other impedimenta so that it can be inserted easily).

A minimum of four people are necessary to apply such a device.

- The ideal device should not 'concertina' during insertion behind the patient. It should not be applied before a semi-rigid cervical collar is in place. There should be an effective cushion component to block out the space between the board and the rear of the collar and head. All straps should be applied and tightened, except the leg straps in the presence of a fractured femur
- Once secured, the patient can be moved in any suitable direction except the vertical. A vertical lift requires the addition of a vertical movement harness
- Some devices have what appears to be a handle at the head end. This must never be used for lifting the patient.

Long spinal board

The technique of choice when using a long spinal board is to bring the device in behind the patient from the rear of the wreckage and to move the patient up the long axis of the spinal board.

This requires removal of the roof of the vehicle. If a rapid extrication is mandated by the presence of a time-critical injury, the patient may be rotated onto a spine board through the adjacent doorway of the vehicle.

The spinal board is used with head immobilisers attached to it which prevent lateral movement.

Helmet removal

The removal of motorcycle helmets is essential even in the presence of a spinal cord injury. Opening the visor is not sufficient to manage the airway.

The occipital portion of all helmets will move the head into flexion, reducing the diameter of the spinal canal.

Helmet removal is essential to obtaining neutral alignment of the cervical spine. Helmet removal is not an emergency if the airway is clear and protected.

Helmet removal should, wherever possible, be undertaken by two people.

- First, undo the chin strap
- One person supports the neck from the front and gradually moves their hands up the back of the neck and head while the helmet is tipped backwards and forwards in the vertical plane to clear the occiput and then the nose

- While the helmet is being removed, it should be carefully expanded laterally
- At every stage, the person holding the neck must have complete control and should ask his colleague to stop if problems arise.

Pressure sores

Pressure sores can start to develop within an hour of a spinal cord injury occurring. In the supine position on the heels, the buttocks, the scapulae and the back of the head.

The scoop stretcher can produce pressure sores even on a short journey. It should only be used as a transfer stretcher and patients should not be left lying directly on it.

Ideally the evacuation of spinal injury patients should be carried out on a vacuum mattress. This device is essential for long journeys or secondary transfers or for aeromedical flights.

- Loosen clothing, including the shoe-laces
- Removed hard objects from pockets where they are next to the skin
- Place padding between the legs
- Pad any additional splintage
- Keep the patient on a spinal board for as short a time as possible, ideally no more than 30 minutes
- Remove the spinal board in hospital at the earliest safe opportunity.

Hypothermia

A paralysed person cannot sweat or shiver. Patients with spinal injuries must be protected from the cold; they must be warmed passively by being wrapped up well.

During the primary journey this is not usually a problem, but because of the large distances between spinal units, it can be a problem on a secondary journey from the receiving hospital to the spinal unit, for which the ambulance service is also responsible.

In hot weather the reverse problem – heat illness – can also occur.

For further information, see Ch. 28 in *Emergency Care: A Textbook for Paramedics*.

CHAPTER 29

Patient immobilisation and extrication

It is crucial that decisions about stabilisation, extrication and subsequent evacuation are taken early on in the rescue. The techniques used for stabilisation must not be viewed in isolation, but should be part of the total rescue activity and should complement the other treatments used.

Principles of immobilisation

In the prehospital setting, the principles of skeletal management are to:
- Prevent further injury
- Ensure neurovascular supply
- Make the patient comfortable.

The overriding importance of managing the airway with cervical spine protection, breathing and circulation (ABC) is fundamental to the treatment of any injury.

With the exception of cervical spine care, fracture management and extrication follow the primary survey unless a 'snatch rescue' is necessary.

The principles of definitive fracture management are:
- Reduction
- Immobilisation
- Preservation of function.

Every piece of equipment will cover or hide the patient to a greater or lesser extent, it is essential that any immediate local treatment and observations are carried out before the immobilisation device is applied.

Wounds should wherever possible be photographed and appropriately dressed before immobilisation.

The benefits of immobilisation are:

- Pain relief
- Reduction of blood loss
- Prevention of neurovascular damage
- Prevention of fat embolism.

Remembering the ABC principles, splinting or extrication devices should never produce any airway, breathing or circulation compromise.

The patient should always feel more comfortable after the splint or device has been applied, so that handling becomes easier.

Always check the pulses distal to an injury before starting treatment

---

Forms of splintage

Box splints

Box splints are simple in design and are useful for some arm, lower leg and ankle injuries and are carried by every front-line ambulance.

The splint forms an oblong box, open along one side with the other three sides able to be folded in such a way as to form a gutter. There may be a foot support at one end. Box splints are available in adult and child sizes.

Application

- Expose the injured leg
- Remove footwear (occasionally, footwear may provide support and should be left in place)
- Apply dressings to any wounds
- Straighten the ankle and check the peripheral pulses
- Raise the leg and pass the splint passed underneath it
- Fold the two sides of the splint so they fit closely against the leg, place the foot support
- Secure with the Velcro straps
- If any strap passes near to an injury, care should be taken that it does not cause pain; if it does, it should be left loose
- Once the splint is applied, the patient should be rechecked – specifically, the pulses in the limb and the distal sensation must be noted and recorded
- Mark the position of a palpable dorsalis pedis pulse with pen once a splint has been applied to the leg.

Traction splints

The primary function of a traction splint is to immobilise the fracture (of a lower limb) in a reduced position

- Following a fracture of the shaft of the femur the muscles of the thigh will shorten the leg, causing the bone ends to override. This increases the radius of the thigh so that it becomes more spherical: this shape has a larger internal volume than a cylinder and so presents a larger space into which blood can fill
- Application of traction will restore the cylindrical shape of the thigh, reducing its volume and reducing the overall blood loss
- Three types of traction splint are found in prehospital care: the Hare® or Trac-3® splint, the Sager® splint and the Donway® splint
- There may be other more life-threatening injuries which must take priority. Patients are far less likely to die from a fracture of the lower limb than they are from a blocked airway
- All compound fractures will need to be explored and cleaned. Therefore the receiving hospital must know that a fracture was compound and if possible a photograph should be taken.

Indications for traction splintage

- Closed (simple) fractures of the femoral shaft
- Closed (simple) fractures of the proximal two-thirds of the tibia and fibula
- Compound fractures of the femur, and the proximal two-thirds of the tibia and fibula.

Contraindications to traction splintage

- Fractures around the knee
- Dislocation of the hip
- Fracture dislocation of the knee
- Ankle injuries
- Simple undisplaced fracture of the lower third of the tibia and fibula (better immobilised with a box splint)
- Fractures of the pelvis.

Complications of traction splintage

- Damage to the neurovascular supply to the leg. This can be prevented by careful examination of the distal limb function
- Absence or change in distal function must be reported to the Emergency Department. If it is found that the distal pulses diminish or are absent after traction has been applied then traction must be gently reduced until the pulse returns
- The pulse oximeter can be used to detect alterations in the blood flow if the probe is placed on one of the toes of the fractured leg.

Hare® or Trac-3® traction splint

This splint can be used with traction to maintain a reduced fracture of the lower limb and can also be used without traction simply for support.

Application

- The splint requires two people to apply it correctly and analgesia should be given as required before manipulating the fracture
- The splint should be set-up as follows:
  - The fracture site is exposed (clothes should be cut if necessary). Motorcycle leathers should not be removed as these can be dramatically effective in the control of lower limb and pelvic fracture bleeding
  - The limb should be examined thoroughly and the footwear removed
  - The pulses distal to the fracture together with the colour and warmth of the limb and sensation and motor function distal to the fracture should also be assessed (the neurovascular examination)
  - Wounds are dressed if required
  - The splint is prepared
  - Select the appropriate ankle hitch
  - The splint is placed by the good leg, measured for length and adjusted accordingly, then laid by the injured leg
  - All the straps are checked; these should be open and placed at the correct intervals down the splint
  - Some of the traction strap should be unwound
  - The foot is straightened and the ankle hitch placed well under the ankle
  - The side straps are then tightly folded over the ankle (not around the foot) and the rings brought together below the foot
  - Finally the strap at the bottom of the foot is firmly grasped: traction must be applied along the longitudinal axis of the femur, not over the dorsum of the foot, which can cause permanent damage to the limb
  - Manual traction is started with one hand while the other hand supports the leg
  - The splint is then put in the correct position. The best method is to roll the patient away from the splint while a colleague slides the splint under the leg
  - The top padded ring must fit under the ischial tuberosity. The patient is then rolled back onto the splint. If the position is still not correct then the patient can be moved down slightly so that he is sitting on the padded ring. Manual traction MUST be maintained THROUGHOUT this procedure
  - The top strap is done up and padding applied if required. The external genitalia should be avoided in males. If correctly positioned, this strap will lie parallel to the crease of the groin
  - The traction hook is then put through the 'D' rings and traction taken up, ensuring that manual traction is not released before the splint's mechanical traction is tightened

- Traction is applied until the limb is comfortable (to a maximum of 7 kg in adults)
- The neurovascular examination is repeated and the oximeter reading rechecked
- The leg is elevated by raising the foot stand
- The Velcro straps are positioned and tightened to support the site of the fracture
- The leg is covered to keep it warm.

En route to hospital

The neurovascular examination should be repeated every 5–10 minutes. The straps should be checked and loosened if required – the leg may swell.

The tension of traction should be checked; as a result of reduced spasm in the muscles, tension can be lost.

To release traction

The two splints (Hare® and Trac-3®) have slightly different release mechanisms
Manual traction is taken up and then the mechanical traction is released after all the supporting Velcro straps have been removed
The Hare® splint has a pull ring which releases the traction suddenly, whereas the Trac-3® has a knob which has to be unwound to release the traction (which is less likely to be accidentally released).

Sager® traction splint

The Sager® traction splint weighs <2 kg and can be used to treat single or bilateral fractures of the lower limb, especially of the femur.

Application

- The shoe and sock are removed and the leg exposed as necessary
- The distal pulses and sensation in the injured leg are assessed
- The cushioned end of the splint is applied between the patient's legs, against the perineum and symphysis pubis (avoiding the external genitalia in males)
- The bridle 'S' strap is applied around the top of the thigh
- The splint is extended so that the ankle hitch lies between the patient's heels or at the level of the normal heel if the fractured leg has been shortened
- The ankle harness is applied beneath the heel and wrapped around just above the malleoli, adjusting the cushions on the strap to fit the size of the leg
- Traction is applied (recommended at 10% of the body weight) until the patient is comfortable
- The leg cravats are applied
- The bridle around the thigh is tightened if necessary
- The cravats are secured
- The foot-binding strap is placed around the feet and ankles in a figure-of-eight
- The foot pulses must be checked following application.

To release traction

Manual traction is taken up. The cravats and ankle hitch are removed. Along the shaft of the splint there is a small sprung piece of metal, which should be lifted to release the tension.

Donway® splint

The Donway® splint employs a different method to achieve traction.

- The fractured leg is cradled by the splint with the foot firmly fixed to the ankle support
- The top strapping is put around the thigh and then, using the pump provided, the two halves of the splint (lower and upper) are pushed apart by increased pressure (like the slide on a trombone)
- Once the patient is comfortable the securing screws are tightened; the pressure in the splint is then released through a valve
- The leg straps are applied and (as with other forms of traction splint) the pulses and sensation in the limb must be checked.

Care must be taken to ensure the ankle hitch is applied in a manner that avoids traction over the dorsum of the foot.

Cervical spine immobilisation

Manual methods

From behind the patient:

- The rescuer's palms are placed behind the patient's ears
- The little fingers should lie just under the angle of the jaw and the thumbs should be extended upwards behind the posterior aspect of the skull
- The rescuer's hands should be adjusted so that the patient's ears lie between the fingers. It is important not to cover the ears: the last thing an anxious patient needs is to be prevented from hearing
- If the head is not in a neutral position, it should be moved slowly and gently into a neutral position. If resistance is felt during this procedure the patient should be managed in the position in which he has been found
- Traction is not applied
- The rescuer should move into a comfortable braced position in order to support their own arms to prevent them from becoming tired.

From the side:

- One hand should be placed behind the patient's head so the occiput lies in its palm
- The other hand should support the jaw between the thumb and second finger The two hands now hold the neck in a similar way to a cervical collar
- The head can be moved into a neutral position. The anterior arm should be braced against the patient's sternum.

From the front:

- The rescuer's hands are placed over the patient's cheeks so that the fingers pass around the neck and the extended thumbs lie just in front of the ears over the temporomandibular joint
- The head may be moved into a neutral position. The anterior arm should be braced against the patient's sternum.

Cervical collars

A number of different types of cervical collars are available. Some are 'one piece' and require a range of sizes to be carried (e.g. the Stiffneck® collar); others come in one piece but are adjustable. The collars have to be sized according to the manufacturer's instructions and then applied correctly while maintaining manual immobilisation.

Collars do not completely immobilise the cervical spine and it is essential to continue manual immobilisation until this is replaced by a short spine board or long spine board and head immobiliser. It is of little use merely to hold on to the collar: the hands have to support the head and should be placed above the collar. A correctly sized collar will reduce flexion and extension and to lesser extent sideways movement, but will not stop rotation – it is rotation that the rescuer's hands or headblock and tape will prevent.

Access to the airway and trachea is available at all times through the gap in front of the collar. The application of a cervical collar, even when correctly sized, will cause a rise in intracranial pressure (through venous compression). It is, therefore, acceptable to release the collar in these circumstances once head blocks and tape have been correctly applied.

Patients who are unconscious should have their cervical spine protected and be fully immobilised. However, patients who are conscious should be carefully assessed to include:

- Consideration of the mechanism of injury
- The presence of drugs or alcohol
- A long bone injury or other distracting injury
- The presence of midline cervical spine tenderness.

The presence of any of these features following an accident with possible cervical spine injury should mandate full immobilisation. Similarly, patients who complain of pain and are reluctant to move their neck of their own volition should receive full immobilisation.

Correct scene and patient assessment will ensure the correct management of the cervical spine.

Log roll technique

Log rolling is a method of turning patients either to inspect their backs or to help put them on to a long spinal board. The object is to keep the whole spine in alignment.

- To log roll a patient, there should be a minimum of four people
  - The patient should lie with his arms by his sides and the palms placed against the legs. Alternatively the patient can place his arms in a crossed position on his chest
  - The cervical spine is stabilised and the patient moved with the neck, shoulders and pelvis kept in the same plane
  - One person takes the head and this person controls the manoeuvre
  - The next person grips the patient's shoulder on the opposite side and also the further arm
  - The third person grips the pelvis
  - The fourth person controls the legs
  - The person at the head calls the instructions and the whole body is rolled over, keeping the spine from twisting
  - The roll should be only as far as is needed to inspect the back or insert a long board underneath the patient
  - A fifth person, if available, should examine the patient's back and perform any necessary treatment (e.g. dressing a bleeding wound).

The patient is then rolled back into the supine position, again controlled by the person controlling the head and neck

The person at the head should inform his colleagues what command will be given before the manoeuvre begins: 'I will say one, two, three, move. Everybody ready? Good. One, two ...'.

Scoop stretcher

The scoop stretcher provides a means of lifting a patient onto a trolley or ambulance cot with minimal movement. The scoop stretcher can be split in half longitudinally and may have a head cushion. The bottom half can be extended to fit the patient

- The scoop should be laid beside the patient and extended to the required length
- The patient should be told what is about to happen
- The halves are slid underneath the patient's body from the sides, taking care not to pinch the body as the halves are brought together
- The patient may have to be rolled slightly to allow each half stretcher to be slid underneath
- Once the stretcher is in place and the halves are locked together, the head cushion is secured and the patient is lifted onto the trolley or cot
- The distance that the stretcher has to be carried should be kept to a minimum and if rough ground or stairs have to be negotiated, restraining straps can be used to increase the patient's security.

Once the patient is on the trolley, the scoop stretcher should be removed to prevent pressure sores developing, unless the transfer time is short and the removal of the stretcher would delay definitive treatment.

Spinal boards

Spinal boards are used to assist in the movement (extrication) of casualties from an accident scene. They provide a secure and stable base onto which a patient may be strapped, so providing full spinal immobilisation

The use of a long board requires many hands and everyone must be aware of his role because teamwork is all-important. Before using a long board, the method of log rolling a patient must be understood (see above).

Long board

- A patient may be rolled onto a long board or lifted onto a board using a scoop stretcher. Depending on the situation of the patient, a cervical collar may be applied before or after placing the patient on the board. Either way, manual in-line cervical stabilisation will be required until the patient is secured to the board
- The head should be supported in a head immobiliser ('headbox'). The straps on the board are applied according to the manufacturer's instructions
- If a child is placed on a long board, because of the relatively larger size of the child's head, a pad may be required below the shoulders to prevent any forward flexion of the neck. Some paediatric boards are formed so as to accommodate the larger occiput of the child
- It is perfectly possible to use an adult board in the prehospital environment to prevent the ambulance having to carry a further piece of equipment. In this situation several blanket rolls will be required to secure the child comfortably on the board.

Extrication

If the roof of the car has been removed, the long board can be slid behind the patient. If the patient is in a front seat, the seat can be reclined as the patient is slid onto the long board and lifted clear

- Otherwise:
  - The front door must be forced open
  - One person maintains in-line cervical stabilisation from the back seat
  - A second applies a cervical collar from the side
  - The third brings the long board, which is placed on the seat under the patient.

Unless a 'snatch' rescue is necessary, a brief assessment should be performed

- Then:
  - The patient's feet and legs are then freed whilst manual in-line cervical stabilisation is maintained
  - The third rescuer, beside the patient in the front of the car prepares to lift the patient's legs across the unoccupied front seat

- The second rescuer assumes the command of all movements, placing one hand on the patient's midthoracic spine and the other hand on the sternum
- The legs are swung onto the seat so that the patient's back faces the open door; this movement should be done in short steps
- A new rescuer may have to control the patient's neck while the first rescuer negotiates the doorpost
- Once the patient is sitting across the front seat, the long board (if not already in place) is pushed onto the seat, and then elevated to meet the patient's back
- The patient and the board should then be lowered together, ideally onto a waiting ambulance trolley. The patient is then slid in small movements up the board
- As the patient is slid up the board, rescuer 1 maintains in-line cervical stabilisation, rescuer 2's hands are placed in the patient's armpits and the third rescuer steadies the hips, pelvis and legs.

All straps should be applied before the head immobiliser is fitted to avoid a moving patient 'hinging' at the neck. Two straps are applied across the thorax, extending over the clavicles and crossing to the opposite pelvic crest. Strap buckles must not rest on the clavicles. A third strap is attached across the pelvis, and a fourth in a figure of eight from the proximal tibia and around the ankles.

- A close fit must be established when applying head blocks, and the forehead strap applied first, tightening both sides together. The chin strap should be applied over the point of the chin and collar, never under the chin, to avoid obstructing the airway.

Vacuum splints

Vacuum splints provide rigid support to the body and can be very comfortable. They are bags of polystyrene beads enclosed in tough plastic. The injured limb or the whole patient can be placed onto the splint, which is actively moulded around the injured part. Suction is then applied to the bag, creating a vacuum: the contents take up a rigid form, supporting and splinting the injury.

- Vacuum splints can be used to immobilise:
  - Limbs (upper or lower)
  - The cervical spine, in conjugation with a semi-rigid collar
  - Other spinal injuries.

The vacuum mattress is applied as follows:

- Lay the splint on the trolley
- Place the patient onto the mattress
- Secure the mattress around the patient's body using Velcro straps or a continuous webbing strap

- Mould the mattress around the patient. Ensure the vacuum mattress is smooth and flat before positioning the patient
- Mould the mattress to support the neck and side of the head
- Create the vacuum inside the mattress using the suction pump provided
- Secure the valve mechanism and remove the pump.

A vacuum mattress is a good immobilisation device but a poor lifting device. It is important therefore to place a long spinal board or scoop stretcher under the vacuum mattress if the patient is to be lifted or carried any distance.

Extrication devices

In current use are the Kendrick Extrication Device (KED)®, the Russell Extrication Device® (RED) and the ED2000®.

The devices are to an extent flexible and can therefore be slipped between the patient and the car seat. Once applied, they offer some protection to the spine and allow the patient to be lifted from the vehicle onto a trolley or other device. The method of application is as follows:

- The cervical spine is immobilised manually and with a cervical collar
- The extrication device is then slipped down behind the patient, making sure the various straps do not become caught on any object
- The device is then positioned correctly in relation to the patient's head and shoulders
- The wings of the device forming the chest sides are drawn together with the chest straps, which are then tightened, in the sequence upper, bottom, middle, ensuring that this produces no respiratory embarrassment or pain
- The leg straps are passed under the patient's legs and then fitted back onto the device. These straps are tightened
- The shoulder straps are placed across the body and fixed to the opposite side of the device; they must not overlap the cervical collar
- The head straps are applied after making sure that any space behind the head is filled in with the padding supplied. These straps will hold the head and cervical spine firmly and the person who has been immobilising the cervical spine can now let go
- All straps are checked for tightness and adjusted so they are even.

The patient can now be lifted out of the vehicle using a long spine board and placed on a trolley. The leg straps must be loosened to allow the legs to extend.

Patient extrication

The basic prehospital approach of primary survey, resuscitation and stabilisation is even more important when dealing with the trapped patient. The <C>ABC principles apply and continuing reassessments will be required during the rescue.

Actual entrapment

Actual entrapment occurs when the victim is physically enclosed or held in a vehicle or area by the structure impinging on his body, e.g. a deformed vehicle following an RTC or a roof fall following building collapse.

Relative entrapment

Relative entrapment occurs when the victim needs help because of his location, the environment or pain preventing extrication. For example, a traffic accident victim may have a fractured humerus. It is the pain that immobilises the patient.

Preparation

Preparation includes training and a knowledge of the rescue teams and other services. It is essential to know the equipment they carry and their potential skills and benefits. The paramedic's own equipment must be checked and kept up-to-date.

Teamwork

If power-operated tools are required then this part of the rescue should be left to the specialists (the fire service). Equally, these specialists should have a clear understanding of what the medical priorities are. That may mean giving early access to the paramedic to allow stabilisation of the casualty. The paramedics can then concentrate on controlling the cervical spine during the rescue and monitoring the patient.

Clothing

Entrapments can be dangerous to the rescue worker and therefore proper clothing should be worn. This should include a helmet and robust footwear that gives protection from sharp metal and glass as well as tough 'debris' gloves.

Safety

Any entrapment scenario will have its associated dangers. Road traffic collisions, for example, are associated with the dangers of moving vehicles. Industrial accidents may well involve unfamiliar machinery or chemicals. In domestic entrapments risks from falling debris, electricity or gas may be present. The movement and actions of fellow rescue personnel and their associated equipment must not be ignored as a potential cause of additional injury.

Assessment

Key features of the assessment include:

- The forces involved in the incident and the energy exchange which took place
- The number of casualties involved
- The clinical priority of the patients (triage)

- Individual casualty assessment
- Communication with the patient and emergency services
- Identification of actual or relative entrapment
- Protection of the casualty from environmental dangers.

Once these early stages of assessment have been completed, the patient's <C>ABC can be assessed, followed by D and then E. Significant fractures are often identified under E. Team discussions can take place on how best to tackle the extrication, allowing for the additional hazards that the environment may pose.

Monitoring

Continual monitoring is essential and must be performed by the ambulance crew who will be close to the patient. Electronic blood pressure monitoring, electrocardiography and pulse oximetry are useful, but none of these replaces clinical observation. Chest auscultation or assessment is almost impossible, so rescue field shutdown is required to enable this procedure to be completed. When there is relative silence, it is important to take the opportunity to check the whole patient. The Fire service will always help but they should not be expected to stop the rescue unnecessarily or more frequently than is needed.

In a hostile environment a rapid extrication may be necessary. There is little point in unprotected paramedics entering smoky or fume-filled environments such as a coal mine or ship's cargo hold. Rescue should be left to specialist crews in protective clothing. In the first instance rapid extrication from a hostile environment is all that can be achieved.

Snatch rescue

Snatch rescue is the retrieval of the casualty from a difficult or dangerous environment with minimal stabilisation and resuscitation until a place of safety is reached.

In civil disturbance or terrorist situations, the rescue workers may be under hostile fire. Both rescuers and casualties are at risk. In these situations, the airway and cervical spine protection, breathing and circulation management must be restricted to the basics, safety of all personnel being paramount. Once the casualty is retrieved to a safer area then the primary survey can be repeated and more advanced <C>ABC techniques used if necessary.

For further information, see Ch. 29 in *Emergency Care: A Textbook for Paramedics.*

CHAPTER 30

Blast and gunshot injuries

Injuries to blast and gunshot are becoming increasingly common in modern Western society.

Basic rules for blast and bomb incidents

- Do not become a casualty yourself. Do not approach the scene until it has been declared safe – risks of secondary explosions, fire and building collapse are high
- Do not disturb or remove objects found in the environment – they may have forensic or other non-medical implications
- Do not disturb obviously dead victims or move body parts
- If there are multiple victims, triage will be necessary so that those most in need are identified, assessed and resuscitated first. This will normally be coordinated by an ambulance incident officer (in liaison with a medical incident officer)
- Care for multiple victims involves teamwork and it may be necessary to summon medical teams to the site – particularly if entrapment of victims is a feature.

Basic rules for gunshot incidents

- Do not become a casualty yourself. Do not approach the scene until it has been declared safe by the police, preferably by a firearms unit
- The management of the gunshot victim follows exactly the same <C>ABC system as any other trauma patient.

A front of high pressure or shock wave is formed which travels through the surrounding environment with a velocity greater than the speed of sound in air.

Behind the shock front is an area of turbulence defined as the dynamic pressure or blast wind.

The magnitude of an explosion is determined to a large degree by the type and quantity of explosive used as well as the environment – whether the explosion occurs in an open space or is confined inside a building.

Other features are the flash from the explosion, the risk of fires developing and the collapse of buildings.

Mechanisms of bomb injury

- Blast shock wave
- Blast wind
- Fragmentation
- Crush
- Burn
- Psychological.

Biological effects of blast

Primary effects

Primary effects result from exposure of the body to the overpressure associated with the shock wave. The most notable effects are in areas of the body where there are air-fluid interfaces:

Ear

The tympanic membrane or eardrum is very susceptible and injury is common but unpredictable. The ear must be correctly aligned to the shock wave for injury to occur.

Abdomen

Injuries range from mild contusion of bowel wall to areas of perforation with faecal spillage and subsequent peritonitis.

Lung

The most significant clinical primary effect is contusion injury to the lungs, which may progress in some cases to 'blast lung'. The problem results from widespread pulmonary bruising with haemorrhage into the alveolar spaces.

Clinical features of blast lung

- Breathlessness
- Acute respiratory distress
- Use of accessory muscles of respiration
- Pneumothorax
- Haemothorax
- Haemoptysis (rare)
- Sudden death (rare).

Secondary effects

The most common serious clinical problems facing paramedics after an explosion are the penetrating and non-penetrating injuries caused by fragments. These may arise from the casing of the exploding device (primary), or from the environment, such as pieces of glass, masonry and wood propelled by the blast wind (secondary).

Size, shape, type of material, velocity and terminal effectiveness vary enormously. Widespread contamination by foreign bodies and mixed bacterial species is common to all.

> Primary fragments – components of the explosive munition or improvised explosive device
> Secondary fragments – energised environmental fragments including body parts.

Tertiary effects

Tertiary effects result from gross displacement of the body by the blast wind. The clinical consequences include traumatic amputation and even complete body disintegration.

Injury may also be caused by a body being thrown onto a hard or irregular surface. Finally, tertiary injury may result from building collapse caused by the blast winds.

Burn injury

Burns are common and may be caused by flash, flame or both. Flash burns occur at the moment of detonation and particularly affect exposed parts such as face, arms and legs.

Flame burn occurs if the surrounding environment ignites.

Psychological injury

Over 40% of those involved in incidents such as terrorist explosions may expect to suffer some form of psychological distress in the aftermath period. For the majority of trained personnel, the outlook is very good, particularly if their efforts were successful in reducing morbidity and mortality. Debriefing and stress counselling may be helpful and is now mandatory for many emergency personnel after exposure to a stressful incident such as a bomb explosion.

Wound ballistics and mechanisms of injury

Wounding missiles, irrespective of type, cause injury by penetrating the body and transferring energy to the tissue. Therefore the wounding capacity of a particular missile wound may be defined by:

- The degree of penetration into the body and the structures directly penetrated
- The capacity of the missile to cause injury to structures surrounding and remote from the missile track.

Wounding missiles

Bullets

- Police handguns (many varieties)
- Military handguns
- Military assault rifles (5.56 mm, 7.62 mm)
- Hunting rifles (many varieties)
- Machine guns.

Fragments

Primary

- Natural (fragments from bomb casing, shells and mortars)
- Preformed (claymore mine, etched wire from hand grenades)
- Flechettes (individual darts preloaded into a carrying munition).

Secondary

- Masonry
- Glass
- Wood
- Metal.

Intrinsic

Body parts.

Gunshot injuries

In the UK, gunshot wounds are mainly caused by handguns and shotguns. Although patients are now being seen with wounds caused by bullets from military assault rifles and other military automatic weapons, these are still, fortunately, rare.

Handguns

If there is no event history, a gunshot wound may be missed.

In general, bullet wound entry and exit wounds give very little information on the patient's condition. Assume serious injury in all cases and arrange rapid transfer to hospital.

Bullets may travel an erratic and unpredictable path and may enter several body cavities. A careful primary survey should detect evidence of intrathoracic or abdominal penetration, which is a particularly ominous feature.

Shotguns

Shotguns have a smooth bore and are designed to fire multiple pellets or shot; some fire large, solid lead or plastic slugs. Pellet size varies from large buckshot to small birdshot.

Wound severity varies enormously and depends on range, body region and size of shot. In general, wounds tend to be extensive, with heavy foreign body contamination, which may include the wadding from the shotgun cartridge.

Military weapons

Assault rifles and automatic weapons are now readily available to criminals and terrorists. It would be sensible to presume anyone wounded by bullets from military weapons to have serious injury until proved otherwise.

For further information, see Ch. 30 in *Emergency Care: A Textbook for Paramedics*.

CHAPTER 31

Burns

The following information should be sought in all cases of burn injury:

- Time of the burn
- Burning agent
- Is the patient complaining of pain?
- Has the patient jumped or been involved in an explosion?
- Was the patient in a confined space?
- Has the patient lost consciousness at any time?
- A brief medical history, drug and allergy history (AMPLE)
- Tetanus status of the patient.

Simple erythema

Simple erythema is a superficial burn with no skin loss, e.g. sunburn. The skin is red and tender; this heals in 5–10 days with no scarring.

Superficial partial-thickness burn

Blisters are thin-walled and the burn is extremely painful. The skin is red and moist with a granular appearance and the germinal layer is not penetrated; an example is a scald from boiling water. Healing takes 10–20 days and there is minimal scarring.

Deep partial-thickness burn

A deep partial-thickness burn can be produced, e.g. by boiling fat; it is deeper than the superficial partial-thickness burn and the blisters are thick-walled. The underlying skin is granular and white in appearance, with pinpoint red mottling; sensation may be dulled. Healing is by migration of epithelial cells from the edge of the wound or skin adnexa, which takes 25–60 days.

Deep full-thickness burn

Full-thickness burns are caused by prolonged contact with the burning agent or dry heat. The appearance is white, leathery or charred. Although the areas of full-thickness burn are painless, the depth of the burn is usually shallower around its margins and these areas will be painful. This burn affects the full thickness of the skin and may extend further into fat, muscle or bone; it does not heal. Treatment includes tangential excision and either skin graft or free flap repair, depending on the depth.

Types of burn

- Wet heat
- Dry heat
- Flash burns
- Chemical burns
- Electrical burns
- Radiation burns.

Extent of burn

It is important to assess the extent of the burn accurately. Methods include:

- The Lund and Browder chart (Figure 31.1) – this is more appropriate for in hospital use
- The rule of nines for adults (Figure 31.2)
- The rule of fives for children and infants (Figure 31.2)
- Using the approximation that the patient's hand (flat with the fingers together) is equal to 1% of the patient's body surface area
- Serial halving. Ask 'Does the patient have 100% burns?' If not, 'Does the patient have 50% burns?' and so on until an estimation is reached that reflects total body surface area burnt (excluding erythema).

As the time of exposure to the burning agent is increased, the severity of the burn increases

---

Burn site

Burn sites with a poor prognosis are:

- Face
- Hands and feet
- Eyes
- Ears
- Perineum.

NAME _____ WARD _____ NUMBER _____ DATE_____

AGE _____ ADMISSION WEIGHT _____

LUND AND BROWDER CHARTS

IGNORE
SIMPLE ERYTHEMA

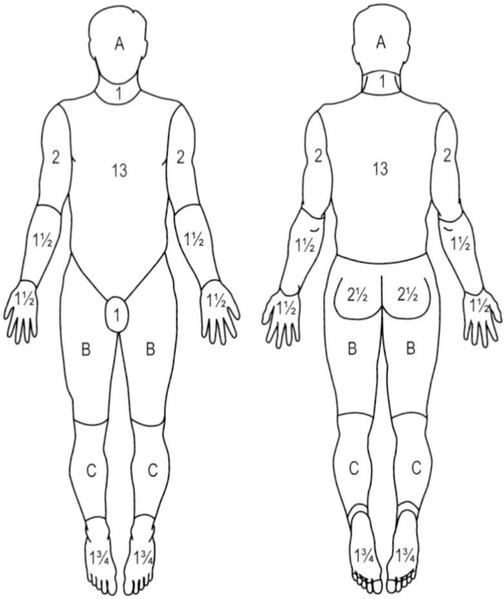

Partial thickness loss (PTL)

Full thickness loss (FTL)

REGION	%	
	PTL	FTL
HEAD		
NECK		
ANT. TRUNK		
POST. TRUNK		
RIGHT ARM		
LEFT ARM		
BUTTOCKS		
GENITALIA		
RIGHT LEG		
LEFT LEG		
TOTAL BURN		

RELATIVE PERCENTAGE OF BODY SURFACE AREA
AFFECTED BY GROWTH

AREA	AGE 0	1	5	10	15	ADULT
A5½ OF HEAD	9½	8½	6½	5½	4½	3½
B5½ OF ONE THIGH	2¾	3¼	4	4½	4½	4¾
C5½ OF ONE LEG	2½	2½	2¾	3	3¼	3½

Figure 31.1 Lund and Browder charts.

Facial burns are often associated with an inhalation injury

Circumferential burns

If there is a circumferential burn to the neck this can cause airway obstruction. Circumferential burns to the limbs produce constriction, causing oedema and distal ischaemia. A circumferential burn to the chest can lead to respiratory failure.

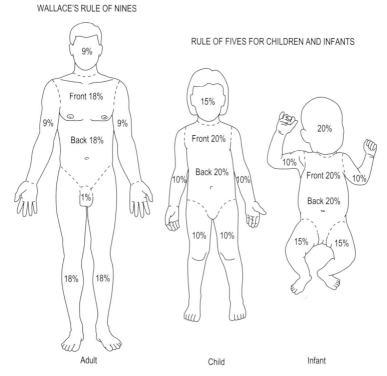

Figure 31.2 The 'rules of nines' (adults) and the 'rules of fives' (children and infants).

Inhalation injury

Inhalation injury is now the major cause of death in burns and occurs in 15% of burn patients who are admitted to hospital.

There are three different pathological processes:

1.   Direct thermal injury from hot gases
2.   Inhalation of smoke containing harmful chemicals
3.   Systemic poisoning from carbon monoxide or cyanide.

The upper airway is damaged by either direct thermal injury or smoke inhalation. This leads to oedema and sometimes obstruction of the upper airway which can have a rapid onset.

The lower airway is damaged by smoke; in addition, superheated steam can produce thermal damage to the alveoli and this has a poor prognosis.

Smoke inhalation can cause sloughing of the airway lining, producing obstruction and inflammation followed by pulmonary oedema and hypoxia.

Inhalation injury should be rapidly assessed and treated promptly.

Mortality will be higher in patients with an underlying respiratory illness.

> If there is any evidence of an inhalation injury or a critical burn, the patient should be given the highest concentration of oxygen available

Features suggestive of inhalation injury

- History of being confined with the fire in a closed space
- History of unconsciousness at the time of the incident
- Exposure to smoke or gas during the incident
- Evidence of burns to the face
- Singed nasal hair
- Cough or carbonaceous sputum
- Blistering or redness in the mouth
- Evidence of laryngeal oedema, e.g. hoarseness, stridor
- Wheezing
- Signs of airway obstruction or respiratory distress
- Full-thickness burns to the nasolabial area of the face or posterior pharyngeal swelling.

Critical burns

Critical burns will normally require specialist management in a burns centre.

Critical burns

- Simple erythema over more than 75% of the body surface area
- Partial-thickness burn exceeding 10% surface area in a child, 15% in an adult and 5% in an elderly patient
- Deep burn over more than 10% of the body surface area
- Inhalation injury
- Burns complicated by a fracture or major soft tissue injury
- Burns in patients with associated medical conditions
- Any chemical or electrical burns.

Safety at the scene

Ensure that the environment is safe. It may be necessary to wait for the fire service to put the fire out or to rescue the burned patient. Simply opening a door or window enhances the oxygen supply to the fire, increasing its intensity or possibly causing a flash-over.

Stopping the burn process

Dry and wet heat

- If the patient's clothes are on fire, force them to the floor and wrap them in a blanket to extinguish the flames
- If the clothes are smouldering or have hot liquid on them, they must be removed quickly
- If the clothing is stuck or burnt onto the skin the clothes must be cut around the adhesive area and soaked with clean cold water to minimise the burn process
- Burns that are extensive from either dry or wet heat (e.g. flame or scald) can be soaked with clean cold water but cold water must not be left on the burn for more than 10 minutes unless it is less than 5% of body surface area
- It is vital to ensure that patients with burns do not become hypothermic.

> Cool the burn; warm the patient

Tar burns

The tar should not be removed but immersed in cold water to cool the area and to stop the burning process.

Chemical burns

- All clothing should be removed from the affected area and any dry powdered chemical brushed off
- The burn should be copiously washed with large quantities of water for up to 10 minutes at the scene. The patient may then be transferred to hospital
- The severity of chemical burns depends upon the agent, the time of contact and the concentration
- Some alkaline substances, such as wet cement, are highly corrosive and will continue to burn until completely removed
- Acid burns usually produce less damage but will continue to burn if left on the skin. An exception to this is hydrofluoric acid which penetrates deeply and produces extensive tissue destruction and pain; these burns require treatment with calcium gluconate applied topically.

Carbon monoxide poisoning

Presentation

If large amounts of carbon monoxide are present, oxygen is displaced from haemoglobin and large quantities of carboxyhaemoglobin are produced.

The binding of carbon monoxide to haemoglobin is much stronger than that of oxygen which reduces oxygen transport and worsens tissue hypoxia.

The half-life of carboxyhaemoglobin in room air is 320 minutes; on 100% oxygen it is 80 minutes and on 100% oxygen at 3 atmospheres (hyperbaric oxygen) it is 23 minutes.

The signs and symptoms of mild carbon monoxide poisoning are:

- Lethargy
- Muscle weakness
- Headache
- Nausea
- Vomiting.

The signs and symptoms of severe carbon monoxide poisoning are:

- Cyanosis
- Coma
- Pulmonary oedema
- Dilated pupils.

Management

Any person with carbon monoxide poisoning should be given 100% oxygen and transferred to the accident and emergency department immediately.

Pulse oximetry will not detect the difference between carboxyhaemoglobin and oxyhaemoglobin and may therefore appear falsely reassuring.

After arrival at hospital, the patient is considered for hyperbaric oxygen if:

- The patient is unconscious at any time
- The carboxyhaemoglobin concentration exceeds 20%
- Neurological signs and symptoms are present
- The patient is pregnant.

Patients with carboxyhaemoglobin levels of 50–60% are comatose and require ventilatory support.

Fluid resuscitation

- Intravenous fluids must be started in a patient with a burn greater than 25% of body surface area or if the transfer time is greater than one hour, as vast quantities of plasma will be lost from the burn
- Look for other injuries as a cause of hypovolaemic shock
- Avoid obtaining intravenous access through burnt skin
- Give 1–2 litres of crystalloid in adults or 10 mL/kg in children.

Analgesia

Partial-thickness burns are extremely painful and either Entonox can be self-administered by the patient or the patient can be given intravenous morphine.

No analgesic drug should be given intramuscularly or subcutaneously in severe or moderate burns, as it will remain unabsorbed owing to poor circulation.

Non-steroidal antiinflammatory drugs are contraindicated due to the risk of gastrointestinal problems or ulcer formation.

> It is essential that hospital medical staff are made aware that opiate analgesia has been given

Dressings

The burned area should be wrapped in clingfilm or sterile towels to reduce pain.

If the burn is less than 5% of body surface area, sterile cold water or saline soaks are placed on top of the clingfilm to reduce contact with the air, reduce pain and cool the burn.

If clingfilm is unavailable, clean sterile towels can be placed on the burn prior to rapid transfer to hospital.

Circumferential clingfilm should never be applied to the thorax or limbs. Individual sheets of cling film should be gently laid on the burned area.

> Under no circumstances should any cream (antibiotic or otherwise) be applied to a burn before hospital assessment

Disposal

All burn patients should be transferred to hospital and there a decision can be taken as to whether the patient needs to be transferred to a burns unit, admitted to the hospital from the accident and emergency department or treated as an outpatient. Critical burns should be sent, wherever possible, to a hospital with a burns unit as long as general resuscitative and treatment facilities are available.

For further information, see Ch. 31 in *Emergency Care: A Textbook for Paramedics*.

CHAPTER 32

Wound management

Definitions

Abrasion – Removal of part of the surface of the skin. There is often oozing from the capillaries on the surface of the dermis. Conventionally referred to as a 'graze'

Avulsion – The forced separation of two parts; with wounding, this is when a flap of skin and associated tissue has been partially or completely removed

Amputation – Removal of a portion of a limb or the complete limb

Closed wound – An internal injury caused by a blunt direct force to the surface of the body. The skin itself is intact but there is injury to the underlying tissues

Cut (incised wound) – A breach of the skin caused by a sharp edge

Contused wound – Loss of continuity of the tissue with surrounding bruising

Contusion – An area of bruising due to the effect of a blunt force

Haematoma – An accumulation of blood due to bleeding beneath the skin as a result of a blunt direct force

Healing by primary intention occurs when the edges of the wound are already adjacent or can be brought together (e.g. with sutures or Steri-Strips)

Healing by secondary intention occurs when there is significant tissue loss from the wound and regrowth of skin cover is required. With secondary intention healing wound contraction is more prominent. This can lead to significant deformity or contractures if the defect has been large

Laceration – A tear of the skin caused by a blunt force; it is usually irregular in shape

Puncture wound – A wound with a narrow path made by, for example, a nail

Wound – Any interruption by violence or surgery of the continuity of the external surface of the body or the surface of an internal organ. *Strictly, a wound is a disruption of the continuity of tissue.*

Factors affecting wound healing

- Age
- Nutrition
- Diseases
- Drugs
- Infection
- Foreign body
- Poor blood supply
- Adhesions, movement and drying
- Ionising radiation
- Hypoxia
- Psychological stress.

Immediate management of wounds

The primary survey comes before dealing with any soft tissue injury.

If there is a penetrating wound to the chest the object must be left *in situ* (if it has not already been removed).

If there is an open pneumothorax, an Asherman® or Bolin® chest seal or a dressing sealed on three sides must be placed over the wound, thus preventing a sucking chest wound.

Control of external haemorrhage

There are three different kinds of bleeding:

- Arterial
- Venous
- Capillary.

Direct pressure

Constant direct pressure is applied to the wound with a clean, large gauze pad (dry or moist). If a gauze pad is not immediately available a gloved hand can be used initially.

Several layers of gauze can then be placed on the wound and a bandage placed over these layers of gauze to secure them in position.

Elevate the injured area above the heart to reduce blood flow to the area.

Indirect pressure

If the wound is still bleeding, the dressing should not be removed but may be reinforced with further dressings.

If the wound continues to bleed through the dressings indirect pressure may be applied to pressure points.

Five important pressure points are:

- The femoral artery in the groin, which can be compressed against the pelvis
- The brachial artery approximately 2 cm in from the medial epicondyle of the elbow, which can be compressed against the lower end of the humerus
- The superficial temporal artery, which can be palpated just anterior to the tragus of the ear and can be compressed against the temporal bone to reduce bleeding from scalp lacerations on that side
- The supraorbital and supratrochlear arteries supplying the forehead, which can be compressed against the supraorbital margin to reduce bleeding from lacerations of the forehead
- The facial artery, which can be compressed against the mandible approximately halfway from the angle of the mandible to the tip of the chin to reduce bleeding from the lower half of the face.

Splinting is also effective in reducing movement of the limb, thereby reducing the amount of bleeding.

Topical haemostatic agents

Topical haemostatic agents such as Quikclot® Hemcon® or Celox® can be used for the control of severe exsanguinating external haemorrhage. All are highly effective but may be associated with exothermic reactions and tissue damage. They are therefore very much second line agents if direct pressure is insufficient to gain control of bleeding. These agents have been widely used in military environments but are seldom used by UK ambulance services.

Tourniquets

Tourniquets are used as a last resort where the patient is exsanguinating from a limb and it must be tight enough to prevent both arterial and venous flow.

If the tourniquet is too loose it allows arterial flow and leads to venous engorgement in the limb and further bleeding.

A commercially produced tourniquets is always preferable to an improvised tourniquet.

- The tourniquet must be placed as distal as possible, close to the wound, in order to preserve as much of the limb as possible
- The tourniquet must be tightened until no further bleeding occurs. This will be very painful for the patient

- The time of application of the tourniquet, the name of the person applying it and its position must be recorded. The tourniquet must never be covered
- The tourniquet may be loosened after 15 minutes to see if haemostasis has occurred and retightened or removed as indicated.

Control of external haemorrhage of an open wound with a sharp object protruding

When a sharp object is protruding from a wound it must not be removed. Pads or thick dressings are placed around the protruding object to support it and reduce unwanted movement. The dressings are then secured firmly in place.

Bites

The most significant risk in the management of bites is the development of infection, especially in human bites, the most common of which is a laceration over the knuckle from a punch to the face which has struck the opponent's teeth.

Bites from large animals (including powerful dogs) may be associated with underlying fractures.

Puncture wounds

These wounds are caused by a sharp point and since the wound closes over, they are prone to infection, especially with anaerobic bacteria. These patients need antibiotic cover.

Environment in which the injury occurred

Wounds which are tetanus prone include wounds more than 6 hours old which have not been thoroughly cleaned, those with a large amount of necrotic tissue present and wounds that have been in contact with soil or manure.

Tetanus prophylaxis can be administered in hospital.

The temperature of the environment is also important; frostbite will reduce wound healing.

Time of injury

The longer a wound is left without appropriate cleaning and dressing, the more likely it is to be infected.

In all traumatic wounds, there is an infection rate of approximately 15%.

The chances of wound infection are reduced by clearing debris from the wound, applying a clean sterile dressing or gauze and transferring the patient to an emergency department so that the wound can be cleaned and treated.

Older wounds are more likely to be contaminated and are usually cleaned and allowed to remain open with an appropriate dressing.

Examination

Prehospital examination of the wound includes observation of the size, shape and depth of the wound and of any underlying structures that have been exposed or are protruding from the wound (e.g. bone, tendons, vessels, nerves or subcutaneous tissue).

At the scene, it is important to note movement and sensation distal to the wound so the examining hospital doctor can assess if distal function has deteriorated.

Wounds at specific sites

Scalp wounds

Replace any skin flaps and to provide direct pressure on the site of the wound with a sterile gauze and secured with a bandage. In the absence of other injuries, these patients are best transferred sitting up.

Neck wounds

Neck wounds may be associated with airway compromise due to pressure from external bleeding or bleeding into the airway, pneumothorax (simple or tension), shock or severe damage to underlying structures. Foreign bodies should be left in situ and a simple dressing applied.

If there is an air leak, an occlusive dressing must be applied to prevent air embolism. Direct pressure may be necessary to control bleeding, but simultaneous pressure on both carotids must be avoided.

Wounds of the palm of the hand

A sterile pad should be placed over the wound, with the patient's fingers over the gauze to apply pressure over the injury. The fingers can then be bandaged down. The limb should be elevated.

Eye wounds

Any contusion, laceration or penetrating wound to the eye should be covered by a sterile dressing and the sterile dressing bandaged *in situ*.

Lacerations to the eyelids should be kept moist with damp gauze.

The bandage should ideally cover both eyes as this prevents any consensual movement of the eye which could cause further damage.

Varicose vein injuries in the lower leg

Direct pressure should be applied to the wound with gauze, the patient should be laid down and the leg elevated during transfer.

Management of specific types of wounds

Flap wounds

It is important to make sure that the flaps are replaced and that a sterile gauze dressing, dry or moist, is placed over the top.

Foreign body wounds

If there is a large impaled object then this should not be removed and a dressing should be applied around the area.

A small foreign body, either glass or grit, on the surface which is not embedded, can be removed.

If small particles of glass or grit are embedded these will be more difficult to remove and a sterile dressing, dry or moist, should be placed over the wound and the personnel at the hospital notified on arrival.

Crush injuries

Fingertip crush injuries are common and cause local tissue damage, often with an underlying fracture and marked swelling.

The injured digit should be covered with either a dry dressing or a moist saline soak, elevated and the patient taken to hospital.

With extensive crush injuries to the limbs toxins may be released once the crush has been released. Before the patient is released (or en route to hospital if this is not possible) fluid resuscitation should be commenced.

If life-threatening thoraco-abdominal bleeding is present, give 250 mL aliquots of normal saline to maintain the presence of a radial pulse.

In the absence of thoraco-abdominal bleeding a patient with a severe crush injury should receive IV fluids (2 litres in an adult, 20 mL/kg in a child).

Intravenous opiate analgesia is likely to be required to control pain.

High-pressure injection injuries

Injuries may occur from a high-pressure oil or grease gun and initially very little injury may be evident. However, these injuries must be seen in hospital as there may be severe damage and necrosis to the tissue underlying the skin. These injuries can lead to extensive loss of soft tissue.

Amputation

When either a limb or a digit has been completely severed there can be massive bleeding, but bleeding is usually limited as the vessels go into spasm and retract into the wound.

The area should be covered with a sterile saline soak or sterile gauze, direct pressure applied and the stump elevated.

The amputated part should be wrapped in a polythene bag. The bag can then be placed in a second bag which can then be placed in iced water.

It is important not to place the amputated part directly in contact with either cotton wool, gauze or ice as this will cause tissue damage or contamination.

Abrasions

The abrasion should be covered with a sterile dressing, preferably moist, and the patient transferred to hospital so that the abrasion can be cleaned adequately under local anaesthesia.

Contusions

Where there are severe contusions to a limb, hand or digit, the injured part should be immobilised in a splint, elevated and, where possible, ice or a cold compress used to alleviate the pain and swelling.

For further information, see Ch. 32 in *Emergency Care: A Textbook for Paramedics*.

CHAPTER 33

Overview of trauma resuscitation

On arrival at an accident, identify yourself to the other emergency services

Safety

The first priority at all times is to be safe: are you safe, is the scene safe, is the casualty safe? It is important to remember that the Fire service has overall responsibility for the safety of an accident scene.

Safety – self, scene, casualty

Assessment

The first role of the paramedic, particularly if the Ambulance service is the first emergency responder to arrive, is a brief assessment of the scene:

- Safety
- Hazards
- Casualties – numbers
- Mechanisms of injury
- Emergency services – present and required.

Communication

Report to ambulance control your arrival (if this is not automatic) and the situation as soon as you have made your assessment.

Patient management

The first and most important part of the management of any trauma victim is the primary survey. This must be performed rapidly, carefully and in a standard manner; it is the basis of all good trauma care.

> Primary survey = identification of life threatening problems + treatment

On approaching the patient, an introduction is essential (and good manners), as is an explanation of what is about to happen.

The primary survey

<C> –Catastrophic haemorrhage must be addressed if present

A – Airway with cervical spine control

B – Breathing with ventilation

C – Circulation with control of overt haemorrhage

D – Disability with neurological assessment

E – Exposure and environment

Management of catastrophic haemorrhage

Obvious heavy external bleeding should be immediately controlled with direct pressure and elevation, pressure dressings, pressure point control and if necessary a tourniquet or haemostatic dressing.

Airway with cervical spine control

Maintain in-line cervical stabilisation from the outset.

If the patient is breathing quietly and comfortably, no other action may be necessary other than to apply oxygen at 12–15 L/min via a face mask with reservoir.

If the patient can speak, however incoherently, it means that the airway is clear and the patient is breathing; otherwise the first step is to assess the airway.

If the airway is at risk, either the insertion of an airway (nasopharyngeal or oropharyngeal) or putting the patient in the recovery position should be considered (remembering the possibility of a cervical spine injury).

If the airway appears obstructed or partially obstructed, any obvious removable obstruction should be removed digitally or by suction and simple airway manoeuvres should applied. These are chin lift and jaw thrust.

All trauma victims require high-flow oxygen

The airway takes precedence over the cervical spine and if it is absolutely necessary to compromise the cervical spine (e.g. by performing a head tilt) in order to achieve a patent protected airway, then this must be done.

Airway takes precedence over cervical spine

---

1. Airway clearance – manual and aspiration
2. Manual airway opening manoeuvres:
   - Chin lift
   - Jaw thrust
3. Oropharyngeal airway
4. Nasopharyngeal airway
5. Oral tracheal intubation
6. Cricothyroid ventilation.

Breathing with ventilation

When – and only when – the airway is patent and protected, it is possible to move on to the assessment of breathing. Assessment of breathing begins with the neck, look for:

- Tracheal shift
- Wounds
- Emphysema (surgical)
- Laryngeal crepitus
- Vein distension
- Swelling.

Penetrating neck wounds should be sealed with an occlusive dressing to reduce the risk of air embolism.

Then the chest must be assessed:

- LOOK for movement, instability, flail segments, wounds
- PALPATE for surgical emphysema, tenderness, wounds, paradoxical movement

- PERCUSSION for resonance or dullness
- LISTEN with a stethoscope for breath sounds.

Hyper-resonance with reduced breath sounds suggests a tension pneumothorax; dullness with reduced breath sounds is indicative of a haemothorax.

If the clinical signs suggest a tension pneumothorax, an intercostal needle thoracocentesis should be performed. Penetrating chest wounds should be covered with an Asherman seal or a dressing sealed on three sides.

Remember to examine the back of the chest

Life-threatening chest injuries (ATOMIC):

A – **A**irway obstruction

T – **T**ension pneumothorax

O – **O**pen pneumothorax

M – **M**assive haemothorax

I – Flail chest

C – **C**ardiac tamponade

Box 33.1 Overview of examination findings in chest trauma

- Chest wall contusion
- Pattern bruising
- Surgical emphysema
- Penetrating object
- Tension pneumothorax
- Rib fractures
- Flail chest
- Open chest wound (sucking)
- Open chest wound
- Simple pneumothorax
- Fractures of the clavicle/shoulder/scapula.

Circulation with control of external haemorrhage

The patient must be assessed for signs of shock; at the same time obvious external haemorrhage not controlled under <C> should be controlled by external pressure. In the trauma patient the causes of shock are:

- Hypovolaemic: due to bleeding, by far the most likely cause of shock in trauma
- Cardiogenic: may result from tension pneumothorax or cardiac tamponade, usually secondary to penetrating injury
- Neurogenic: (rare) never assume that shock is neurogenic, since any accident severe enough to cause spinal injury is also likely to be capable of producing haemorrhage from other associated injuries
- Septic shock: unlikely to be a problem in the trauma victim unless rescue is particularly prolonged (e.g. following a natural disaster such as an earthquake).

Table 33.1 Classification of hypovolaemic shock (adult)

	Class I	Class II	Class III	Class IV
Blood loss (mL)	Up to 750	750–1500	1500–2000	>2000
Blood loss (%BV)	Up to 15%	15–30%	30–40%	>40%
Pulse rate	<100	>100	>120	>40
Blood pressure	Normal	Normal	Decreased	Decreased
Pulse pressure (mmHg)	Normal or increased	Decreased	Decreased	Decreased
Respiratory rate	14–20	20–30	30–40	>35
Urine output (mL/h)	>30	20–30	5–15	Negligible
CNS/mental status	Slightly anxious	Mildly anxious	Anxious and confused	Confused and lethargic
Fluid replacement (3:1 rule)	Crystalloid	Crystalloid	Crystalloid and blood	Crystalloid and blood

The **golden hour** is defined as the time from injury to definitive surgical treatment

Hypovolaemic shock

Haemorrhage may be divided into:

- External
- Internal.

Significant external haemorrhage is likely to be obvious but this is not always the case and an appropriate search should be made. The location of internal (concealed) haemorrhage may be:

- Chest
- Abdomen
- Pelvis
- Thigh.

Brief palpation of the abdomen and pelvis will aid the location of bleeding. Significant haemorrhage into the chest should already have been identified during the assessment of breathing. Severe shock may result from bleeding into the thighs from femoral fractures.

All patients with significant trauma should have an intravenous cannula inserted and should receive fluid replacement in order to maintain the presence of a radial pulse.

> Intravenous access must never delay patient transfer

Isolated head injury is not a cause of shock in adults (shock occasionally occurs in babies due to bleeding into the layers of the scalp).

Disability

The patient's conscious state is classified as follows:

A – **A**lert

V – Patient responds to **v**oice

P – Patient responds to **p**ain

U – Patient **u**nresponsive

Check the pupils and make a brief assessment of limb movement and sensation.

Exposure and environment

The degree of exposure of the patient that is appropriate depends on the clinical situation. Exposure of the chest is always necessary for assessment of B and other exposure must be performed as necessary to ensure that no significant injury is missed.

Motorcycle leather trousers should only be removed after very careful consideration, as they may act to tamponade significant lower limb bleeding from pelvic or long-bone fractures.

Don't ever forget to check glucose (DEFG) and record the patient's temperature.

> If the patient deteriorates, repeat the primary survey from the top

The secondary survey

It is seldom appropriate to complete a secondary survey in the prehospital environment. A brief check is however necessary to identify scalp lacerations, limb fractures and other injuries not found in the primary survey.

The secondary survey should follow a logical order, starting at the head and working towards the feet.

Examination of the limbs should include an assessment of neurovascular status.

> *Remember:* chest injury + leg injury = abdominal injury

Having completed the secondary survey, all the findings (positive and negative) must be recorded.

> If it isn't written down, it wasn't done

Preparation for transport

Transfer of the patient will begin before the secondary survey, at a time when only the primary survey has been completed and major injuries have been identified.

Major fractures, dislocations and soft tissue injuries should be identified during **E** of the primary survey and not during the secondary survey.

Whenever preparations for transport are made the principles remain the same.

Airway

The patient's airway must be safe and secure during handling. The patient should continue to receive high-concentration oxygen and should be moved in such a way that the risk of spinal injury is minimised.

Breathing

The patient must be breathing or, if not, supported respiration must be in progress and maintainable during transfer. Cannulae or chest drains must be fastened securely.

Circulation

During transit, it is essential that the patient's condition can be observed and that a central pulse is easily to hand. During short periods of transfer drips should be switched off and the fluid bags placed against the patient; alternatively infusion bags may be carried at shoulder height and handed into the vehicle.

Always tape a loop of the IV giving set to the patients arm to reduce the risk of the cannula being inadvertently pulled out.

Disability

Assessment of AVPU and pupillary reactions should be repeated as soon as the patient is in the back of the ambulance.

Exposure

The patient should be reasonably covered during transfer. It may be appropriate to remove clothes or blankets during transport to facilitate observations. Keep the back of the ambulance warm.

In hospital

Only the paramedic can give details of the accident and, most importantly, of the mechanism of injury. The ambulance service report form should be given (ideally) to a doctor or to the senior nurse involved with the case. A brief verbal handover is essential and hospital staff should have the courtesy to remain silent and listen.

The MIST system can be used as a basis for the handover:

M – **M**echanism

I – **I**njuries

S – **S**ymptoms and signs

T – **T**reatment given

For further information, see Ch. 33 in *Emergency Care: A Textbook for Paramedics*.

CHAPTER 34

The paediatric history

A paediatric history is made up of two elements:
- The account of what has happened
- Background information about the child which might affect the current or future situation.

The AMPLE format

If there is very little time to take a full history then the mnemonic AMPLE should be the basis of a very brief history:

A – Allergies

M – Medicines

P – Past medical history

L – Last food and drink

E – Events leading up to the current problem

Allergies

It is especially important to know about allergies if any drugs may be given. Occasionally, an allergic reaction to medicines or foods is the cause of the illness.

Medicines

The list of regular medication gives much information about known medical problems and the current state of health.

Past medical history

The medical history has a major bearing on the current problem. At this stage, just a list of important past illnesses is required. Even in young children, the past history can be surprisingly complicated.

Last food and drink

The presence of food and drink in the stomach is a major risk factor for regurgitation. This may lead to airway and breathing problems. To be forewarned is to be in a position to take action if necessary.

Events leading up to the current problem

Brief details of the course of an illness or the mechanism of an injury together with the nature of the present complaints are extremely helpful.

The story from the scene

At a child's home, the normal living environment reveals much about the child's daily life. The family's social circumstances and habits may give useful clues as to the current problems. The apparent health and wellbeing of the other children in the household are also important.

The carer's tale

Children are unique in often having someone in close proximity who is looking after them. This person, who is usually a parent but may be a relative, friend or teacher, can usually give a good account of what has happened.

What the bystander saw

People at the scene of an incident often give valuable information. Such people may include passers-by, neighbours or professionals such as police officers and fire-fighters. After the incident, all these people disperse and this part of the history may be lost for ever.

The child's own account

Children often respond very well to appropriate questions. Their account of events can be extremely accurate. It should not be assumed that an adult's story of events is any more credible than an older child's.

The full medical history

The full history can be structured as follows:

- Presenting complaint and history of presenting complaint – why have they called an ambulance?
- Past medical history – past illnesses and operations
- Social history – the environment and the people that the child lives with
- Family history – medical problems of other family members
- Medications – the child's current and past medication and known allergies
- Review of systems – a checklist of the different body systems involving inquiry into possible problems with each.

> Never delay urgent treatment to collect unnecessary data

Relevant immediate questions

The depth of enquiry should vary with the immediacy of the situation and the questioning should be directed to the most appropriate person, be that the carer or the patient.

Breathing problems, fits, pain, injury and general symptoms of infection are responsible for the majority of paediatric emergencies. A systemic consideration of some useful urgent questions is helpful. These questions make up the **E** (events) and some of the **P** (past medical history) of AMPLE. The following lists are not exhaustive, but can be used as a guideline for questioning:

A – Airway

B – Breathing

C – Circulation

D – Disability

E – Environment

F – Fits

G – Glucose

I – Immediate needs.

Airway

Diagnosis of the problem

- When did the problem start?
- Is there reason to suspect an inhaled foreign body?

Severity of the problem

- Has the child been distressed?
- Has the child been drooling?
- Can the child eat and drink?

Breathing

Diagnosis of the problem

- When did it start?
- Has it ever happened before?

Severity of the problem

- Has the child been responding normally?
- Has the child been distressed?
- Has the child ever needed steroids?
- Has the child ever been admitted to hospital with breathing problems before?
- If admitted, has the child ever been on an intensive care unit?

Circulation

Diagnosis of the problem

- When did it start?
- Has the child any heart problems?
- Does the child have a rash? Meningococcal septicaemia causes purpura (bruises)
- Has the child had any diarrhoea or vomiting?

Severity of the problem

- Has the child been responding normally?

Disability

- When did it start?
- Has the child been responding normally?
- Does the child have a rash?
- Has the mother (or other carer) noticed any agitation or an odd cry or affect?

Environment

- In what position is the child most comfortable?
- Is the child too hot or too cold?

Fits

Diagnosis of the problem

- Has the child ever had fits before?
- Has the child been generally unwell in any way before the fit?
- Has the child had a raised temperature?
- Have the child's eyes rolled up at the time of the attack? (Mothers often notice this)
- Was the child playing when he or she went limp and collapsed? Febrile convulsions often occur with minimal tonic/clonic activity.

Severity of the problem

How long did the fit last?

Glucose

Diagnosis of the problem

- Does the child have diabetes?
- Has the child had his or her normal insulin dose?
- Has the child been eating and drinking normally?

Young children have limited stores of glucose. Always check blood sugar in seriously ill children and correct if evidence exists of hypoglycaemia, regardless of whether or not the child is diabetic.

> Hypoglycaemia in any child is a life-threatening emergency

Severity of the problem

Has the child been behaving and responding normally?

Immediate needs

- Where does it hurt?
- How bad is it?

Further background questions

In the situation of immediate care, extensive consideration of the child's background is often irrelevant and may be counterproductive.

Maternal health and pregnancy

The health of the mother may affect the development of the fetus and health of the newborn.

Birth problems

A difficult birth (caesarean section or forceps delivery) may later manifest itself as developmental problems or fits. Did the baby spend time on the special care baby unit (SCBU)?

Development

The continuing rapid development of a child distinguishes it from the adult. Questions should be asked about relationships, behaviour, play, school, sports and activities.

Immunizations

Children in the UK benefit from a planned programme of immunisations. The immunisations received by the child should be ascertained.

Siblings

The health of brothers and sisters may give useful information concerning a child's illness.

Exploration of the current problem

It is important to listen to the story told by the child or the carer. Direct questions will involve expanding on the AMPLE format and the systematic A–I approach above. The particular complaints that are common in children may also involve:

- Raised temperature or shivering
- Lethargy or drowsiness
- Headache and neck stiffness
- Aches and pains
- Cough, cold, sore throat and earache
- Feeding problems
- Diarrhoea and vomiting
- Reduced or increased urine output (are there normal wet nappies in a small child?)
- Difficulty sleeping.

Sometimes the worries of the parents and other carers predominate over the symptoms of the child and these problems must also be explored.

Early suspicions of child abuse

Several different types of child abuse are now recognised.

- Physical abuse (non-accidental injury)
- Emotional abuse

- Neglect
- Sexual abuse
- Organised or ritual abuse.

There are patterns of physical signs for some types of abuse, but the history and the context in which the events occurred are the most important first indicators to alert the health worker. The following features of a history of injury might point to abuse:

- Inappropriate delay in seeking help and advice after a significant injury
- Previous history of frequent accidents
- The history of the accident is not a likely mechanism for that injury
- Vague or absent history of an accident
- Different carers give different explanations for the same injury
- The child gives a different history
- The injury is supposed to have been sustained in a way that is inconsistent with the child's development, e.g. a fall before the child has started walking
- The adults with the child are either unconcerned or hostile during questioning.

Suspicions of child abuse, in whatever form, should not be voiced in the prehospital environment. Such concerns should be brought to the attention of a senior doctor after arrival in hospital. It is also the individual responsibility of paramedics to ensure any concerns are reported to the relevant social services department. All ambulance trusts should have a child welfare policy in place that details the correct procedure.

How to hand over the history to the hospital

Good communication is vital at the point where the care of the patient is transferred from the prehospital workers to the hospital. It should include both handing over the written records of the history and some direct discussion. What happened after the ambulance arrived and during the journey to the hospital is now part of the history.

For further information, see Ch. 34 in *Emergency Care: A Textbook for Paramedics.*

CHAPTER 35

Assessment of the paediatric patient

The aim of the prehospital assessment is management of the child's condition rather than specific diagnosis.

The age of a child is usually known but the weight must sometimes be approximated by the formula:

Weight (kg) = (Age in years + 4) × 2

This works well between the ages of 1 year and 10 years.

The average birthweight of a full-term infant is 3.5 kg; this has usually doubled by 5 months of age and tripled by 12 months.

Table 35.1 Estimating a child's weight

Age	Weight (kg)
2 months	5
6 months	7.5
1 year	10
3.5 years	15
6 years	20
10 years	30
13 years	40
14 years	50

The SAFE approach should be used. Children are usually easy to move to a safer place.

Airway

Check for responsiveness. Failure to respond indicates a significantly lowered level of consciousness and therefore an airway at risk. There may be a need for airway opening manoeuvres and action to protect the airway.

Partial upper airway obstruction is suggested by snoring, rattling or gurgling.

Stridor is heard best in inspiration – this differentiates it from wheezing, which is usually loudest in expiration. Stridor suggests obstruction at the level of the larynx and upper trachea and can be caused by a foreign body or by infection (usually associated with fever).

> Do not examine the throat with any instrument in children with stridor or suspected partial airway obstruction – doing so may convert the problem to complete obstruction

Drooling, the inability to swallow saliva, suggests blockage at the back of the throat.

> Cyanosis and reduced haemoglobin saturation readings on a pulse oximeter are very late signs of airway obstruction

All children will benefit from high-concentration oxygen therapy. Only a small group of infants with congenital heart disease need controlled oxygen therapy.

> It is not worth struggling to make an unwilling child wear an oxygen mask

If a child's airway can be maintained by simple manoeuvres, an oropharyngeal (Guedel) airway is best avoided. This is because retching is easily induced in children and may be followed by laryngospasm or aspiration.

Box 35.1 **Airway and endotracheal tube sizes**

- Oropharyngeal airway size = the distance from the centre of the lips to the angle of the jaw
- Nasopharyngeal airway size = the distance from the tip of the nose to the tragus of the ear
  Endotracheal tube size:
  - Internal diameter (mm) = $\dfrac{\text{age in years}}{4} + 4$ (neonate 3–3.5 mm tube)
  - Oral tube length (cm) = $\dfrac{\text{age in years}}{2} + 12$

Assess the need for cervical spine protection before any airway intervention

---

Breathing

Look, listen and feel for breathing. The absence of breath sounds indicates the need to follow procedures for cardiorespiratory arrest.

Look for:

- Difficulty in talking – a child who is unable to speak because of laboured breathing is very unwell
- An abnormal respiratory rate – usually fast, laboured breathing. Very slow respiratory rates may occur just before respiratory arrest or in children poisoned with narcotic drugs
- Recession of the chest wall – the indrawing of the elastic tissues of a child caused by increased respiratory effort
- Wheezing and rattling, grunting and panting
- Nasal flaring and use of the shoulder and neck muscles during breathing
- Unequal or diminished breath sounds.

Table 35.2 Respiratory and pulse rates in children

Age (years)	Respiratory rate (breaths/min)	Pulse rate (bpm)
Under 1	30–40	110–160
1–5	25–30	95–140
6–12	20–25	80–120

> Absence of breath sounds means that the movement of air in the lungs is so diminished that it cannot be heard

All the above suggest that the child is struggling to achieve normal respiration. Failure to adequately oxygenate the blood and hence the tissues, is shown by:

- Tachycardia – the hypoxic nervous system is stimulating the heart
- Cyanosis – a late sign
- Irritability, confusion or reduced responsiveness mean that the brain is short of oxygen – this is an extremely worrying sign.

> The oxygen saturation shown by the pulse oximeter should be close to 100% in a normal, healthy child

All wheezy children will benefit from nebulised bronchodilators, whether they are known to be asthmatic or not. Agitation, tachycardia and tremor may be signs of salbutamol overdosage. Ventilation is indicated as an emergency procedure for respiratory insufficiency in a child in the same way as in an adult, suggested ventilator settings for children are:

- Tidal volume 10 mL/kg
- Minute volume 100 mL/kg.

Circulation

Check for a central pulse (over 10 seconds). The brachial or femoral pulses should be used in infants rather than the carotid pulse. The absence of a central pulse (or a rate of less than 60 bpm in infants) indicates the need to follow procedures for cardiorespiratory arrest.

> In a child with ventricular fibrillation and no obvious precipitating factors, the cause could be poisoning with tricyclic antidepressants

A fast or slow heart rate

The worst cause of bradycardia is severe hypoxia (or hypovolaemia) and, in this case, cardiac arrest is imminent. Occasionally, bradycardia is seen with poisoning and severe head injury.

Abnormal systolic blood pressure

This varies with age.

Estimation of normal blood pressure:

Systolic blood pressure (mmHg) $= 80 +$ (age in years $\times 2$)

Blood pressure can be difficult to measure in young, restless children and requires a cuff of the correct size. It will not fall until very late in shock.

A raised capillary refill time
It should be less than 2 seconds if the circulation is satisfactory. May be prolonged in a cold patient.

Pallor and coolness of the skin
The body diverts blood away from the skin when there are circulatory problems.

Active bleeding

> A child's blood volume is approximately 80 mL/kg

Inadequate circulation will reduce tissue oxygenation and thus may also cause a raised respiratory rate or altered level of consciousness. The ECG is rarely as helpful in making a diagnosis in children as it is in adults, except for arrhythmias. A cardiac monitor does, however, provide constant information about the heart rate.

The need for venous access and the site should be assessed carefully. Use IO access if necessary.

Give the minimum IV fluids required to achieve improvement, start with small boluses of fluid up to a maximum of 3×20 mL/kg in all patients.

Bolus fluid therapy

Excessive fluid therapy runs the risk of causing heart failure and may be counter-productive.

Dehydration is shown by a dry, non-elastic skin or sunken eyes. In infants, a floppy anterior fontanelle is a useful, if late, sign of severe fluid loss. Diarrhoea and vomiting can quickly dehydrate a small child. Wet nappies confirm urine output in young children.

Disability

The AVPU scoring system is as useful for children as for adults:

A – **A**lert

V – **V**oice elicits a response

P – **P**ain elicits a response

U – **U**nresponsive.

> Consider hypoglycaemia as a cause for a reduced level of consciousness

Signs of an intracerebral problem

- Reduced level of consciousness – even sleepy children should be rousable
- Abnormal pupils – dilated, fixed or uneven pupils
- Abnormal posture and limbs movement – never assume an abnormality is congenital

- Airway obstruction
- Respiratory depression
- Bradycardia and hypertension.

Table 35.3 The Glasgow Coma Scale in children	
Response elicited	**Score**
Best eye opening response	
Open spontaneously	4
React to speech	3
React to pain	2
No response	1
Best motor response	
Moves normally and spontaneously or obeys commands	6
Localises pain	5
Withdraws in response to pain	4
Flexes abnormally to pain (decorticate movements)	3
Extends abnormally to pain (decerebrate movements)	2
No response	1
Best 'verbal' response	
Smiles, follows sounds and objects, interacts	5
Cries consolably or interacts inappropriately	4
Cries with inconsistent relief or moans	3
Cries inconsolably or is irritable	2
No response	1

Exposure and environment

Look for:

- Cold extremities
- Shivering
- Wet clothing
- Pyrexia and clamminess
- The position in which the child is most comfortable
- The proximity of the mother or other carer.

Because of their large surface area relative to their small body volume children will lose heat much faster than adults. Attention to these details early on can radically change the wellbeing (and demeanour) of a child. A child may well need clothing removed to facilitate assessment. However, children easily become cold and embarrassed.

Fits

Look for:

1. Frank tonic or clonic activity
2. Spasmodic twitching
3. Postictal drowsiness
4. Gurgling, rattling or other signs of airway obstruction
5. Cyanosis – during a fit there is a very high demand for oxygen, coupled with respiratory inadequacy
6. Signs of head injury
7. Signs of other injury caused by a convulsion (e.g. a bitten tongue and intraoral bleeding)
8. Reasons to consider hypoglycaemia.

It is very difficult to assess or manage a fitting child. Hence termination of the convulsion must be an immediate aim.

Glucose

Children use their glucose reserves very quickly. Glucagon will therefore be less consistently effective than in adults.

Look for:

- Restlessness, agitation or other mental change ('jitteriness' in a neonate)
- A reduced level of consciousness
- Signs of insulin usage (all diabetic children will be on insulin; oral hypoglycaemic drugs are generally only used in adults. This does not mean, of course, that a child cannot take someone else's drugs and become hypoglycaemic)
- A low blood glucose level on testing with a reagent strip
- Convulsions – can be caused by hypoglycaemia.

Glucose: 5 mL/kg of 10% dextrose solution

Immediate needs of the child

The relief of suffering is of paramount importance. Assess:

1. The need for analgesia
2. The need for limb splintage
3. The tolerance of cervical and spinal splintage.

The needs of the parents

Parent and carers will need reassurance and sometimes need medical treatment themselves. Parental anxiety should not be dismissed as it may be the only sign of serious illness in a child.

Poisoning

Bizarre symptoms and signs and unexplained combinations of findings suggest poisoning. Younger children may ingest substances accidentally; older children may experiment with drugs. Look for the most common signs:

- Confusion, agitation and drowsiness
- Tachycardia
- Dilated pupils
- Evidence at the scene (which is of enormous help to hospital staff).

Other important findings

- Raised temperature – a hand on the abdomen may reveal an obvious pyrexia. This often accompanies a fit. Febrile convulsions are common between 5 months and 5 years of age. Children with epilepsy are more likely to have a fit during a pyrexia
- Neck stiffness indicates inflammation of the meninges, i.e. meningitis. This is often accompanied by pyrexia, headache and drowsiness; however, the diagnosis can be difficult
- Rashes usually indicate systemic infection, allergy or specific skin disease. Purpura is the most worrying skin sign (suggesting possible meningococcal septicaemia or other cause of vasculitis)
- Drawing up of the knees suggests pain in the abdomen
- Signs of congenital abnormality – children with congenital problems are often prone to fits and chest infections
- The relationship and interaction with the parents and the other family members is always important.

Signs of child abuse

Signs suggestive of non-accidental injury

- Unexplained head, facial, chest or limb injuries – especially in children who are not able to walk and thus fall (few children walk before the age of 11 months)
- Multiple bruising
- Injuries of different ages
- Unusual burns (e.g. those of a 'glove' or 'stocking' distribution)
- Unusual cuts and bruises – imprints of hands, sticks, cords, shoes, belts and teeth may be present.

For further information, see Ch. 35 in *Emergency Care: A Textbook for Paramedics.*

The sick child

Children tend to be treated with a greater sense of urgency than adults. This reflects both the instinct that most adults have to protect the young and the correctly held view that children can 'go off' quickly. While urgency is important, at no stage must a sense of panic prevail. The most important skill that comes with experience is recognising that a child is ill. Rapid and safe transport to hospital can be life-saving.

Recognition of serious illness

Health workers with a great deal of paediatric experience will intuitively recognise a very sick child. A systematic approach can be used following the familiar <C>ABC pattern, which is difficult to forget, even under pressure.

Assessment of the airway

- The airway may be patent or obstructed, protected or unprotected. Obstruction may be partial or complete and protection may be secure or insecure
- Any child who has anything other than an open and securely protected airway is seriously ill
- If the child is conscious, then a simple question such as 'How are you?' or 'What's wrong?' should start the assessment and if you get a reply, then you have confirmed that the airway is patent, that they are breathing and that they have at least enough circulation to perfuse their brain
- In an unconscious child, an appropriate airway-opening manoeuvre should be performed and then breathing assessed.

The airway is at risk in any child who is not fully conscious

Assessment of breathing

The respiratory rate should be counted by exposing the chest. Exposure will also reveal recession. Recession is the appearance of indrawing of the chest wall that occurs while it is expanding during inspiration. It can be seen in a number of areas: intercostal (between the ribs), subcostal (below the ribs) and sternal.

Table 36.1 Normal respiratory rates in children

Age (years)	Respiratory rate (breaths/min)
<1	30–40
1–5	25–30
6–12	20–25

Wheezes (during both inspiration and expiration) indicate that respiratory work is raised because of the increased pressure associated with narrowing of the airways. Severe upper airway obstruction (such as that caused by a foreign body) can result in stridor. It is important to note that the loudness does not correspond to the severity of the problem. Silence in a previously noisy chest may indicate either exhaustion or total obstruction.

Hypoxia (reduction in oxygenation – <90% on air or <95% on oxygen) initially causes the heart rate to rise as the body attempts to deliver more blood to the tissues to make up for the lower concentration of oxygen. Eventually, however, the heart rate falls to below normal levels: this is a very serious sign and usually indicates imminent death. Hypoxia will also affect conscious level. First of all, the child becomes agitated but as the low oxygen delivery continues, drowsiness and then unconsciousness will ensue.

Bradycardia in a sick child or infant is a critical sign

Assessment of circulation

Palpate a large artery (carotid or femoral in a child or brachial in an infant) for 5 seconds to see whether any pulse is present

Decreased capillary refill time and increasing peripheral pallor and coolness are early signs of a failing circulation in children. The capillary refill is measured by applying gentle pressure (enough to squeeze out the blood) over the forehead or sternum for 5 seconds, then releasing the pressure and counting the time in seconds that it takes for the blood to return. The normal time is less than 2 seconds.

Pulse rate and blood pressure vary with age. In addition, the equipment needed (blood pressure cuffs) will be different depending on the size of the patient. This makes analysis of the blood pressure difficult.

Table 36.2 Normal pulse rate and systolic blood pressure in children

Age (years)	Pulse rate (bpm)	Systolic blood pressure (mmHg)
Newborn	160	60–80
<1	110–160	70–90
1–5	95–140	80–100
6–12	80–120	90–110
13+	60–100	100–120

Assessment of disability

Disability assessment involves a rapid evaluation of conscious level. Children with a reduced conscious level for whatever reason should be classed as seriously ill and treated accordingly. AVPU should be used initially, and whenever possible calling the child's name is recommended. The painful stimulus should only be applied if there is no response to voice. An examination of the pupils for size and reactivity should be carried out at this stage.

Appropriate treatment

Performing procedures on children can be practically difficult and emotionally draining for the professional involved. Since the circumstances of most prehospital care are not ideal, resuscitative procedures should be limited to those necessary for safe transportation.

Airway

Opening and maintenance of the airway are both essential. Simple opening manoeuvres should be performed first – head tilt, chin lift and jaw thrust can be used in children. The head should be kept in the neutral position in infants (>1 year old), since overextension may cause deformation of the soft trachea with consequent airway obstruction.

Oropharyngeal airways can be used as simple adjuncts to airway opening. The appropriate size can be found by selecting the size that reaches from the angle of the jaw to the level of the incisor teeth.

The selected airway should be inserted the 'right way up' by depressing the tongue (using a tongue depressor or a laryngoscope blade) and slipping the airway into the mouth until the flange lies at the lips. Attempts to insert an airway using the adult twisting technique may cause considerable damage to the soft palate and may compromise the airway as bleeding occurs. Nasopharyngeal airways are not routinely used in children.

Do not interfere with a child who has severe stridor who is managing to maintain their own critically threatened airway. These children often wish to sit up during transport and should be allowed to do so. Forcing a child with stridor to lie flat may precipitate a respiratory arrest. Transport the child calmly to an advanced facility (preferably warning that facility of one's imminent arrival so that appropriate preparations can be made).

Breathing

All children with inadequate breathing should be given oxygen in the highest possible concentration. Paediatric oxygen masks with rebreathing bags can achieve an inspired concentration of 85% with high gas flow rates. If respiratory support is required it can be given either by using a bag-valve-mask system or by intubating the child and using a self-inflating bag or ventilator.

An appropriately sized mask can be quickly selected by considering the size of the child's face; the mask should cover both the mouth and nose. Three sizes of self-inflating bag are available – infant, child and adult. If there is any doubt, the larger bag should be used.

Attempts at intubation are only indicated in apnoeic children and then only once other avenues have been exhausted. Intubation may be unsuccessful and critical time should not be lost to failed attempts. However, if the decision to intubate has been made then the correct equipment must be selected and the correct technique used which will depend on the age of the child.

Internal diameter (mm) = (age in years/4) + 4

Intubation technique in children

Infants and very young children have a long, floppy epiglottis and this cannot be elevated sufficiently to allow the cords to be seen if the standard intubation technique is used. Consequently, it is necessary to directly lift the epiglottis with the laryngoscope. This is achieved by passing the laryngoscope almost to the oesophagus and slowly withdrawing it in the midline. As the laryngoscope is withdrawn, the epiglottis will remain elevated and the cords will come into view. A tube can then be passed through the cords and ventilation commenced. Adult blades can be used but straight paediatric blades will make this easier.

Once intubated, ventilation should be started and the position of the tube checked by listening with a stethoscope and observing chest movements. Adequacy of ventilation is judged by looking for rise and fall of the chest.

Circulation

If circulation is present, then circulatory resuscitation is rarely necessary in the prehospital phase of care. Gaining intravenous access can be extremely difficult in children and time should not be wasted unless access is essential.

If immediate vascular access is required (usually because of progression or imminent progression to cardiorespiratory arrest) then a vein should be identified and the area prepared as usual; if standard techniques do not work within *90 seconds* then the procedure should be abandoned and an intraosseous line should be inserted. This is usually achieved in the medial surface of the upper tibia using a specially designed intraosseous needle. Both drugs and fluid can be introduced through this route.

For further information, see Ch. 36 in *Emergency Care: A Textbook for Paramedics*.

CHAPTER 37

Paediatric cardiac arrest

Introduction

Cardiorespiratory arrest in children is a much rarer event than in adults. Unfortunately, the outcome for children is much worse. In children the underlying event is usually hypoxia followed by a respiratory arrest and it is easier to prevent paediatric respiratory arrest than to treat it. For the youngest children (i.e. infants) the most common clinical cause is sudden infant death syndrome. For older children, the underlying cause is hypoxia which is secondary to severe sepsis, drowning, poisoning, aspiration and trauma.

Basic life support

Infants (aged under 1 year)

- For infants, basic life support (BLS) starts with checking for responsiveness by shaking while shouting for help
- The next step is to open the airway by tilting the head and lifting the chin
- When this is achieved, the presence of breathing is assessed by looking, listening and feeling for any signs of respiration
- If breathing is found to be absent deliver five rescue breaths. When this has been performed, the next step is to check for a brachial pulse.

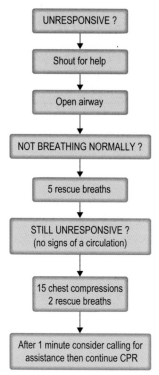

Figure 37.1 Paediatric basic life support (Resuscitation Council UK). The authors are aware of impending changes in resuscitation guidelines (late 2010). Refer to: www.resus.org.uk for further up-to-date information.

In infants check the brachial pulse

- If the pulse is absent or the infant is found to be significantly bradycardic (i.e. the pulse rate is less than 60/min) then chest compressions should begin
- To achieve this, two fingers are placed on the lower sternum, a finger's breadth beneath the nipple line. The chest is compressed by approximately one-third of its depth and five rapid compressions are administered
- Alternatively, use the encircling technique. Place both thumbs, side by side, on the lower third of the sternum with the tips pointing towards the infant's head,

encircle the lower part of the rib cage with the fingers and depress the rib cage with the thumbs by *at least* one-third of the depth of the chest.

- If the pulse is below 60/min, commence basic life support
- Ratio of: 15 chest compressions : 2 rescue breaths
- Rate 100–120 compressions per minute.

The paramedic crew attending such a call should continue basic life support measures while more advanced life support techniques are considered.

Children (aged over 1 year)
- For children over 1 year old, the same algorithm is followed with some slight differences
- Cardiac output can be established by feeling the carotid pulse
- Chest compressions can be given with the heel of one hand or with a two-handed technique, whichever is the most effective for the size of the patient
- In both instances the heel of one hand is placed on the lower sternum, one finger's breadth above the xiphisternum, and the chest compressed by one-third of its depth.

Advanced life support

Basic life support should not be interrupted while advanced life support equipment is prepared. The patient should be placed on cardiac monitoring and the underlying rhythm determined. Intubation may be required. Intravenous or intraosseous access should be obtained in order to give drugs.

The size of the endotracheal tube used for intubation and the dosage of the drugs used in arrest depend on the age and size of the child. Two important formulae will assist the paramedic to choose correctly. To estimate the weight of the child, 4 is added to the child's age in years and the result doubled. For instance, a 4-year-old child will weigh approximately 16 kg.

Weight (kg) = (age in years + 4) × 2

To estimate the endotracheal tube size (internal diameter in mm), the age is divided by 4 and 4 added:

Endotracheal tube size = (age in years/4) + 4

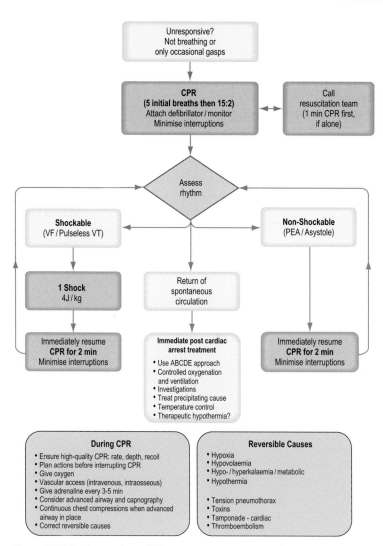

Figure 37.2 Paediatric advanced life support (Resuscitation Council UK).

For example, a 6-year-old child would require an endotracheal tube of 5.5 mm.

Arrest algorithms

When the child is placed on a cardiac monitor, the first decision, as in adult practice, is to determine which arrest rhythm the child is suffering from.

Asystole

- Asystole is by far the most common rhythm found in paediatric cardiac arrest
- The treatment is intubation and ventilation with supplemental oxygen to try to give an inspired oxygen content of 100%. Circulatory access should then be gained as rapidly as possible

Table 37.1 Adrenaline doses for children

Age	Dose (µg)	Volume (mL)
11 years	350	3.5
10 years	320	3.2
9 years	290	2.9
8 years	260	2.6
7 years	230	2.3
6 years	210	2.1
5 years	190	1.9
4 years	160	1.6
3 years	140	1.4
2 years	120	1.2
18 months	110	1.1
12 months	100	1.0
9 months	90	0.90
6 months	80	0.80
3 months	60	0.60
1 month	44	0.44
Birth	n/a	n/a

n/a, not applicable.

- Once access is achieved, adrenaline in a dose of 10 µg/kg is administered. Pre-filled syringes of 1 mg adrenaline in 10 mL should be used (1:10 000)
- Consider giving the child a fluid bolus, normally 20 mL/kg of normal saline, particularly if the history suggests hypovolaemia.

Pulseless electrical activity

PEA can be found in paediatric practice. The treatment is as per the algorithm:

- Intubation
- Ventilation with 100% oxygen
- Intravenous or intraosseous access
- Adrenaline 10 µg/kg every 3–5 minutes
- IV fluid bolus 20 mL/kg
- CPR in 2-minute cycles
- Consideration of underlying cause of EMD
  - PEA is usually secondary to some known cause, such as profound hypovolaemia, tension pneumothorax, cardiac tamponade, drug overdose or hypothermia
  - Since hypovolaemia is common, it is reasonable to administer a challenge of 20 mL/kg of fluid such as normal saline for this particular arrest rhythm unless it is specifically contraindicated.

Ventricular fibrillation

- VF in paediatric cardiac arrest occurring out of hospital is rare
- VF may occur typically with some poisons, such as with tricyclic antidepressant drugs, and also with drowning in cold water and hypothermia
- A shock should be delivered immediately at 4 J/kg. As for adults, the 2 minute cycle of CPR should be completed before reassessing for output
- 2 minute cycles should be continued with one shock per cycle as necessary
- The patient should be intubated and ventilated
- Access should be gained and adrenaline administered every 3–5 minutes (Table 37.1)
- If unsuccessful after three cycles, consider the use of amiodarone, in a dose of 5 mg/kg.

Automatic external defibrillators

- The energy delivery from most automatic defibrillators (AEDs) is fixed at that which is appropriate for adults
- Purpose made paediatric pads, or devices/programs which attenuate the energy output of an AED are recommended for children between 1 and 8 years
- An adult AED can still be used in all patients over the age of 1 year if there is no other option.

Continuation of care

If an output is achieved then begin post-resuscitation care, otherwise transport to hospital must be carried out without any break in CPR. It is vital to warn the receiving hospital so that they can assemble a paediatric resuscitation team for your arrival.

For further information, see Ch. 37 in *Emergency Care: A Textbook for Paramedics.*

CHAPTER **38**

The injured child

Differences between children and adults

Children differ from adults in the following ways:

- **Size** – smaller size means that a child sustains more injuries than an adult would sustain from the same force
- **Shape** – the child's relatively large head means that more forces may be applied through the neck during deceleration. A falling child tends to land head first
- **Skeleton** – the skeleton in children is very elastic, the child may sustain internal organ damage without overlying fracture; lung contusion may occur without overlying rib fracture because the ribs are more pliable
- **Surface area** – the larger surface area relative to body size in children means more rapid heat loss can occur.

Psychological problems

A careful and gentle approach is needed to the assessment and treatment of a frightened child who is in pain. Children almost invariably find the presence of a parent calming and although they may not understand what is said, continuous quiet speech is also reassuring. Under stressful circumstances, the child may regress to a younger age and may not behave as might be expected for the chronological age.

Equipment

Appropriately sized and designed equipment must be available in order to allow appropriate treatment.

Specific differences

Airway

- Relatively large tongue and easily damaged soft palate. This is why oropharyngeal airways are inserted the right way up instead of rotating them during insertion
- Relatively large epiglottis which should be picked up directly by the laryngoscope blade to allow better visualisation of the vocal cords
- Relatively short trachea. When inserted, the black vocal cord marker near the tip of the endotracheal tube should be placed at the level of the cords. After placement it is essential that intubation of the right main bronchus has been excluded
- The narrowest part of the upper airway is below the level of the cords at the level of the cricoid, cuffed ET tubes should be avoided to avoid necrosis of the wall of the trachea
- The larynx is more difficult to visualise
- Surgical cricothyroidotomy should not be performed in children; only needle cricothyroidotomy is appropriate.

Breathing

- Children have low oxygen reserves and their metabolism uses oxygen very quickly, so if ventilation is impaired, cyanosis rapidly ensues
- Children breathe rapidly, if ventilatory support is needed, then the rate of ventilation should be around 20 breaths/minute for a child and 40 breaths per minute for an infant. The volume of the ventilation is best judged by watching the child's chest move
- Children do not tolerate tension pneumothorax well. This is because the mediastinum is very mobile and it can be pushed across to compress the other lung by the increased pressure within the injured hemithorax. Repeated assessment of air entry in the ventilated child and early needle cricothyrotomy are therefore of paramount importance.

Circulation

- The heart rate in children is faster than in adults
- In children under 1 year old, the minimum acceptable normal systolic pressure is 70 mmHg
- In children older than 1 year, the expected systolic pressure can be worked out by the formula:

  Systolic pressure (mmHg) = 80 + (age in years × 2)

- The circulating blood volume of a child is approximately 80 mL/kg, which means that the total blood volume of a neonate is likely to be around 240 mL

- A child's first response to a decrease in blood volume is a tachycardia. The next response is usually cool skin at the peripheries, with a drop in blood pressure as a late sign. The absence of low blood pressure does not exclude the diagnosis of shock
- In the majority of cases, immediate evacuation to hospital for fluid therapy and possible surgical intervention is the most appropriate course of action. In cases of prolonged transfer or entrapment, however, prehospital fluid administration may be required
- Try the antecubital fossa or in a child under 1 year old, the dorsum of the hand or foot and have a low threshold for switching to intraosseous access.

Table 38.1 Mean heart rate in children

Age	Mean heart rate (bpm)
Newborn–3 months	140
3 months–2 years	130
2 years–10 years	80
More than 10 years	75

Disability (neurological status)

- Children frequently sustain head injuries because of the relatively large size of their head. Vomiting once or twice after head injury is common and does not necessarily imply increased intracranial pressure, however persistent vomiting will require admission for observation and possible investigation
- As with adult head injuries periods of hypoxia or hypovolaemia must be avoided
- Infants can lose a large proportion of their circulating volume from scalp lacerations or into haematomas within the scalp. Head injuries do not otherwise cause hypotension
- The key to optimum management is the prevention of secondary brain injury by paying attention to the airway, breathing and circulation. This, combined with rapid evacuation to definitive care, is far more important than attempts at neurological assessment
- The AVPU assessment can be used in children but the Glasgow Coma Scale has to be modified for children younger than 4 years of age.

Table 38.2 Glasgow Coma Scale verbal response for children under 4 years old

Verbal response	Score
Smiles, follows sound and objects, interacts	5
Cries consolably or interacts inappropriately	4
Cries with inconsistent relief or moans	3
Cries inconsolably or is irritable	2
No response	1

Non-accidental injury

Healthcare professionals have a responsibility for the protection of children. It is important that a child who is being deliberately abused is identified and protected from further injury. All healthcare professionals need to be aware of the features of non-accidental injury. Suspicion should be aroused by:

- A history that does not fit the apparent injuries
- A delay in seeking help
- An inappropriate response from the child or carers
- Inconsistent history of the injury.

Injuries that are especially associated with a non-accidental cause include:

- Injuries around the mouth
- Injuries around the genital area
- Long-bone fractures in children under 3 years old
- Bizarre injuries such as cigarette burns or rope burns.

It is important that prehospital personnel pass on any suspicions to the healthcare professionals to whom the case is handed on at the hospital.

For further information, see Ch. 38 in *Emergency Care: A Textbook for Paramedics.*

CHAPTER 39

Care of the elderly

The proportion of the population that is over the age of 70 is rising.

Old age may bring a combination of factors rendering the old person especially vulnerable to an acute breakdown in their capacity to cope:

- Social isolation
- Poor housing
- Low income
- Precarious functional capacity
- Dependency on others.

Many old people are fiercely proud and independent and may fail to recognise or acknowledge their increasing vulnerability.

Negative attitudes to old age (ageism) must be avoided by healthcare professionals.

The nature of acute illness in old age

Acute illnesses in old people often fail to present with convenient and characteristic symptoms or physical signs:

- A myocardial infarct may not present with crushing central chest pain but rather with a fall, acute onset of mental confusion or simply breathlessness
- Acute infections may fail to mount the response of an immune reaction (raised white cell count) or a raised body temperature.

Acute illnesses in old people arise in the context of a general background of failing health such as:

- Memory loss and impairment of intellect. The elderly brain is especially susceptible to the toxic effects of any acute illness, so that acute onset of mental confusion may be a presenting symptom
- Failing eyesight or hearing
- Increase in postural sway so that acute illnesses may present as falls

- Impaired central control of bladder function so that acute illnesses may present with urinary incontinence
- Perhaps most importantly, an accumulation of other diseases; for example, a fairly trivial acute illness may arise in a person already compromised by heart failure and further limited by impaired mobility following an operation for a fractured neck of femur.

Acute illnesses in old people often arise in a situation of precarious social circumstances in which the support network for the individual is already stretched.

The paramedic called to an emergency must be aware that an apparently minor illness in an old person can have very different consequences from the same illness in a young person.

Major health problems in old age

Intellectual disorder

In simple terms, intellectual disorder is of two types: due to disease outside the brain (extrinsic) and due to intrinsic brain disease (dementia).

Extrinsic causes

Mental impairment may be caused by:

- Drugs
- Infections
- Hypoxia
- Dehydration
- Electrolyte disorders
- Disturbances of carbohydrate metabolism
- Renal or hepatic failure
- Hypothyroidism and vitamin B_{12} and folate deficiency (rare)
- Head injury.

The intellectual dysfunction associated with these extrinsic causes is usually short-lived, unless there is co-existing intrinsic brain disease.

Two cardinal features distinguish this type of mental disorder from dementia:

- Acute onset (and usually rapid resolution)
- Disturbed or fluctuating conscious level.

Intrinsic causes

Dementia is a pathological state characterised by diffuse loss of brain tissue. When brain tumour and other focal conditions have been excluded, the usual causes are Alzheimer's disease, multifocal vascular disease and a mixture of the two. Dementia also occurs in Parkinson's disease, Huntington's chorea and other rarer brain diseases.

Alzheimer's disease is a slowly progressive disease with a 10-year course on average. Most cases appear in the 8th and 9th decades.

Vascular brain disease, also called multiinfarct dementia, occurs in hypertensive patients who suffer progressive loss of brain tissue, with or without focal neurological signs. Many of these patients die from cardiac disease or stroke.

The history

Patients may give a very misleading history of the illness as they are unable to assess their current state, but may be able to talk convincingly and positively of their past life. Be very wary of patients who make even the slightest lapse from consistency of accuracy in answering questions and seek information from relatives who have watched them over a period of time.

Eventually a crisis occurs, which carers can no longer accept and this fracture of sound support may masquerade as a medical emergency.

Indicators of intellectual disorder in the elderly

- An increased use of the telephone, especially in the middle of the night
- Frequent losses of key, pension books, money, jewellery
- Accusations that others have stolen these
- Burning out kettles
- Leaving the gas on unlit
- Resistance to bathing and changing clothes
- Changes in sleep–wake patterns
- Soiling of clothes and neglect of personal appearance
- Leaving the house and getting lost
- Repeatedly asking the same question
- Misidentifying or failing to identify near relatives
- Speaking of the past as if it were the present and of dead people, e.g. parents, as if they were still alive.

Immobility

Immobility can be defined as an inability to occupy space (the life-space, ranging from anywhere in the world to the confines of an upstairs bedroom).

What are the consequences of immobility?

Loss of choice:

- Being able to go where we want to be and thus be able to do what we want to do
- Being alone or with others
- Having the TV on or off (look around any hospital ward or old people's home).

Loss of capability:

- Getting to the toilet in time, answering the door or getting upstairs
- Social responsiveness
- Worsening physical dependency.

An old person's world may thus contract and after becoming housebound, he (or more often she) then becomes restricted to the lower half of the house and eventually perhaps to one room.

Barriers to maintaining mobility in old age

Physical barriers (often more than one):

- Joint problems, especially osteoarthritis of knees and hips
- Neurological deficit: impaired balance, stroke, Parkinson's disease
- Previous falls
- Sensory deprivation: deafness, impaired vision
- Cardiovascular and respiratory diseases.

Mental barriers:

- Reduced expectations of an active life
- Loss of adaptability and creativity
- Introversion with reduced social contact
- Anxiety and fear of going out (or of allowing others to).

Social barriers:

- Retirement brings with it dangers of reduced social contact and a drop in income
- Living alone: an epidemic problem in ageing women
- Nowhere to go – insufficient outside interests or activities.

Incontinence

Anyone can become incontinent if not able or not allowed to have access to proper toilet facilities. The elderly are more vulnerable because of poor mobility and frequency and urgency of micturition. Any acute illness is likely to be associated with deterioration in continence but usually, this is transient. Any change of environment such as admission to hospital may also lead to a temporary period of incontinence.

Extrinsic causes

Common causes for incontinence in old people include:

- Faecal impaction – easily diagnosed by rectal examination and quickly cured by enemas
- Chronic brain failure – partly due to a diminished response to sensation of bladder filling

- Following the removal of indwelling catheters
- Urinary tract infection.

The problem may be exacerbated by:

- Diuretics
- Hypnotics and sedatives (especially at night)
- Anticholinergic drugs such as antidepressants
- Antiparkinsonian drugs and verapamil can cause urinary retention with overflow.

Intrinsic causes

Intrinsic causes include disorders of the bladder, sphincter or their nerve supply. Incontinence may be caused directly because of over- or underactivity of the bladder itself or the sphincter.

Instability
Balance

Under normal circumstances, the body undergoes oscillations around a fixed point known as the 'sway path'. As these balance mechanisms deteriorate with increasing age, sway increases.

Ocular mechanisms

Under normal circumstances, visual cues are constantly used to correct minor deviation from the fixed point. In old people, visual acuity is frequently reduced, as is the threshold for light stimulation.

Vestibular mechanisms

The vestibular apparatus is mainly involved with rotatory movements of the head and neck, whereas the otolith organ is involved with acceleration and deceleration. With advancing age, these mechanisms are relatively inefficient.

Proprioceptive mechanisms

Sensory information from proprioceptors in the spine and major weight-bearing joints may be impaired with ageing and arthritis. Failure of these mechanisms leads to an increased likelihood of falls.

Falls

About 20% of elderly men and 40% of elderly women will give a history of a recent fall and the liability to fall rises with age; the probability going up from 30% chance of falling at 65 years to 50% at 85 years. Fall is one of the most common causes of emergency admission to an acute geriatric ward, often after a prolonged period lying on the floor unable to get up.

Where and when do falls occur?

Most falls occur indoors or very close to the house, in the daytime. Falls on stairs are more likely to occur when the person is descending.

What are the clinical features?

Falls may be divided into two broad categories: extrinsic and intrinsic.

- *Extrinsic* falls are those in which an external factor is responsible, e.g. tripping or accident. This type of fall occurs in a younger, fitter person and the vast majority are unreported and cause no serious injury
- *Intrinsic* falls are those in which the dominant cause is failure of balance for the reasons described above and in which one or more precipitating causes may play a part. In this case, the patient is older and more frail.

Precipitating causes for falls

Change of posture

Getting out of a chair – an unstable situation requiring strength and coordination in antigravity muscles – is a typical precipitating cause.

Extended movement

In falls due to extended movement – the person reaches out or up, which puts the centre of gravity outside the ground base but owing to a slowing of postural reflex movements, is unable to compensate by moving the feet quickly enough to prevent a fall.

Illnesses

Any acute illness such as cardiac disease or arrhythmias may lead to a fall, as may poor vision.

Drugs

Diuretics, hypnotics and drugs for hypertension are particularly implicated in falls in the elderly and reducing multiple drug therapy is the most powerful preventive measure that can be taken.

Consequences of falling

- Fractures (7–10% of falls), usually wrist, hip, pelvis, upper humerus and ribs. The most serious, proximal hip fracture, has a mortality up to 40% and serious morbidity including loss of mobility in survivors
- Other injuries: soft tissue injuries (5–10% of falls), including bruising, subdural haematoma and dislocations, can occur. Inability to rise from the floor after a fall can result in pressure sores, incontinence and hypothermia and even death

- Psychological effects: fear of falling often results in delay in re-establishing mobility and a re-setting of postural mechanisms which cause a temporary tendency to fall backwards after standing up
- Institutionalisation: recurrent falls are a particularly powerful reason why patients may lose the confidence to live independently.

What is the prognosis?

About one-quarter will die within a year of their index fall. If they have lain for more than 1 hour, half will be dead in 6 months.

Visual impairment

Visual handicap remains grossly underreported both to doctors and registering authorities. Failing vision dramatically increases the burden of other handicaps.

Eye diseases

The four major diseases of the eye in old age are:

- Cataract (clouding of the lens of the eye)
- Macular degeneration (deterioration in central vision)
- Glaucoma (increase in pressure of fluid within the eye)
- Diabetic retinopathy (visual failure due to small vessel disease of the retina).

Changes in the ageing eye

Cornea
The cornea becomes more opaque with slight scattering of light and reduction in light transmission, especially at the ultraviolet end of the spectrum. Specific diseases rather than age itself are responsible for any visual handicap.
Lens
The largest contribution to the visual consequences of the ageing process is made by changes in the lens: it becomes thicker, stiffer, denser and more yellow (filtering out blue and violet). The main consequence is presbyopia or reduced ability to accommodate.
Ciliary apparatus
Thickening of the ciliary apparatus may lead to closed angle glaucoma.
Retina
The blood vessels of the retina become narrower. Macular deterioration reduces spatial discrimination, black and white contrast and colour perception.

Hearing impairment

Deafness is a common problem in the elderly which increases in prevalence with age, 30–40% of people over 75 years having some degree of hearing loss.

Pathology

Acquired causes are either conductive or sensorineural deafness and are super-imposed upon an age-related sensorineural hearing loss termed *presbyacusis*. Presbyacusis is characterised by a predominantly high-tone hearing loss caused by degeneration and atrophy of the sensory cells and neuronal connections within the cochlea.

Symptoms

Difficulty understanding speech is the most distressing and common consequence of hearing impairment. Frequency discrimination, sound localisation and reaction time are also impaired. In some patients, distressing tinnitus (whistling or ringing) and abnormal loudness perception may add to their problems.

Hearing aids

Hearing trumpets are still available and, although they may appear outdated, are still effective. Postaural and body-worn aids are readily available; these aids have a volume control and settings marked 'O' for off, 'M' for on (microphone) and 'T' for use with telephones fitted with an induction coupler (telecoil) loop, which cuts out background noise. Some public buildings and phones are also fitted with coupler loop systems. Bone conductor aids are available to patients with severe middle ear disease causing profound conductive deafness.

Social consequences of deafness

- Difficulty in hearing speech during group conversation (early stages)
- Loss of independence
- Social isolation
- Irritation and unhappiness
- Clinical depression
- Suspicion
- Paranoid ideas.

Depression

Depression is both a subjective mood state and an objective psychiatric illness. The psychiatric illness of depression is characterised by low mood, unaffected by external circumstances, feelings of unworthiness and helplessness. Suicidal ideas may be present. Depression in the elderly is characterised by:

- Appetite disturbance
- Weight loss
- Sleep disturbance (early wakening)
- Poor concentration
- Decrease in normal interests

- Delusions and hallucinations
- Hypochondriasis.

Masked depression

Hypochondria or anxiety symptoms predominate and there is no complaint of depression, although symptoms are present and can be revealed by questioning.

Pseudodementia

Pseudodementia is the term given to a syndrome that presents with poor self-care and poor cognitive ability. This change in function is brought about by a retarded depression. All the features mentioned above may be present; lack of interest will result in poor self-care and cognitive function. These patients will often answer 'don't know' to questions rather than confabulate. The history of onset of the illness is weeks or months rather than years, as in a true dementia. There may be a family or previous history of affective disorder.

Adverse drug reactions

The paramedic called to see an old person should (with permission) search for all medications (both prescribed and 'over the counter') and bring them with the patient to hospital. They may be crucial in assisting diagnosis, especially when the patient is unable to give an accurate history.

Table 39.1 Drugs that may cause problems in elderly patients

Drug group	Symptoms and signs
Diuretics	Falls, confusion, dry mouth, dehydration, postural fall in blood pressure, urinary incontinence
Compound analgesics	Drowsiness, confusion, falls, constipation
Tricyclic antidepressants	Greater risk of anticholinergic effects: urine retention, constipation, dry mouth, postural hypotension and confusion
Digoxin	Reduced renal excretion. Increased risk of side-effects such as sickness, diarrhoea, slow pulse rate and other heart rhythm disorders causing dizziness, fainting or falls
β-blockers	Falls, confusion, heart failure, slow pulse, postural hypotension, asthma attacks, cold limbs
Hypnotics	Increased and prolonged effects. Confusion, drowsiness, staggering and falls (especially at night)

Communicating with old people

Medical problems and the effects of social isolation may cause problems in communicating with old people. Simple measures such as ensuring that a hearing aid is switched on and that dentures are worn, may help. In people with impaired hearing, ensure good lighting and that the patient can see your face clearly to assist with lip-reading.

1. *Introduce yourself.* Patients do not know who you are and it is a simple courtesy to tell them
2. *Shake hands.* This friendly action provides information on the patient's vision (does the patient see and attend to the hand? Does he miss it when he reaches out his own hand?) and on the strength of grip, the temperature and moisture of the palm and the general feeling of eagerness or apathy
3. *Sit down close to the patient.* It is off-putting to be asked questions by someone who is towering over you. Get down to the patient's level both physically and psychologically. Speak clearly, have your face in a good light and never put your hand over your mouth
4. *Don't waste questions.* Have a clear purpose in mind with every one you ask
5. *How well does the patient hear you?* Watch the movement of the head, the facial expression and the response to questions, rather than directly asking if the patient hears you.
6. *How credible is the patient as a witness?* Begin by asking name, address, date of birth and current age. Check these against your own information. Discrepancies are very significant
7. *How good is the patient's memory?* Avoid or postpone 'formal' tests of cognitive function. You will obtain just as much information, without risking upsetting the patient, by asking about family: the name of spouse (including wife's maiden name where appropriate), the names of sons, daughters, sons-in-law, daughters-in-law and grandchildren
8. *How well is the patient oriented?* Establish first orientation by saying, 'You know who I am, of course, don't you?' and following with, 'Well, who am I?' and 'What is my job?' If you are still in doubt about orientation, continue with, 'You know what place this is, don't you?' Orientation for time is best tested by asking about the month or the time of year, rather than the day of the week. Knowledge of the time of day is also a good guide; but do not ask more questions than you need.

The home environment: clues to aid diagnosis and management

The major illnesses of old age often leave environmental clues to give assistance to the hospital or primary care team. This investigative role of the paramedic is especially crucial when the patient is a recluse, perhaps not well known to neighbours or to the primary care team, or is reluctant to go to hospital and may deny that problems exist.

Consider who initiated the emergency call; was it:

- The patient? (probably wants help – consider fear and loneliness as well as genuine illness)
- A neighbour? (consider antisocial behaviour or genuine concern about failure of the patient to cope)
- Relatives or carers? (consider severe dependency and carer stress. Has the general practitioner been involved? If not, why not?)

Clues in assessing a patient:

- *The garden and outside of the house* – is it well maintained? If so, by whom? If not, is this because of low income, lack of interest or lack of ability?
- *Access to the house* – if this is difficult, is the patient a voluntary recluse or socially isolated or is it because of neglect of maintenance, fear of assault or burglary? Check with neighbours
- The patient who is *slow or unable to answer the door* may be deaf, immobile or ill. Alternatively, the doorbell may not work
- *The letterbox test* – lift the flap and sniff! If the smell is unpleasant, consider severe neglect, urine or faecal incontinence of cats or dogs as well as humans
- *The general state of repair, maintenance and cleanliness* inside will give clues to the person's general level of household competence. Is the house well heated? If there is central heating, is it used? If the house is clean and tidy, who does it? At the other extreme, the visitor's feet may stick to the carpet and there may be extreme neglect and squalor. A not uncommon condition is what geriatricians call the 'senile squalor' (or Diogenes) syndrome. An elderly person (or occasionally a young person) lives in utter squalor, often surrounded by piles of junk or magazines to the extent that movement within the house is almost impossible. Surprisingly the person is not demented or ill and may often have a middle-class background and have lived alone for many years. Usually they function reasonably well. People with long-standing psychiatric problems or alcoholism may also live in such squalor
- The *life-space* (see section on immobility) – how much of the house does the person occupy? Are there walking aids or grab rails? Does the person go upstairs? Where are the toilet and bathroom? Are they used? Is there a commode? Does the person sleep in a chair? Can they get up and walk safely? Problems in these areas point to difficulties with mobility, recent or previous falls
- The *kitchen* – is there food around? Is there a refrigerator? If so, is there fresh food in it? Has the person been eating? Who prepares the food? Is the person capable of using the kitchen?

Abuse of older people

Abuse may be physical, sexual, psychological or financial; it may be due to neglect by relatives, carers or (it could be argued) by the welfare state which leaves many old people on very low incomes or insufficiently supported in their own homes.

Injuries such as finger-mark bruising (especially on the upper arms), cigarette burns (which may not be self-inflicted), bruising around the head and neck and on non-extensor surfaces may be due to assaults and should be carefully documented. Usually they are blamed on falls and in direct confrontation, the old person will often deny abuse, which is often from a stressed carer on whom the old person depends. Physical abuse most often occurs within a caring relationship in which the carer, often inadequately supported, is dealing day and night with a person who is mentally or physically very dependent. Management of the situation demands care and treatment not only for the abused person but also for the carer.

For further information, see Ch. 39 in *Emergency Care: A Textbook for Paramedics*.

CHAPTER 40

Hypothermia

Hypothermia is defined as having a core temperature below 35°C. Clinically, it can be divided into three categories:

- Mild: 32–35°C
- Moderate: 30–32°C
- Severe: below 30°C

and into three groups according to circumstances:

- Immersion – patient has been in water
- Dry – patient is on dry land but has been exposed to low air temperatures
- Urban – such as elderly patients who fall in their home.

The underlying clinical effects are broadly the same for each group.

Heat loss

Heat loss occurs from the body via conduction, convection, radiation and evaporation.

The surface area over which heat is lost is important. Children have a larger surface area for their weight than do adults and hence tend to lose heat more quickly.

The temperature of the human body is normally regulated within strict limits around an average core temperature of 37°C.

Clinical recognition of hypothermia

Cases will be missed unless specific consideration is given to its possible presence. It should be remembered that where hypothermia has occurred in one member of a party, the others will also be at risk and further cases may occur unless corrective action is taken.

Table 40.1 Clinical features of hypothermia

Core temperature (°C)[a]	Clinical feature
36	Sensation of cold, stumbling, personality changes, mild confusion
35	Slurred speech, incoordination. Amnesia of events (on recovery)
34	Development of arrhythmias – typically atrial fibrillation
33	Shivering lost – replaced by muscular rigidity
31	Pupils become dilated. Loss of consciousness
30	Insulin ineffective. Risk of spontaneous ventricular fibrillation – often unable to defibrillate
26	Major acid-base disturbance
24	Significant hypotension
23	Apnoea
18	Asystole

[a]These temperatures are a guide and will vary between individuals.

History

The history frequently gives an indication of the likely presence of hypothermia and may well be the only indicator. The following questions should be asked:

- Has the patient been immobile for a prolonged period (after a fall or entrapment)?
- Is the patient wet (rain or immersion)?
- Are they adequately clothed for the conditions?
- Has the patient been exposed to the wind?
- Has the patient got open wounds, increasing heat loss?

Examination

There are few consistent signs other than the patient's skin feeling cold.

If a temperature is taken, it should be performed with a low-reading thermometer. Axillary temperatures are unreliable, but will at least give an indication of the degree of hypothermia.

The best guide is a rectal temperature, which is usually not practical prehospital.

Clinical signs of hypothermia:

- *Shivering* – disappears around 33°C
- *Pulse* – initially raised, then falls (but other factors interfere, e.g. hypovolaemia and raised intracranial pressure). The pulse is difficult to feel and weak. It may be irregular owing to cold-induced arrhythmias
- *Breathing* – slow and shallow (although initially the rate may be raised)
- *Breath* – fruity, acetone smell due to incomplete metabolism
- *Mental state* – confusion through to unconsciousness (but other factors interfere, e.g. hypovolaemia and raised intracranial pressure).

The patient who is thought to be hypothermic must be examined for signs of injury or medical illness which may be masked by the effects of the hypothermia. Hypoglycaemia should be specifically excluded.

Treatment

The initial management of the patient is aimed at reducing further heat loss. The patient must therefore be provided with protection against the elements. This involves:

- Insulating them from the ground using a foam mat
- Removing and replacing wet clothes
- Covering the head
- Applying blankets (including a 'space' blanket)
- Providing a windproof outer layer
- Providing shelter
- Providing warm drinks if the patient is conscious (alcohol must be avoided as it causes peripheral vasodilation)
- Careful handling as sudden manoeuvres can precipitate cardiac arrhythmias. (insertion of an oral airway may precipitate bradyarrhythmias or cardiac arrest and should be carried out carefully)
- Administering oxygen (ideally warmed and humidified)
- Where possible, administering warmed intravenous fluids.

The main prehospital danger is that the patient may suffer a cardiac arrest. This is most likely to be due to ventricular fibrillation.

The protocols for treating arrests should be followed, but it must be appreciated that it may be impossible to defibrillate successfully if the core temperature is below 30°C.

The relative protective effect of severe hypothermia on the brain gives rise to the edict that 'no one is presumed dead until they are warm and dead'. Thus, resuscitation should be continued until the patient is adequately rewarmed.

> No one is dead unless they are warm and dead

No attempt should be made to actively warm the hypothermic patient prehospital by other means, such as hot-water bottles or heaters. This causes peripheral heating, with opening of the skin and splanchnic blood vessels, resulting in the washing out of metabolites that have built up in the hypoxic tissue. When these arrive at the heart they can induce fatal arrhythmias.

> Careless handling of hypothermia victims may precipitate fatal arrhythmias

Active rewarming

Active rewarming involves actively reheating the patient. There are a number of methods used in hospital:

- Warm humidified oxygen
- Warmed intravenous fluids
- Thoracic cradle heating
- Peritoneal lavage
- Oesophageal warming
- Extracorporeal rewarming using cardiopulmonary bypass
- Immersion rewarming in a bath (only used in immersion hypothermia).

For further information, see Ch. 40 in *Emergency Care: A Textbook for Paramedics.*

CHAPTER 41

Near drowning

'Wet' drowning

The individual aspirates water into the lungs, after an episode of breath holding until the victim cannot hold the breath any longer. On inspiration, much of the water is probably swallowed, but a proportion is inhaled. This inhaled water blocks the airways, only a proportion of it getting as far as the alveoli. The result is hypoxia, which after a short period results in hypoxic cardiac arrest and hence death. It only requires 10 mL of inhaled water per kilogram of body weight to be fatal.

Fresh water in the alveoli is absorbed, resulting in haemolysis of red blood cells and haemodilution. Sea water, being hypertonic, causes withdrawal of water from the blood and no haemolysis.

'Dry' drowning

No (or very little) water actually enters the lungs. This may be because of laryngeal spasm but is more likely to be because of primary cardiac arrest due to stimulation of the vagus nerve by cold water. It is this mechanism that causes the death of people who drop into cold water. It is likely that this is the cause of death in 'spray drowning' – deaths that occur in people on the surface of rough water. Vagal sensitivity is increased by hypothermia which occurs rapidly in cold-water immersion.

'Dry' drowning accounts for between 10% and 25% of drowning deaths.

In the UK, drowning is the fourth leading cause of death in men under the age of 35 years and the second leading cause of death in children, with 40% of all drowning deaths occurring in children under the age of 5 years.

> 'Near drowning' is the term applied to a survivable drowning episode

Effects of immersion in cold water

> Box 41.1 **Cardiac and respiratory effects of near drowning**
>
> - Sudden rapid deep breath
> - Rapid shallow breathing at maximal lung capacity
> - Reduced ability to hold the breath (very low temperatures)
> - Peripheral vasoconstriction
> - Reduction in circulating volume
> - Fluid shifts between compartments
> - Sudden fall in BP on removal from the water in a vertical position.

> Hypothermia is routine in patients removed from the water

The diving reflex

The diving reflex occurs in many mammals but its significance in adults is doubtful. It does seem to be more developed in children and probably explains why young children can survive prolonged cold-water immersion.

A reflex bradycardia occurs when cold water stimulates areas of the face and neck. This bradycardia, associated with the rapid cooling caused by cold-water immersion, can be protective of the victim by rapidly reducing the oxygen requirements of the brain and other tissues with a high metabolic requirement.

Other effects

The cold water, partly by producing hypothermia and partly by a direct cold effect on the pharynx, causes intense vagal stimulation, which results in a severe bradycardia or asystole. For this reason, manipulation of the airway in a near-drowned person can cause cardiac arrest.

Effects of near drowning

The effects of near drowning are variable and depend on a number of factors: the temperature of the water, the length of time immersed and the amount of inhaled water. There is little difference between salt and fresh water.

Initial (primary) effects

Victims progress through:

- Hypoxia
- Confusion
- Lethargy
- Unconsciousness.

Patients frequently report that they experience a 'high'. Several divers have described this phase as being 'pleasant', in that they no longer cared what would happen to them. If the hypoxia continues, then cardiac arrest will occur as a result of hypoxic myocardium. The victim will also suffer the associated problems of hypothermia and the loss of hydrostatic pressure (as described above). In very cold water an asystolic arrest can occur owing to intense vagal stimulation.

Delayed (secondary) effects

Water inhaled into the lungs causes damage; this is multifactorial and includes the development of pulmonary oedema and a reduction in the amount of surfactant. As a result, the subject may initially have few symptoms but may develop marked respiratory problems over several hours (usually 4–8). This problem is known as *secondary drowning*.

The other secondary problem is infection. Victims will have swallowed and inhaled water that may well contain microorganisms from sewage effluent or rat urine contamination (common in canals). Thus, consideration should be given to the development of infectious illness such as Weil's disease.

Diagnosis

The diagnosis would seem to be easily deduced from the circumstances; however, the picture is more complex, as the patient is likely to be hypothermic and may have other injuries associated with a fall or dive into water or sustained while in the water. The classic injury to the cervical spine occurs in the person who dives into shallow water thinking that it is deeper than it actually is.

The clinical picture may vary from a cardiac arrest (which may be ventricular fibrillation or asystole) to a conscious patient with few signs or symptoms but who is at risk of secondary drowning.

Airway

Airway findings are variable. The airway may be totally patent, it can be obstructed by the tongue owing to unconsciousness or it may be obstructed by water in the oropharynx.

Breathing

Breathing may be normal, but the chest should be auscultated as the presence of crepitations may indicate that secondary drowning is likely to occur. Breathing may be absent, either with or without cardiac arrest.

Circulation

The pulse is highly variable; many of the changes will be cold related. A profound bradycardia may occur in relation to vagal stimulation.

Treatment

Removal from the water

It is very important that the patient should be kept as horizontal as possible when removed from the water because of the loss of hydrostatic pressure to the body. This is especially important if the patient is hypothermic and it is this combination that has frequently led to deaths in the past.

Airway and breathing

The airway should be checked and cleared with care being taken to maintain the neck in midline immobilisation if cervical spine injury cannot be ruled out. Protecting the neck is difficult while in the water but an inflated life-jacket (not a buoyancy aid) gives some neck protection.

- Suction of the oropharynx may be used to clear the airway, but it must be remembered that in the hypothermic patient, any airway manipulation could cause vagal stimulation or laryngeal spasm
- It is impossible to remove water from the smaller airways because of the capillary attraction between the wall and the water. This water will be absorbed if the patient survives
- The patient should not be put in the head-down position, as this does not help remove water from the lungs and will raise the intracranial pressure, which may already be elevated from the preceding cerebral hypoxia
- Chin lift and jaw thrust should be used but head tilt avoided, if there is a possibility of neck injury. Guedel or nasal airways can be used, but care is needed as vagal stimulation can occur
- In the apnoeic patient, ventilation should be commenced. This is best undertaken via an endotracheal tube or laryngeal mask, as bagging via a mask tends to blow air into the stomach, which usually contains water, and thus increases the risk of regurgitation of stomach contents
- The breathing patient may be placed in the recovery position if spinal injury is excluded, the combination of hypoxia and swallowed water being a good stimulus for vomiting.

Circulation

In the absence of a palpable central pulse, cardiopulmonary resuscitation should be commenced and the appropriate cardiac arrest protocol followed. It should be appreciated that ventricular fibrillation may not be 'shockable' if the core temperature is below 30°C. Cardiopulmonary resuscitation on its own can occasionally cure the patient by correcting the hypoxia (this has been recorded a number of times in children).

Bradycardias should be treated with caution. If caused by vagal stimulation their treatment improves the situation, but in the severely hypothermic patient, it is frequently detrimental. A variety of other arrhythmias may be present due to hypothermia. Hypothermia, the loss of hydrostatic pressure and the presence of other injuries all contribute to a relative hypovolaemia. Intravenous access and warmed fluids are therefore required.

Ventricular fibrillation may not be 'shockable' if the core temperature is below 30°C.

Hypothermia

The near-drowned patient is frequently hypothermic. Once the patient is out of the water, wet clothes should be taken off as early as possible, otherwise continued heat loss will result from evaporation. First-aid measures must be aimed at preventing further heat loss.

Associated Injuries

The possibility of injuries must be considered and appropriate measures taken. The presence of hypovolaemia from a significant haemorrhage considerably complicates the clinical picture.

Further treatment in hospital

In the patient with cardiac arrest, continued resuscitation will take place until the patient is warm but still not responding. Immersion hypothermia can be treated by rapid rewarming, in which the patient is placed in a bath at 40°C with legs and arms dangling out. This should only be done where the cooling has been rapid. This treatment is only practicable and safe if the patient is conscious and sufficiently alert to cooperate. It should not be used for the unconscious patient. If a bath is unavailable a shower is an alternative, but is less efficient and requires even greater cooperation from the patient.

The patient should be kept under observation owing to the risks of secondary drowning and should not be discharged home unless the blood gases and chest X-ray are normal and the patient is free from any symptoms, with a clear chest on auscultation.

For further information, see Ch. 41 in *Emergency Care: A Textbook for Paramedics.*

CHAPTER 42

Heat illness

Heat illness does occur in the summer months and is frequently associated with strenuous activities such as sport or military exercises.

As with other environmentally produced disorders, there is a range of problems progressing through minor conditions (e.g. muscle cramps) to the life-threatening illness of heat stroke.

Physiology

The centre for heat regulation is sited in the hypothalamic region of the brain. Heat is produced through metabolism, either as a byproduct (e.g. of muscle contraction) or directly as a heat-producing mechanism.

In humans, the core temperature is regulated to remain constant at around 37°C.

Table 42.1 The physiological response to heat

System	Effects
Respiratory	Increased respiratory rate – with increased fluid loss[a]
Cardiovascular	Dilated skin capillary beds Increased heart rate[a] Increased cardiac output[a] Relative or actual hypovolaemia Reduced renal blood flow
Fluid and electrolytes	Dehydration Hyponatraemia (especially if fluid loss replaced by water only)

Table 42.1 The physiological response to heat—cont'd	
System	**Effects**
Skin	Warm and red – increased blood flow Increased sweating
Other	Decreased liver function Impairment of coagulation

ᵃExercise-related condition.

Acclimatisation

Prolonged exposure to a hot environment results in acclimatisation. Many of the changes that occur with this process are an attempt to reduce salt loss.

Types of heat illness

- Heat cramps
- Heat syncope
- Heat exhaustion
- Heat stroke.

Heat cramps

Heat cramps usually occur in the muscles of the lower limbs and are related to exercise. They occur in people in whom significant fluid losses due to sweating have been replaced with fluid with an insufficient salt content. As a result the individual becomes hyponatraemic and it is this electrolyte disturbance that is thought to cause the muscle cramps. Adequate salt replacement relieves the problem.

Heat syncope

Fainting related to the heat is not infrequently seen in Emergency Departments during hot weather. Elderly people seem particularly prone to this condition.

The probable mechanism is a degree of dehydration from sweating, combined with peripheral vasodilation.

If the person then stands for a long period, there is pooling of blood in the lower limbs (loss of the calf muscle pump) resulting in a drop in blood pressure and a subsequent syncope. Injuries can occur as a result of the fall.

The patient should be rested and provided with an oral fluid intake. In the elderly patient this diagnosis should only be made after other, more serious, diagnoses have been excluded.

Heat exhaustion

Heat exhaustion is a condition caused by water or salt depletion. It typically occurs in subjects who are not acclimatised and who undertake vigorous exertion, e.g. in military training.

Symptoms and signs

The following symptoms and signs may develop.

- Headache
- Dizziness
- General weakness
- Fainting
- Normal or mildly elevated core temperature ($<40°C$)
- Tachycardia
- Orthostatic hypotension.

It is very important that the patient is treated at this stage as, if left untreated or allowed to progress, heat stroke will occur.

Treatment

The patient should be placed in a cool environment and an oral electrolyte solution provided. Care needs to be taken when cooling the patient as the traditional tepid sponging and fanning can increase core temperature by causing capillary shutdown in the skin and by stimulating a shivering response. This is a particular problem with younger children. Cautious cooling with a fan is appropriate.

In patients who have significant symptoms, intravenous fluid and electrolyte replacement is required.

Heat stroke

Heat stroke is a serious life-threatening condition and requires rapid treatment. The condition normally occurs in hot, humid conditions where there is little wind and it can occur in the absence of exercise.

The condition occurs when the heat-regulating systems fail to keep up with heat production, are unable to function effectively or fail (e.g. loss of sweating).

It is recognised that there are two clinical forms of heat stroke: classic and exertional

- *Classic heat stroke* occurs during a period of sustained high environmental temperature and humidity. It tends to occur in older or debilitated people
- *Exertional heat stroke* is caused by overproduction of heat as a result of exertion and occurs primarily in young, fit subjects. Some people seem to be genetically prone to this condition.

Exertional heat stroke differs from classic heat stroke in that rhabdomyolysis and hypoglycaemia are a frequent problem. From the prehospital perspective, the conditions are very similar.

Symptoms and signs

The diagnosis is primarily clinical. The symptoms and signs are:

- Temperature usually 41°C or greater
- Skin is hot and dry, although sweating may still be present
- Weakness
- Nausea and vomiting
- Confusion progressing to lethargy and eventual coma
- Tachycardia and hypovolaemia
- Clotting abnormalities, including disseminated intravascular coagulation
- Hepatic damage – jaundice seen after 24 hours.

Treatment

Early initiation of treatment in the prehospital phase is very important as heat stroke, if not corrected, will result in rapid death due to damage to the central nervous system. This has been likened to frying eggs – the heat causes the protein to be denatured and irreversibly changed.

- Cool the patient carefully
- Remove clothes
- Consider immersion in water if there is likely to be a significant delay in transfer of the patient to hospital
- Otherwise rapid cooling can be commenced after urgent transfer to hospital
- Give high flow oxygen
- Protect the airway is consciousness is obtunded
- Give intravenous fluids
- Check BM stix and correct hypoglycaemia.

Immersion rapidly cools the individual owing to the high specific heat capacity of water (its ability to remove heat rapidly). Care needs to be taken if the conscious level of the patient is altered and in the unconscious patient protection of the airway is mandatory while performing this procedure. It is important to avoid the production of hypothermia.

Fits can occur and treatment is primarily aimed at airway control and maintaining oxygenation. Hospital management is usually undertaken on an intensive care unit. Cooling needs to be continued and electrolyte levels and the clotting status monitored.

For further information, see Ch. 42 in *Emergency Care: A Textbook for Paramedics.*

CHAPTER **43**

Electrocution

- Approximately 20% of reported electrocution injuries are fatal
- Generated electricity accounts for over 90% of the deaths, the rest being due to lightning strike
- Children account for 33% of all victims of electrical injury.

The effects of electrical passage are generally worse with alternating current (AC) than with direct current (DC).

The current follows the line of least resistance within the body. Skin has a high resistance when dry, followed by bone, muscle, blood vessel and nerve. The higher the resistance, the greater the damage produced.

The points at which the electrical energy actually enters and leaves the body are marked by burns: the entrance and exit wounds.

Alternating current in the domestic setting produces entrance and exit wounds of approximately the same size.

In an industrial environment, direct current is the most common cause of injury and produces a small entrance wound and a much larger exit wound.

At the time of injury, ventricular fibrillation may have been precipitated by the electric shock.

The greatest threats to life following electrical injury are a consequence of tissue damage, resulting in the release into the circulation of potassium and a product of muscle breakdown, myoglobin. These may cause cardiac arrhythmias and renal failure respectively.

Remember the possibility of secondary blunt injury, which may have resulted from the victim being thrown by the electrical contact. In any unconscious patient, therefore, cervical spine injury must be assumed and closed head injury suspected.

Alternating current is generally more dangerous than direct current at any given voltage because it is more likely to induce ventricular fibrillation.

- Above 10 ma tetanic contractions may make it impossible for the patient to release the electrical source

- Above 50 ma tetanic contraction of the diaphragm and intercostal muscles leads to respiratory arrest
- Above 100 ma primary cardiac arrest may be induced (defibrillators deliver approximately 10 A)
- Above 50 A massive shocks cause prolonged respiratory and cardiac arrest and severe burns.

> Suspect secondary injury (including to the cervical spine) in electrocution incidents

At the scene

- When dealing with electrical injury, the first consideration must be personal safety

> Safety first!

- Ensure that the current is switched off before attempting to touch the victim or remove the victim from the electrical source
- If the current cannot be switched off, the victim may be separated from the current using a non-conductive object, such as a dry broom handle
- A victim may be unable to release an electrical source. The only course of action will be to interrupt or discontinue the source of electricity, since separation of the victim from the source will be impossible
- In electricity pylon accidents, it will be necessary to telephone the electricity board to prevent them reconnecting an interrupted source, which they will do as a matter of routine after only 20 minutes, since the cause of most temporary interruptions is bird strike, which is generally not investigated
- When a worker on a utility pole is electrocuted, expired air ventilation can often be initiated by rescuers on the pole, with chest compressions if needed as soon as the victim can be lowered to the ground
- Even if there is no loss of consciousness, a victim of high-voltage electrical shock should receive cardiac monitoring and transport to hospital because of the danger of delayed cardiac arrest from life-threatening arrhythmias.

Railway accidents

Many electrical injuries occur on railways, a significant proportion of which are suicide attempts. Railway-related electrocution may be AC or DC; many lines are electrified on the 25 000 Volt AC overhead system, whereas others are electrified on a 750 Volt DC third rail system or the 630 Volt DC fourth rail system, which is used by the London Underground.

The railway is a hazardous environment; it is important not to go onto a rail track unless you have to. One should be aware of warning signs which indicate 'Reduced Line side Clearance' or 'No Refuge'. At all times, one should face oncoming traffic and a high-visibility tabard must be worn.

Telephones are clearly marked at crossings and signals and provide direct communication with Network Rail Control. Permission must be obtained from Network Rail before going on to the track and an official railway lookout should be requested using the trackside phones or through your ambulance control. Overhead line structure numbers, signal numbers or mile-post numbers can be used to identify the exact location.

Using the line side phones, the current isolation procedure and procedure for stopping trains is as follows:

- State:
    1. 'Emergency call'
    2. Name
    3. Location
    4. Why the current needs to be switched off
- Then wait for assistance!

It is important to assume that the electricity supply (whether overhead or a third or fourth rail system) is live until definite assurance that it has been switched off has been received from Network Rail. If it is not possible to switch the current off, expert advice from railway personnel must be followed at all times.

Management

After the safe extrication of the patient at the scene of an injury, immediate management follows basic principles with an evaluation of <C>ABCDE:

- Emergency intervention and resuscitation will occur as for any victim of trauma, to control severe external bleeding, achieve and secure an airway, establish adequate ventilation and provide fluid resuscitation. Accepted conventional algorithms for cardiac resuscitation should be followed in the case of cardiac arrest following electrocution
- Electrical shock victims with no signs of life should receive the most immediate treatment
- In any unconscious patient who has been electrocuted the cervical spine should be immobilized and the patient placed on a spine board
- High flow oxygen should be administered immediately
- Intravenous access should be obtained via a large-bore (14 or 16 gauge) cannula in the antecubital fossa *en route* to hospital. If there is any suspicion of tissue damage, in the absence of intrathoracic or abdominal bleeding, a fluid bolus of 2 litres of normal saline (20 mL/kg in children) should be given

- If non-compressible haemorrhage is also suspected, IV fluids should be restricted to 250 mL aliquots titrated against the maintenance of a radial pulse
- Cardiac monitoring is essential, as there is a significant incidence of delayed arrhythmias following electrocution
- A brief search should be made for any entrance or exit wounds, which should be covered with a clean, simple dressing during transfer to hospital
- All pregnant electrocution victims should be transferred urgently to a hospital with obstetric facilities, regardless of the type, voltage or ampage of the shock.

Lightning strike

Unlike other forms of electrical injury, lightning strike rarely produces exposure long enough to cause breakdown of the skin, the primary insulator of the body to current flow. The current instead passes over the outside of the body: the 'flashover' phenomenon. The majority of the current thus passes outside the body. If the victim is wet, the flow of current may cause secondary burns as the fluid is turned into steam. Because of the flashover phenomenon, true entrance and exit wounds are uncommon.

The almost universal cause of death is respiratory arrest. Lightning acts as a massive DC countershock, sending the heart into asystole that is normally temporary in the otherwise healthy young adults that are most often its victims. Unfortunately, the respiratory arrest that often accompanies cardiac arrest may last significantly longer than the cardiac event and ventilatory support will be required in these patients.

Patients who do not arrest immediately have an excellent chance of recovery: the victim who is moaning and groaning has a degree of stability of the vital signs and recovery is the rule.

For further information, see Ch. 43 in *Emergency Care: A Textbook for Paramedics*.

Chemical incidents

Chemical casualties may be generated from a wide range of incidents including explosions, fires, leaks, spills or through the ingestion of contaminated water. This can result in casualties suffering from a multitude of injuries including:

- Burns (thermal, chemical or both)
- Trauma
- Environmental effects (hypothermia)
- Acute poisoning
- Fire and explosion.

However, the direct effects of exposure to chemicals may result in:

- Acute or chronic poisoning from the absorption of the chemical through the lung, skin or digestive tract
- Direct tissue damage to the skin or lungs.

The severity of these injuries will depend on a number of factors including:

- The strength of the chemical
- The prevailing environmental conditions
- The length of time an individual is exposed to the chemical.

The first priority is to remove the casualty from the main area of chemical exposure (the hot zone) and then second, to decontaminate the casualty as quickly as possible.

Hazard warning symbols

The standard diamond-shaped hazard warning symbols indicate to both the emergency services and the public the primary hazard present. Symbols represent hazards including flammable solids or liquids, flammable or toxic gases, compressed gases, oxidising agents and corrosive substances. On multiloads, the hazard warning diamond simply contains an exclamation mark.

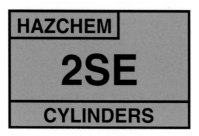

Figure 44.1 Conventional hazard warning signage.

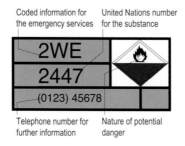

Figure 44.2 A HAZCHEM plate.

The HAZCHEM action code system

The HAZCHEM code system is a set of code numbers and letters displayed on a vehicle carrying hazardous substances which gives information about the appropriate fire-fighting methods and personal protection needed to deal with a spill.

HAZCHEM also gives guidance as to whether or not the substance can be safely washed into drains and whether evacuation of surrounding areas should be considered.

The HAZCHEM plate displayed on vehicles will also show the diamond warning sign, the United Nations (UN) number for the chemical carried and a contact number for specialist advice from the manufacturer.

ADR Kemler code

The ADR system is the European road transport system of hazardous load markings. Vehicles must bear a 40×30 cm label on both front and rear. The label is in two parts: the upper bears the Kemler code and the lower the UN substance number.

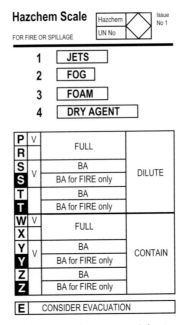

Figure 44.3 HAZCHEM code system *aide-memoire* card (front).

Notes for Guidance

FOG
In the absence of fog equipment a fine spray may be used.

DRY AGENT
Water **must not** be allowed to come into contact with the substance at risk.

V
Can be violently or even explosively reactive.

FULL
Full body protective clothing with BA.

BA
Breathing apparatus plus protective gloves.

DILUTE
May be washed to drain with large quantities of water.

CONTAIN
Prevent, by any means available, spillage from entering drains or watercourse.

Figure 44.4 The HAZCHEM code system *aide-memoire* card (back).

The Kemler code comprises two or three digits which indicate the properties of the load carried. The first digit describes the primary hazard and the second and third digits the secondary hazards. If the same number is repeated, this indicates an intensified hazard. An 'X' in front of the UN substance number indicates that it must not be brought into contact with water. There is no provision in the ADR system for any words to be placed on the warning plate.

Table 44.1 Kemler code system

First digit – primary hazard	Second/third digit – secondary hazard
2 Gas	0 No meaning
3 Inflammable liquid	1 Explosion risk
4 Inflammable solid	2 Gas may be given off
5 Oxidising substance	3 Inflammable risk
6 Toxic substance	5 Oxidising risk
7 Radioactive substance	6 Toxic risk
8 Corrosive	8 Corrosive risk 9 Violent reaction risk X Do not use water

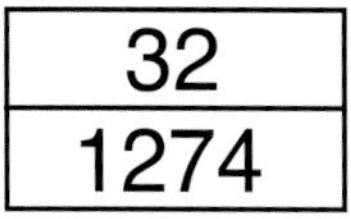

```
┌─────────────┐
│     32      │
├─────────────┤
│    1274     │
└─────────────┘
```

Figure 44.5 Kemler plate.

Transport emergency cards

Transport emergency (TREM) cards exist for road and rail transportation of hazardous loads. For road transport, the TREM card is a standard A4 size; it is kept in the cab of the lorry and should be changed each time the load is changed. This card gives details of the hazard, protective clothing necessary and action to be taken in the case of spillage or fire. The card will also carry first aid information for contaminated casualties and specialist contact details.

The information gathered at the scene from the above hazard warning systems can be supplemented and verified by the use of CHEMDATA. This is a database of many thousands of chemicals and the emergency actions required following exposure provided by the National Chemical Emergency Centre at Harwell.

The role of the Fire service

Most fire brigades now have specialised vehicles and personnel trained in the management of chemical incidents. They will have appropriate gas-tight clothing and breathing apparatus to allow them to work in a toxic and contaminated area. The fire brigade will also provide decontamination facilities for their personnel, usually in the form of portable showers.

The role of the Ambulance service

Ambulance services now have responsibility for the decontamination of chemical casualties. All UK ambulance services therefore must have rapid access to personal protection equipment (PPE) and decontamination equipment suitable for use on contaminated persons who are not wearing personal protective equipment. The Fire service have equipment for the decontamination of large numbers (>50) of *uninjured* survivors.

Management

The management of hazardous materials (HAZMAT) incidents is generally dealt with under the following headings:
- Prevention
- Preparedness
- Response
- Recovery.

Prevention

The responsibility for prevention of chemical incidents normally lies outside the ambulance service, although senior management will normally have been engaged with the risk assessment process within their own service area.

Preparedness

The paramedic dealing with such incidents must be confident about the use of PPE and undertaking clinical procedures, including decontamination while wearing these systems.

Response
Command and control
The incident area will be divided into a series of zones.

Hot zone
Only those personnel with the right level of PPE and training will be allowed to enter; normally this is the Fire service. Hazardous Area Response Teams (HART) may assist in treating casualties in the hot zone.

Warm zone
The warm zone extends from the hot zone to the inner cordon and is where the triage and decontamination of casualties and decontamination of all emergency service personnel is carried out.

Cold zone
This final zone extends out from the inner cordon to an outer cordon (this will be put in place by the police) and is an area free from contamination. While direct contamination should not be a hazard in this zone, vapour, particularly if the wind direction changes, may cause a problem and therefore respiratory protection (only) may be required by personnel working in this area.

Information gathering
At the scene of any incident involving chemicals, it is important to gather intelligence about the chemicals involved, their quantities, toxicity and the countermeasures that may be necessary. Paramedics should be able to gain enough information to determine whether special chemical precautions are required.

Safety at the scene
In relation to the hazard information, the appropriate level of PPE should be worn. If there is any doubt, it is important to start with the maximum level of protection and work downwards as more information becomes available.

Therefore, rescuer safety consists of ensuring that:

- The appropriate level of PPE is worn (this will be dictated by local policies) and once a task is finished effective personal decontamination takes place
- Casualties are appropriately decontaminated (this stops further injury and prevents contamination of other healthcare personnel)
- If the chemical is unknown a maximum level of PPE is the most appropriate initial response which can be downgraded as more information becomes available.

Triage of chemical casualties

Chemical incidents may produce a large number of casualties with a wide range of problems, but they tend to produce patients in the ratio of:

- Seriously injured (P1) 10%
- Moderately injured (P2) 20%
- Mildly injured/worried well (P3) 70%.

Walking casualties should be moved upwind near the inner cordon emergency service entry/exit gate whereas P1/P2 stretcher casualties should be taken to the casualty decontamination area.

Casualties who are heavily contaminated with chemicals should be triaged for urgent decontamination.

Treatment

Hot zone

Minimal treatment. The Fire service will extract casualties rapidly to the triage area while providing rudimentary airway protection.

Warm zone

Once a casualty has been triaged:

- P3 casualties should be encouraged to self-decontaminate (which is achieved by simply removing their clothes in most cases) before further management in the cold zone
- P1/P2 (stretcher) casualties should be taken to the patient decontamination area and simultaneously the:
  - Face should be rapidly decontaminated by washing with water and detergent followed by the appropriate management of the airway using simple airway techniques
  - Patient should receive 100% oxygen via a mask with a reservoir
  - Rest of the casualty should be decontaminated using the technique described in the section below
  - Patient should receive any other basic life support procedure which is necessary, such as the control of external haemorrhage.

Cold zone

The casualty, once decontaminated, should then be handed over the inner cordon onto a patient trolley and any scoop stretchers (or similar devices) should be handed back into the warm zone. Full resuscitation techniques can now be used. The use of antidotes at this level is questionable, the exception being if a specific acute poisoning (or poisonings) is clearly recognised and the antidotes are easily to hand.

Patient decontamination

Avoid taking contaminated casualties to hospital as this may well necessitate the closure of an emergency department to all other casualties. The decontamination team carrying out decontamination must wear appropriate PPE. Avoid hypothermia and protect the patient's dignity as much as possible.

Equipment required:

- A water source, preferably warm, but with no delay if warm water cannot be found
- A bucket
- Detergent, approximately 10 mL to one 10 L bucket of water
- A soft bristle brush.

Procedure:

1. If the casualty is non-ambulant, he should be placed on either a spinal board or aluminium scoop stretcher
2. Decontaminate the facial area before any ventilation equipment is applied. Once the airway is secured, should this be required, the remainder of the acute care procedures can be carried out
3. Remove all items of clothing unless medically contraindicated. Clothing and valuables should be retained in a sealed plastic bag and the police service consulted regarding their evidential value before disposal
4. Having exposed the patient, rinse the affected areas. This first rinse helps to remove particles and water-based chemicals
5. 'Vigorously clean' the affected areas with a soft brush using the detergent solution. This first wipe helps to remove organic chemicals and petrochemicals that adhere to the skin
6. Rinse for a second time. This second rinse removes the detergent and the chemicals. The whole process should not take longer than 5 minutes
7. Repeat steps 5 and 6
8. When decontaminated, the casualty should be passed over the clean/dirty demarcation line onto a clean trolley. Any equipment used during the decontamination process should not pass over the demarcation line.

Evacuation

The casualties in the cold zone should now be a minimal contact hazard. However, chemicals may continue to be 'off gassed' from the casualty's skin or hair or exhaled from the lungs. It would therefore be prudent to ensure that there is effective changeover of air within the back of the ambulance; for some chemicals, respirators may have to be worn.

The emergency department

A decontamination facility and appropriate PPE should also be available at the Emergency Department.

Recovery

If staff are exposed to the chemicals, they should be followed-up in the emergency department and subsequently by the service's occupational health system. All equipment used in the warm zone will need to be thoroughly decontaminated or destroyed (if decontamination is not an option). Finally, the incident should be internally reviewed and the lessons learned used to change local standard operational procedures and protocols.

For further information, see Ch. 44 in *Emergency Care: A Textbook for Paramedics.*

CHAPTER 45

Nuclear and radiation incidents

In the emergency response to an incident involving radioactivity, the principles of casualty care remain the same:

- Rapid assessment
- Administration of life-saving procedures
- Stabilisation
- Evacuation.

All of these procedures should be carried out without risking the safety and health of the paramedic team who must be sure that they are not placing themselves or the casualty at unnecessary risk – or that the risk is acceptable.

The hazards to which paramedics may be exposed are:

- Penetrating radiation
- Contamination.

Ionising radiation cannot be detected by the human senses but at the levels likely to be encountered in plausible accidents, there is little risk, and simple precautions will promote safe management of the radiological aspects of the injury.

The hazards

Radioactive sources are widely used in the UK, in:

- Industry
- Hospitals
- Further education establishments
- Nuclear power stations
- Research establishments

- Military bases
- During transport (air, road, sea and rail).

Where radioactive materials are processed on a large nuclear site, there will be contingency plans in the event of an accident, which may require the support of ambulance, fire and local authority agencies as well as the employer's own response team.

> Substances are said to be radioactive when they give off radiation

Types of radiation

α-Radiation

Alpha particles travel a very short distance in air and are stopped by a sheet of paper, clothing, blood or dressings. Ingestion or inhalation must be avoided as the particles can damage more sensitive internal organs. Examples of substances that emit α particles are uranium, plutonium and radon.

β-Radiation

β-Radiation is stopped by a thin sheet of aluminium or heavier clothing. It can penetrate the skin surface and therefore damage the epidermis and dermis to produce radiation burns. The hazard is greatest when the β emitter is in direct contact with the skin. Examples are iodine and tritium.

γ-Radiation, X-rays and neutrons

γ-Rays, X-rays and neutrons all travel great distances in air and are only stopped by thick concrete or lead. These forms of radiation can pass through the body, depositing energy and causing damage as they proceed. They are therefore still a hazard at some distance from the casualty or incident. Examples are industrial radiography sources, caesium and cobalt.

Risks of exposure

Ionising radiation can affect a part of the body or the whole body, causing localised effects (radiation burns) or systemic effects (radiation syndrome).

Loose particles of radioactive material (dust, aerosol or liquid) are known as contamination.

The material will emit radioactivity but in addition, it can easily be inhaled or ingested and precautions are needed to prevent this.

There are three scenarios involving exposure to radioactive materials that the paramedic will have to consider in the immediate care situation:

- The exposure to γ-rays or X-rays from a source near to the patient
- The presence or spread of contamination onto skin, hair and clothes of the patient

- The inhalation or ingestion of contamination by the paramedic or patient during rescue, resuscitation and removal.

In each case, simple precautions can be taken to reduce the risk to paramedic personnel and patients.

Figure 45.1 Nuclear hazard warning sign.

There may be useful clues available, such as a radiation identification mark on the package or vehicle, bystander knowledge or an unusual military or police presence.
   Remember:

- Any radiation dose to the attendants is likely to be small
- Simple precautions will reduce risk to personnel.

The principles of ABC (airway, breathing and circulation) still apply and must not be delayed on account of possible radiation exposure.

Patient overexposure to penetrating radiation

A patient who has been exposed to a large dose of penetrating radiation is not radioactive (just as patients who have had a clinical X-ray are not radioactive) and therefore *presents no hazard to the medical personnel*. Such an incident may arise with exposure to an industrial radiography source.

External contamination

If there has been a spread of radioactive materials, then the patient may be contaminated; this contamination may present a hazard to the patient and the paramedic, so it has to be dealt with safely. Most of the contamination is likely to be on the patient's clothes.

Internal contamination

There may have been a release of radioactivity which the patient has inadvertently swallowed, inhaled or absorbed through the skin, e.g. if the casualty has been exposed to smoke in a fire involving radioactive substances. Simple procedures can be used to protect both paramedic and patient.

Contaminated wounds

Treatment of the injury and associated bleeding is of prime importance, but care must be taken to avoid spread of contamination around the site of the wound.

Dealing with an incident

In order to reduce potential exposure to external penetrating radiation and reduce contamination, some simple procedures need to be followed.

- Assess the risks from other hazards, e.g. buildings, traffic, smoke or chemicals
- Position the ambulance upwind from the accident site
- Carry out the initial survey, check ABC, institute immediate care and prepare the patient for movement
- Assume contamination is present and reduce the risk of self-contamination by following the guidelines below
- Keep the time at the accident scene to a minimum.

If there is a continued risk from radiation exposure the patient should, after resuscitation, be moved away 10 metres from the source to reduce the dose to an acceptable level. If this is not possible, paramedics or other ambulance staff can take it in turns to monitor the patient, thereby sharing any radiation dose. Preferably, an attempt should be made to reduce the level of radioactivity coming from the source. This is known as *shielding* and can be achieved by using lead or concrete but if these materials are not available then rubble, heavy stones, sand or earth can be used.

Protection

It is quite possible that personnel will have no prior knowledge of the presence of radioactive materials, but simple precautions of the type used against chemical or biological hazards will help to reduce the spread of contamination and subsequent risk to personnel.

- Always assume that contamination is present when dealing with a casualty affected by an incident involving radioactivity
- Wear a simple surgical face mask and gloves. This will prevent spread of contamination to hands and face. If the clinical condition permits, a face mask can be placed on the patient
- Keep disturbance of the area to a minimum as this reduces the likelihood of air-borne contamination. This should not interfere with resuscitation and other emergency procedures
- Cover open wounds with simple dressings. This prevents contamination entering wounds or contaminated blood spreading from the wound onto surrounding skin
- Remove external clothing (leaving underwear) carefully, if practicable, and place in large, sealable plastic bags. Wrap the patient in a blanket or contamination control envelope, as this helps to prevent spread of radioactive materials
- Do not eat, drink or smoke until checked for contamination by medical physics personnel.

Management of patients

Overexposure to penetrating radiation is unlikely to result in any specific symptoms and other injuries will dictate the management.

- The onset of nausea or vomiting may indicate a significant overexposure and the accurate recording of the time of onset is important for future hospital management
- Erythema may be visible on exposed skin and its distribution should be noted.

A list of hospitals in the area prepared to accept contaminated casualties should be available to the paramedic. The clinical condition of the patient may make it necessary to go to the nearest Emergency Department and then it is essential that warning is given so that suitable preparations can be made.

Movement in the ambulance should be kept to a minimum and staff can expect to be directed to a specific parking area for unloading, where they should remain until screened for contamination, a task likely to be undertaken by medical physics personnel.

It is recommended that the patient be placed in a contamination control envelope, thereby allowing containment of any residual contamination on the patient while permitting observation of wounds, dressings, skin colour and bruising.

Rapid onset of nausea or vomiting or the presence of erythema suggest significant radiation exposure.

Radiation advice

The police will be able to give information on the availability of hospital advice on irradiated or contaminated casualties under the *National Arrangements for Incidents Involving Radioactivity* (NAIR). The NAIR scheme is coordinated by the *National Radiation Protection Board* (NRPB) to provide advice in the event of a nuclear incident if advice from major plant operators (*British Nuclear Fuels Ltd, Scottish Nuclear* and *Nuclear Electric*) is unavailable.

Follow-up

After the patient has been transferred to hospital, it may be discovered that the emergency personnel are contaminated with radiation. Decontamination is a simple process, but may need to be carried out in a special area. This could cause concern to some individuals and requires explanation:

- Contaminated clothing is identified and discarded in sealable bags
- All clothing is then removed
- Monitoring is carried out by medical physics personnel using radiation monitors (Geiger counters)
- Areas of skin contamination are identified by skin markers

- Decontamination is carried out by washing with soap and water
- Areas of contamination that are difficult to remove will require a mild abrasive such as dry soap powder or industrial skin cleanser
- Continued cleansing of the skin must be done with care to avoid inflammation
- If air-borne spread is a possibility then it is necessary to check for inhalation and this is normally done by checking counts on nasal swabs or nose blows
- Personnel will be asked to produce biological samples (faeces and urine) which will be monitored for radioactive substances.

Antidotes

If it is suspected that any intake has occurred, it is unlikely to require treatment, but therapy does exist and has been used for many radioactive substances; examples are: diethylenetriaminepentaacetic acid (DTPA) for plutonium exposure; Prussian blue for caesium exposure and potassium iodate for iodine exposure.

For further information, see Ch. 45 in *Emergency Care: A Textbook for Paramedics*.

The sports arena

Sport-related deaths

Most deaths that occur at sporting events are from natural causes such as myocardial infarctions. Occasionally, congenital heart diseases such as hypertrophic cardiomyopathy can affect young athletes.

Table 46.1 Fatal accidents in sport (UK statistics for 1 year)

Sport	Fatalities per year
Air sports	13
Horse riding	12
Mountaineering	11
Motor sports	10
Ball games	6
Water sports	6
Winter sports	5
Athletics	4
Cycling	1
Shooting	1

Nature of injuries in sport

Most sports injuries are soft tissue injuries. Injuries to the lower limbs are most common, followed by the upper limbs, head and face, and finally the chest and abdomen. The majority are minor and self-limiting; however, serious injuries such as ligament and tendon tears, fractures, spinal and head injuries and damage to viscera do occur.

Paramedics must decide whether the problem must be dealt with in hospital immediately or whether the patient can be left to arrange independently for treatment at hospital or by a general practitioner later in the day. Many injuries do not require medical intervention and can be readily treated with rest, ice, compression and elevation (RICE), plus analgesia:

- **R** – **R**est
- **I** – **I**ce
- **C** – **C**ompression
- **E** – **E**levation

Athletics and field sports

- The majority of athletes suffer soft tissue injury and sprains. Overuse predisposes them to chronic muscle and ligament problems that may be suddenly exacerbated in competition
- High jumpers and pole vaulters are liable to neck injury if they land badly
- Heat exhaustion is frequent during hot conditions.

Combat sports

- Of greatest concern in combat sports are head and neck injuries as a result of direct blows or from falls following throws. Facial fractures and eye injuries are also common
- Soft tissue injury and fractures are features of the martial arts.

Football

- The majority of association football injuries are to soft tissues, with strains and complete tears of leg muscles and tendons being most common
- Severe knee and ankle injuries occur less frequently and fractures to the lower limb are relatively rare
- Head and neck injuries can occur in bad falls or clashes of heads.

Hockey

- Hockey players are prone to the same injuries as footballers; they also run the risk of being hit by a stick or a very hard ball travelling at high speed
- Facial injuries are commonly caused by follow-through of a stick.

Horse riding

- Falls and head injuries may lead to as many as 50% of riding-related deaths

- Kicking injuries and involvement in road traffic accidents also cause serious injury
- Severe injuries to the head, neck and spine are common
- Maxillofacial injuries arising from kicks can be severe and airway care may pose major problems
- Crushing injury can occur if a horse rolls onto its rider, causing severe blunt chest and abdominal injury.

Motor sports

- The speeds involved in motor racing and motorcycle racing can lead to life-threatening multisystem injury
- Extracting the casualty from the wreckage may be prolonged and difficult
- Burns, fractures and head and neck injuries are common and crash-helmets can lead to problems with management
- Spectators are at risk from flying debris and wheels or from direct contact with vehicles whose drivers have lost control
- Rescuers too are at risk as, unless the track is dangerously affected, the race will continue.

Mountaineering and hill walking

Strains, sprains and minor fractures are the most common injuries in these sports. They take on a greater significance when they occur many miles from help in hostile terrain. The weather poses significant problems and the risk of hypothermia and frostbite is ever present. Falls can lead to significant multiple injuries. Hill walkers often have medical conditions and the most common cause of death on the hills is myocardial infarction rather than trauma.

> Remember intercurrent medical illness

Racket sports

Soft tissue sprains and strains are the most common injuries. The upper limb is more often injured in these sports. Facial injury from contact with a racket can occur. Of greatest concern in this group is eye injury. Squash balls and shuttlecocks can produce severe damage if they strike a player's orbit at close range.

Rugby football and American football

Players suffer upper limb problems with fractures to the hand, arm and clavicle; lower limb problems include meniscal tear and knee ligament injury, ankle ligament damage (sprain) and fractures of the tibia and fibula. These fractures are often spiral, resulting from a twisting injury on a planted foot. Head injury with lacerations and fractures to the facial bones can be associated with concussion and loss of consciousness. Neck sprains are common and severe neck injury can occur. The majority of severe neck injuries occur in collapsed scrums or in head-on tackles where hyperflexion of the neck combined with axial loading of the spine is common. Crush injury in the regular 'pile-ups' of rucks and mauls may also occur with resultant damage to chest and abdomen.

Scuba diving

Sudden pressure changes can then lead to major problems with barotrauma or the 'bends' (decompression sickness).

Faulty technique on descent can lead to significant ear problems, with rupture of the tympanic membrane: cold water rushes into the middle ear and disequilibrates the balance mechanism and as a result, the diver loses all sense of direction, with drowning being a real risk.

Too rapid an ascent can lead to overdistension of the lungs and air spaces, resulting in barotrauma to these areas, as the enclosed air expands rapidly with the reduction in ambient pressure. Pulmonary barotrauma can lead to pneumothorax. Air embolus can also occur. Decompression sickness develops because nitrogen bubbles are released from solution in the blood when a diver ascends too quickly. Symptoms include:

- Pain, especially in the joints
- Itchy skin (the 'creeps')
- Headache
- The feeling of being strangled (the 'chokes')
- Neurological abnormalities including spinal cord problems (the 'staggers').

Nitrogen narcosis (euphoria and loss of judgement) occurs in air divers who go too deep.

Divers can develop the bends many hours after a dive, especially if they fly in an aircraft, when the ambient pressure is further reduced. This results in an enhanced release of dissolved nitrogen; any diver who exhibits strange symptoms after a flight that closely follows a dive should be viewed with concern.

Helicopter aeromedical evacuation poses theoretical risks to injured divers, although with transport at altitudes of less than 1000 feet, the pressure changes will not be clinically relevant.

> Injured divers must never be given Entonox

Water sports

Hypothermia is possibly the greatest risk in water sports in the UK. Many sailors, windsurfers and canoeists are ill prepared for sudden changes in the elements. Drowning is an ever-present risk. Head and neck injuries are common in those who dive into shallow water. Sailors can receive head injuries from flailing booms and suffer limb injuries in falls on wet decks. Jet-skiing predisposes to head and neck injury as a result of high-speed falls and collisions.

Powerboat racing poses similar risks to motor racing with multiple injuries and the extra risk of drowning for unconscious or incapacitated drivers.

Drugs and the athlete

Many competitive athletes are governed by strict rules about the use of drugs.

It is incumbent upon medical personnel who attend competitors to ensure that they do not inadvertently provide them with banned substances in the course of treating an injury or illness.

Table 46.2 Banned products

Type of drug	Examples
Stimulants	Ephedrine and pseudoephedrine in cold products Adrenaline
Narcotics	Co-proxamol Co-dydramol Nalbuphine Diamorphine and morphine Kaolin and morphine
Anabolic steroids	
β-blockers	
Diuretics	
Peptide hormones	Corticotrophin (ACTH) Human chorionic gonadotrophin Erythropoietin

Box 46.1 **Restricted products**

- Alcohol
- Marijuana
- Local anaesthetic agents
- Corticosteroids (inhaled, topical or intra-articular administration is allowed).

For further information, see Ch. 46 in *Emergency Care: A Textbook for Paramedics.*

CHAPTER 47

Rescue from remote places

Rescue teams require specialist training, equipment and physical conditioning for working in the remote or austere environments. Paramedics must be fully trained team members, otherwise they may become a liability, placing the other team members at risk. At other times, such as on expeditions, paramedics may have to work alone using their own resources.

> Your medical skills are of value only if your physical fitness and specialist training are appropriate

Remote locations

- Mountain rescue
- Cave rescue
- Ski patrolling
- The Lifeboat service
- Search and rescue helicopters
- Remote industrial and agricultural sites
- Expeditions.

Box 47.1 **Conditions commonly seen in remote rescue situations**

- Environmental injuries: hypo- and hyperthermia
- Dehydration
- Fatigue
- Any physical illness including myocardial infarction
- Near drowning
- Multisystem trauma resulting from falls
- Limb fractures and knee/ankle sprains
- Spinal fractures
- Skull fractures
- Burns.

Planning

A risk analysis and review of any previous audit or reports will help to identify the most common problem areas that a paramedic may face in a particular environment.
Find out:

- The precise location of the incident
- The type of incident and its cause
- Any potential or real hazards
- Access to the casualty with possible approach routes
- Number of casualties.

Much of the planning process used in the Major Incident Medical Management and Support (MIMMS) system of incident management is still applicable to remote rescue.

Box 47.2 **Planning factors in rescue situations**

- Command and control
- Safety
- Communication
- Assessment
- Triage
- Treatment
- Means of evacuation (transport).

Mountain rescue in this country is undertaken by teams of volunteers, many of whom will possess advanced first-aid skills

- A doctor may or may not take part in the actual rescue work but will frequently provide advice to the team via radio
- Mountain rescue teams will usually provide or perform:
  - Cervical, full-spinal and limb splintage
  - Intravenous access
  - Control of external haemorrhage
  - Intravenous fluids
  - Wound dressings
  - Monitoring
  - Oxygen
  - Analgesia including administration of morphine
- Whenever conditions permit, the patient will be evacuated on a special mountain rescue stretcher; UK devices include the McInnes mark 5 and Bell stretchers
- The MIBS stretcher is finding favour because of its portability and relatively compact design
- If the team carries a vacuum mattress the patient should be enclosed in this before being put into the mountain rescue stretcher
- The handover to the ambulance crew will be the first opportunity for a more detailed patient survey
- Special consideration should be given to the possibility that the patient may be hypothermic, since rough handling can induce a cardiac arrhythmia
- Sufficient clothing should only be removed to allow the necessary examination, lest further lowering of core temperature results
- A hypothermic patient cannot be certified dead until they have been taken to hospital and rewarming attempted.

Altitude

When deploying to altitudes of 10 000 feet (3000 m) and above, altitude sickness is a potential problem. Prevention is easy to achieve and the paramedic should be actively involved in the planning of trips to altitude.

The rate of ascent should be no more than 300 m (1000 feet) per day, preferably with a rest day every 3 days. The aim is to climb high during the day and sleep low. If chemoprophylaxis is desired then acetazolamide (Diamox) should be taken, 250 mg slow release daily. Paraesthesia is a common side-effect. There are three forms of high-altitude illness:

1. Acute mountain sickness (AMS)
2. High-altitude pulmonary oedema (HAPE)
3. High-altitude cerebral oedema (HACE)

- HACE can be considered the endpoint of untreated AMS
- HAPE is usually considered a separate illness, but can be preceded by AMS
- AMS commonly affects otherwise fit and healthy individuals who ascend rapidly to altitude. In general, the symptoms will disappear after 5 days provided no further ascent is made
- HAPE occurs in up to 10% of those ascending very rapidly to 4500 m. It typically presents with dyspnoea on exertion and reduced exercise tolerance. Symptoms may progress to dyspnoea at rest and particularly at night
- AMS precedes HACE and the typical feature is ataxia and confusion. Any ataxic and unwell person at altitude should be considered to be suffering from HACE until proven otherwise
- If altitude sickness is suspected, no further ascent should be made. Typically, symptoms settle after 24–48 hours of rest. If symptoms progress or there are any symptoms of HAPE, descent is essential
- Oxygen, nifedipine, dexamethasone and recompression bags all have a useful place in management, but descending back below the level at which symptoms began is the only effective treatment.

Symptoms of acute mountain sickness (AMS):

- Headache
- Nausea
- Vomiting
- Lethargy
- Disturbed sleep.

Cave rescue

Many of the difficulties encountered in mountain rescue also apply to cave rescue. Additional complications arise because of the physical environment: narrow tunnels, waterfalls, sumps, flash floods and underground lakes.

These dangers, combined with navigation difficulties, low temperatures and the total absence of ambient light, make cave rescue especially hazardous.

- Common problems include falls and the medical complications of diving
- Hypothermia is frequent and patients should be left in their wetsuit and wrapped in an exposure bag before being put on a suitable stretcher such as a Stokes litter or a Neil Robertson stretcher
- Remember that an injured person who has been diving should not be given nitrous oxide/oxygen mixtures (Entonox).

The injured diver must never be given Entonox

Ski patrolling

The first layer of planned medical provision on ski slopes is provided by ski patrollers.

In the UK, such persons may well be members of the British Association of Ski Patrollers and this organisation runs courses in advanced first aid.

- Hypothermia and fractures and soft tissue injuries of the lower limb are prevalent
- Extremities showing signs of possible frostbite should not be actively rewarmed during the transportation phase.

The lifeboat service

Rescue around the coasts and seas of the UK and Ireland is efficiently organised by a combined operation involving statutory organisations, voluntary bodies and the armed forces.

- The Royal National Lifeboat Institution (RNLI) responds to approximately 6000 calls per year
- Each lifeboat station has a lifeboat doctor known as the station honorary medical adviser (SHMA)
- The SHMA undertakes a variety of duties, including advising on the health of the crew and first-aid training, and is encouraged to attend regular exercises and go to sea as part of the lifeboat crew
- Provision is also made for any member of a lifeboat crew who has paramedical skills to have access to appropriate equipment and to make use of these skills when on a rescue
- Special reference is given to prolonged care and monitoring of the rescued as it may take a considerable time for such persons to reach hospital
- Lifeboats usually carry a basket stretcher and a Neil Robertson stretcher.

Search and rescue helicopters

Search and rescue (SAR) helicopter services are currently provided in the UK by the Royal Navy and Royal Air Force, although civilian contracts are likely in the future.

- Requests for helicopters are usually made via the police
- The crewman and winch operator will have had advanced first-aid training
- When carrying out SAR over mountainous terrain, helicopters may be used to deliver mountain rescue personnel to the accident location

- Equipment available on air–sea rescue helicopters:
  - First-aid kit
  - Drug box
  - Laerdal suction apparatus
  - PneuPAC-type ventilator
  - Nitrous oxide inhalation (Entonox)
  - Traction splints
  - Pneumatic anti-shock garment (PASG).

Remote industrial or agricultural sites

Certain types of work such as quarrying, oil drilling, fish farming, forestry and estate management take place in remote areas, requiring a lengthy journey to hospital.

- Different sites and companies will have a wide variation in their provision of on-site medical support
- Sites with special hazards, e.g. oil rigs, will have a nurse or paramedic with extended skills directed to the particular problems of their working environment
- These sites will have access to equipment such as survival bags, stretchers, splints, rigid cervical collars, resuscitators, nitrous oxide (Entonox), oxygen and manual suction equipment
- If cyanide is used a dicobalt edetate (Kelocyanor) kit should also be available.

For further information, see Ch. 47 in *Emergency Care: A Textbook for Paramedics.*

CHAPTER 48

Aeromedical evacuation

Medical aviation is now extremely sophisticated and can be conveniently divided into *primary casualty evacuation* and *secondary patient transfer*. The expertise and equipment required for each are different.

> *Primary casualty evacuation* is the transport of a patient from the site of injury to a receiving hospital

This requires a medical crew which is expert in resuscitation, familiar with pre-hospital hazards and practised in cooperation with other emergency services. Equipment must be robust and specific for urgent interventions which may be required. The level of medical expertise determines the range and type of possible medical intervention. This, in turn, determines the nature of the medical equipment carried and varies greatly between systems. The flexibility of a helicopter system makes it ideal for the primary role, allowing the medical team to take the best possible medical care to the patient's side. The helicopter can be reconfigured to take account of the specific requirements of its role.

> *Secondary patient transfer* is the movement of a patient between hospitals

This requires a medical crew expert in the use of intensive care equipment, monitoring and drugs. Often, transfers occur over long distances and it is usually quicker and more cost-effective to use fixed wing aircraft rather than helicopters for this purpose. This is a specialised subject suited to the intensive care physician and is not normally the province of the paramedic.

Helicopter systems vary widely. Their emphasis may be on patient transport or on medical care or a combination of the two.

Transport

The emphasis is on moving the patient from one location to another. Usually the casualty requires transfer from an incident scene that is remote by virtue of distance or terrain. There may be little medical expertise available (or required by the patient) and the system is cost-effective because it obviates the use of long and difficult land transport.

Treatment

A helicopter can bring together a rare clinical event and the required care provider, e.g. a severe head injury and a neurosurgical unit combining high-quality prehospital care with advanced medical skills, delivered by experienced doctors and paramedics.

Triage

Medical services have seldom been planned logically according to the needs of the resident population. Specialist units may have arisen as a result of historical accident or the enthusiasm of individuals. Aeromedical evacuation may offer the opportunity of ensuring the transfer of a patient to the most appropriate clinical receiving facility.

The medical crew

The crew required depends on the aims and use of the system.

- A team that includes an experienced doctor and paramedic will generally provide all the skills required
- The paramedics contribute their experience in the prehospital environment, familiarity with other emergency services and their procedures and experience in providing medical treatment outside hospital
- The inclusion of an appropriately trained doctor contributes advanced assessment skills and allows critical interventions that may be instantly required to treat the patient, including advanced anaesthetic and surgical skills.

The Helicopter Emergency Medical System (HEMS) is a set of criteria laid down by the Civil Aviation Authority on the operational safety of primary retrieval helicopters. It includes the requirements on training for HEMS crew-members.

Training required of HEMS crew members

Duties in the HEMS role

- Navigation (map reading, flight planning, navigational aid principles and use)
- Operation of radio equipment
- Use of onboard medical equipment
- Preparing the helicopter and specialist medical equipment for subsequent HEMS departure
- Basic understanding of the helicopter type in terms of location and design of normal and emergency systems and equipments
- Crew coordination
- Practice of response to HEMS callout
- Conducting refuelling and rotors running refuelling
- HEMS operating site selection and use
- Techniques for handling patients, the medical consequences of air transport and some knowledge of hospital casualty reception
- Marshalling signals
- Underslung load operations as appropriate
- Winch operations as appropriate
- The dangers to self and others of rotor running helicopters, including loading of patients
- The use of the helicopter intercommunications system.

Helicopters may fly with medically trained personnel who are not HEMS qualified. They are accounted for under CAA regulations and are termed *medical passengers*.

Areas of knowledge required of medical passengers

- Familiarisation with the helicopter types(s) operated
- Entry and exit under normal and emergency conditions for both self and patients
- Use of the relevant onboard specialist medical equipment
- The need for the commander's approval prior to use of specialist equipment
- Method of supervision of other medical staff
- The use of the helicopter intercommunication systems
- Location and use of onboard fire extinguishers.

Safety in helicopter operations

The primary danger when working close to a helicopter comes from the moving blades of the main rotor and the tail rotor. The distance from the ground of both the main rotor blades and the tail rotor varies between helicopter types, with some helicopters having blades that dip at the front and do not allow access. Rotor wash is a further hazard, throwing dust and debris into the air and blowing over light objects.

- Only approach when the rotor blades have completely stopped turning
- Stand apart in front of the helicopter and wait for the 'thumbs up' signal from the pilot before approaching
- If a helicopter must be approached while the rotor blades are still running, it is mandatory to wait well outside the reach of the rotor blades for a direct and unequivocal instruction from the flight crew
- Duck while approaching and do not hold any object such as a drip above shoulder height or carry anything that might blow away
- If you are standing within the rotor wash, turn away and close your eyes.

During starting or slowing of the rotor, the blade tips tend to droop closer to the ground and this effect may be enhanced in high winds. This is always dangerous and a helicopter should never be left or approached during this time. Unequivocal instruction from the pilot is essential. If a helicopter is on a slope, the rotor blades are closer to the ground on the uphill side. The medical team can assist the pilot in maintaining aircraft safety during flight and landing by watching out for hazards. Dark wires stretched across a dark background are particularly difficult to see. *The more pairs of eyes that are on the lookout, the better.*

> Never approach a helicopter until instructed to do so by the aircrew or the rotors have completely stopped turning

Medical teams must be well versed and practised in aircraft safety and evacuation. They must wear suitable fire-retardant clothing and approved flight helmets. Seatbelts or harnesses must be worn throughout the flight and only released when the pilot gives the medical team clearance to leave the aircraft.

Aviation medicine

- Helicopter systems involved with primary casualty evacuation in the UK are unlikely to fly at more than 450 metres and at this sort of altitude, pressure changes have few clinical effects
- Some transport systems do go through large altitude changes, under which circumstances the medical crew must be appropriately trained (e.g. to fill endotracheal tube balloons with water and to treat air-filled cavities prior to flying) and know and watch for the effects of pressure changes
- This is a specialist area (usually involving fixed wing repatriation flights), which is usually practised by an intensive care doctor
- Many subtle physiological changes are produced when a patient travels by helicopter, mainly in the cardiovascular system
- Acceleration and deceleration will act on the patient's blood volume, especially if they are hypovolaemic. These changes are mitigated by adequate fluid resuscitation prior to flying
- The loading of a patient may be affected by the nature of their injuries. A helicopter flies 'nose down', which has the effect of raising the patient's

feet if loaded with the head forwards. This may increase intracranial pressure, therefore head injury patients may be best transported with their feet forwards, to elevate the head.

Working in the helicopter

- Internal space is very limited and access to the patient is difficult
- Noise is usually >90 decibels. Ear protection is mandatory for crew and patient
- Vibration, movement and air sickness. All contribute to crew fatigue
- Helicopters are fragile. Even minor damage may render the helicopter inoperable.

Selection of receiving hospital

- The helicopter can cover large distances in a short time so the prehospital team are able to pick the most appropriate hospital destination for each patient
- Clearly the choice of destination is limited by the availability of landing sites
- Patients with isolated head injury can be taken to a neurosurgical centre thus decreasing the time to neurosurgery (particularly critical in cases of traumatic extradural and subdural haematomas)
- Patients with multi-system trauma should be taken to specialist trauma centres
- Medical problems such as myocardial infarction or stroke are increasingly being dealt with by specialist centres.

For further information, see Ch. 48 in *Emergency Care: A Textbook for Paramedics.*

CHAPTER 49

Childbirth

Childbirth is frequently successful without any intervention from healthcare professionals. The time when a paramedic may have to become involved is in the established second stage of labour, when the journey to hospital is too long to complete before delivery is expected.

> From fertilisation to delivery is normally 266 days or 38 weeks and thus the time from last menstrual period (LMP) to delivery is 280 days or 40 weeks

Definitions

- *Parity* is the number of times that a woman has carried a pregnancy to 24 weeks
- *Gravidity* is the number of times a woman has conceived and been pregnant, regardless of the outcome
- A *primigravida* is a woman who is pregnant for the first time
- A *nullipara* is a woman who has never delivered and a *multipara* (or multip) is a woman who has had two or more deliveries.

> In the third trimester, the inferior vena cava is compressed when the mother lies in the supine position. This must be addressed by manual displacement of the uterus or positioning the patient

Inferior vena cava compression syndrome

In the supine position, the inferior vena cava compression syndrome reduces venous return by as much as 40% and fully efficient basic life support only gives at best 30% of the cardiac output. Thus, the pregnant woman should be nursed in the left lateral position and must be resuscitated in that position. The left lateral position may be achieved by placing a cushion or pillow under the right hip or by a human wedge. The uterus can also be manually displaced to the left.

The normal process of labour

- At any time from 37 weeks to 42 weeks' gestation, labour is said to be at *term*
- Prior to 37 weeks, the labour is *premature* and after 42 weeks, the pregnancy is *prolonged* (*postmature*). Full-term is 40 weeks
- Rupture of the membranes, loss of the mucus plug from the cervix or a 'bloody show' in addition to regular painful uterine contractions constitutes a diagnosis of true labour for the purposes of operational paramedic practice.

Duration of labour

Labour falls into three stages. If in the first stage of labour, there is usually enough time to transport the patient to a maternity unit.

Table 49.1 The stages of labour

	Nulliparous woman	**Multiparous woman**
Stage 1	8–12 h	4–8 h
Stage 2	1–2 h	30–60 min
Stage 3	A few minutes to 1 h	A few minutes to 1 h

The normal delivery

The three stages of labour

First stage

- The first stage of labour takes several hours, during which the cervix (neck) of the uterus effaces and then dilates
- Full dilation is 10 cm and marks the end of the first stage of labour
- The forewaters may rupture, liberating 50 mL or more of watery fluid
- The contractions increase in frequency, rising from one every 20 minutes to one every 4 or 5 minutes.

Second stage

- The second stage of labour lasts from full dilation of the cervix to delivery of the baby
- During the second stage of labour, the baby's head descends into the pelvis and positions itself for delivery, this manifests itself externally as 'crowning'

- The occiput is the first part to deliver, followed by the vertex, forehead and then face
- Just after delivery of the face, the head 'restitutes'; in other words, the neck untwists itself so that the head is in the neutral position relative to the shoulders
- As the shoulders deliver, so the second phase of rotation occurs. The anterior shoulder is the first to deliver followed by the posterior shoulder
- The rest of the trunk follows on by lateral flexion of the spine.

Third stage

- The third stage of delivery is from the delivery of the baby until delivery of the placenta is complete
- It is at this stage that the greatest risk of haemorrhage occurs.

Management of labour

- Make an initial decision whether to transport to hospital: if the baby's head is about to deliver then this will not be possible
- Pay attention to all those factors that can be effectively dealt with, namely: airway, breathing with oxygen, circulation with posture, analgesia with nitrous oxide and oxygen (Entonox)
- The biggest threat to the mother is haemorrhage, so be prepared to obtain intravenous access and administer fluids if necessary
- Obtain a brief history. Many women now carry their own complete maternity record with them. The layout varies from district to district
- Establish the patient's estimated date of delivery (EDD) and ask if her waters have broken or whether she has had a 'bloody show' (signs of early labour)
- Details of her pains should be sought, asking specifically:
    1. How long have you had the pains?
    2. Where are the pains?
    3. Are the pains getting worse or staying the same?
    4. Are the pains becoming more frequent. If so, how frequent are they?
    5. Are the pains lasting longer each time there is a pain?
- This should allow you to diagnose true labour and the stage
- Any urge to defecate indicates rectal compression from late second-stage labour
- Useful past medical history includes whether she has had previous caesarean sections and how long previous deliveries have taken
- Permission should be sought to examine the woman's abdomen and to inspect (*not* palpate) the woman's perineum, while giving an explanation of what is going on (e.g. palpation of the abdomen for contractions and observation of the perineum for evidence of the waters having gone or any evidence of crowning)

- Unless the woman is in the later stage of labour, plan to transport her to hospital swiftly in the left lateral position.

Prolonged transfers

In remote situations, it is important to think laterally. There may be alternatives to delivering in the back of the ambulance, so call for help and arrange an alternative destination as soon as possible if there is sufficient time to move the mother but not enough time to reach a district general hospital. There are many possibilities for providing somewhere in which to conduct a delivery that is more spacious, warmer and better lit than the back of an ambulance. There are also many potential sources of experienced staff. Medical and midwifery back-up should be arranged via ambulance control. Helicopter ambulances are unsafe for delivery so should not be used. The partner or a female friend can be assigned the task of chaperone and assistant.

Preparation for delivery

1. **Call for help** – a local doctor or community midwife may be available to help
2. **Preparation of the environment** – somewhere warm and private, locate the maternity pack and some absorbent pads. Keep the mother warm and have towels available to dry the baby
3. **Preparation of the equipment** – bring the maternity pack, paramedic case, oxygen and Entonox from the ambulance. Consider pre-emptive cannulation of the mother
4. **Personal preparation** – the arms should be bare below the elbows and washed. Put the gown on if it is provided in the pack and wear sterile gloves
5. **Preparation of the mother** – position the mother supine, if possible the perineum should be washed with soap and water or chlorhexidine 0.1%. The mother should be draped with sterile towels leaving the perineum exposed. Brief her on the use of Entonox.

The delivery

- While preparing, and in order to slow the delivery, the woman should be instructed to pant during pains as this will prevent her from bearing down. If she wishes to use her hands to pull her knees back onto her chest, this can be beneficial
- Because of the pain, the woman should be encouraged to use the Entonox
- If delivery of the head is not controlled, there is a risk of perineal tears (a doctor trained in obstetrics or a midwife may consider performing an episiotomy to prevent uncontrolled tears of the perineum)
- Taking a gauze pad, preferably soaked in antiseptic, hold it against the anus, allowing the first web space of the right hand to support the perineum with the thumb and forefinger each lying in a groin crease

- Careful gentle pressure on the perineum will allow the head to deliver in a slow, controlled manner with the aim of the head delivering between labour pains
- Once the head has delivered, it should be quickly supported and the neck felt to see whether the umbilical cord is wrapped around the neck. If it is, the first thing to do is to try to slip the loop of cord off over the head. If this fails, the cord should be clamped twice, cut between the clamps and unwound from around the neck
- Do not put traction on the baby's head. Wipe the baby's nose and mop fluid from the mouth. At the next contraction, the baby's head should be gently guided downward. This is more of a lowering manoeuvre, causing the anterior shoulder to deliver
- Then, the baby is raised and the posterior shoulder will deliver rapidly, followed by the rest of the trunk and legs
- The baby should be allowed to lie on the bed and be wrapped in a towel
- Once the baby has cried and the cord has ceased pulsating, the umbilical cord is clamped twice and cut between the clamps, close to the opening of the vagina
- If the baby requires resuscitation, this should be carried out immediately. If the baby is pinking up well and breathing, it must be dried off to prevent heat loss, wrapped in a dry towel which covers the head and given to the mother.

Syntometrine

- Paramedics who have completed emergency domestic obstetrics training may administer intramuscular Syntometrine which contains oxytocin 5 units and ergometrine 0.5 mg
- The oxytocin provokes marked uterine contraction after approximately 3 minutes but is short-lived
- As its effects begin to wear off, the ergometrine begins to act and provides longer-lasting uterine contractions, reducing the risk of postpartum haemorrhage.

Managing the third stage

- The third stage of labour is from the delivery of the baby to delivery of the placenta and usually takes 5–20 minutes
- A delay beyond 1 hour is by definition a retained placenta, which is an obstetric emergency requiring a transfer to an obstetric unit where anaesthetic services are available
- The mother will usually expel the placenta which should be put into a polythene bag for inspection by the doctor or midwife or at hospital, who will check to confirm it is complete. It is at this stage that the risk of haemorrhage is greatest in the absence of Syntometrine administration, hence it is advisable to have an IV line *in situ*

- After the placenta has delivered, bleeding may occur from either the uterus or the perineum or from damage to other structures in the birth canal. A clean pad should be placed over the vagina. If the arrival of a doctor or midwife is not imminent, there is a clear case for moving the woman to hospital but there is no great urgency unless she continues to bleed
- If there is postpartum bleeding, then administer Syntometrine, as it is an effective method of haemorrhage control. Start IV fluids and transfer urgently to hospital.

Other birth presentations

- 3% of all deliveries are breech (bottom first)
- 0.3% of all deliveries are shoulder presentation
- 0.3% are face presentations
- 0.1% are brow presentations.

Malpresentations almost always require the skills of an obstetrician.

Breech presentation

- If you are forced to deliver a breech presentation, the initial approach is exactly the same
- Having called for help, two intravenous lines should be inserted and the mother helped into the supported squatting, kneeling or standing position
- Gravity can be used to assist a more exhausting process of delivery. If left to nature, the baby will normally deliver quite easily and should not be interfered with except to support it when free of the birth canal
- Keep watch for a prolapsed cord where the umbilical cord drops out ahead of the baby
- The baby should be allowed to deliver without interference until the nape of its neck clears the pubic arch. The baby is then grasped by the feet with one hand and lifted vertically upwards and the head will deliver
- The third stage of labour is unchanged
- Transfer to an obstetrician is preferred as the delivery may require instrumentation such as forceps or become obstructed.

Multiple delivery

Twins occur in about 1 in 80 pregnancies. Complications are much more likely, so every effort should be made to get to an obstetric unit. Each twin can be delivered independently as above but do not administer Syntometrine until the second twin is delivered.

Prolapsed umbilical cord

- Prolapsed umbilical cord is an obstetric emergency and occurs when the cord drops out of the uterus into the vagina or even outside the body ahead of the presenting part
- The blood supply to the fetus is likely to be cut off
- Often cord prolapse occurs for one of the following reasons:
  - Unusual fetal presentation, e.g. footling breech or transverse lie
  - Premature or abnormal fetus
  - Multiple pregnancy
  - Polyhydramnios (a condition where there is excessive amniotic fluid)
  - Placenta praevia
- Obtain either gauze pads or towels soaked in warm saline and gently replace the cord as far into the vagina as possible, with the minimum of handling. It may be possible to apply pressure against the fetus if it is compressing the cord
- Pressure with a gloved hand should be maintained all the way to hospital
- The most practical manner of transportation will be with the patient in the left lateral position.

Cord rupture

- This may be as a result of a short cord (<40 cm) or excessive traction on the cord
- Cord rupture can result in an exsanguinating haemorrhage for the baby
- If a rupture does occur, place a cord clamp between the tear and the baby.

Shoulder dystocia

- This is a very serious but fortunately rare adverse event that can occur during the second stage of labour. Following delivery of the head, labour fails to progress and the neck and shoulders do not become visible
- This is a time-critical emergency, as the baby can die within 10 minutes if delivery cannot be completed. It should be managed according to 'the rule of twos' with respect to the number of contractions between each step. If delivery of the shoulders does not occur within *two* contractions of delivery of the head:
  1. Get a message to the obstetric unit and inform them that you are managing a patient with suspected shoulder dystocia
  2. Place the patient on her back with her knees drawn upwards as far as possible and turned outwards (McRobert's position)
  3. If the delivery does not progress after *two* contractions in the McRobert's position, apply suprapubic pressure with the aim of pushing/rotating the anterior shoulder under the pelvic arch:

a. Keeping the mother in McRobert's position, position yourself vertically over the patient's abdomen at their left side
b. Keep your elbows locked straight, with the heel of one hand over the symphysis, with the other hand on top
c. Push down firmly and away from you (but do not administer a blow)
d. Discontinue suprapubic pressure if labour does not progress with *two* further contractions but maintain McRobert's position.

4. You must now decide on the most rapid way for getting skilled obstetric help for the mother; either transportation to the hospital or waiting at the scene for the midwife/GP. Regardless of your decision, contact the *senior* on-call obstetrician for further advice, *en route* to hospital if necessary.

Primary postpartum haemorrhage

Primary postpartum haemorrhage (PPH) is defined as blood loss of 500 mL or more within 24 hours of delivery. It occurs most commonly with delivery of the placenta. The common causes of PPH are atony of uterine muscle, which prevents the process of vascular constriction after separation of the placenta; retained placenta (or placental parts) and trauma to the genital tract.

Tears should be managed by direct pressure. If bleeding is severe and is secondary to uterine atony or suspected retention of placental tissue, give Syntometrine. High concentration oxygen should be administered and IV fluid replacement considered.

For further information, see Ch. 50 in *Emergency Care: A Textbook for Paramedics*.

CHAPTER 50

Emergencies in pregnancy

Pregnancy should be considered in any woman of reproductive age. Not every woman will admit, or even realise, that she is pregnant. There are medical conditions and emergencies specific to the pregnant state as well as general emergencies such as asthma or epilepsy that can occur in any patient.

Vaginal bleeding and abdominal pain in early pregnancy

- Consider pregnancy in any woman of childbearing age
- If the LMP was more than 4 weeks prior to the current date, then the patient should be considered to be pregnant until proven otherwise
- Measure the pulse, blood pressure and respiratory rate to assess whether the patient is clinically hypovolaemic and if so, obtain IV access and administer fluids
- The most frequent cause of vaginal bleeding, with or without abdominal pain, early in pregnancy, is miscarriage
- The most dangerous cause of vaginal bleeding and abdominal pain is ectopic pregnancy and this should be considered in any woman of reproductive age complaining of abdominal pain, especially if this is associated with collapse.

> Abdominal pain and vaginal bleeding in early pregnancy: think of miscarriage and ectopic pregnancy

Miscarriage

- Approximately 10–15% of confirmed pregnancies end in miscarriage
- This occurs most often at either 8 weeks or 12 weeks from the first day of the LMP
- Miscarriage may rarely cause significant uterine bleeding, resulting in hypovolaemic shock
- Avoid the term *abortion* as this may be misinterpreted by the parents:
  1. Threatened miscarriage – vaginal bleeding with cramping abdominal pain, however the cervix remains closed and the pregnancy may continue
  2. Incomplete miscarriage – vaginal bleeding may be heavy, the cervix is open and abdominal pain is caused by uterine contractions, which have begun to expel the products of conception
  3. Complete miscarriage – products are completely expelled through an open cervix.

Management

- Gentle handling and reassurance are very important during the initial assessment
- Transfer to hospital for more detailed examination and management
- Manage hypovolaemia if present
- In hospital, the patient will likely have an ultrasound arranged to check the viability of the pregnancy.

Ectopic pregnancy

- Ectopic pregnancy is the most life-threatening of the early complications of pregnancy
- The incidence of ectopic pregnancy is approximately 1% of all pregnancies and is increasing. Ruptured ectopic pregnancies account for 13% of maternal deaths
- An ectopic pregnancy normally occurs in one or other of the fallopian tubes.

Symptoms and signs

- Most tubal ectopic pregnancies present 5–8 weeks after the LMP
- Pain is typically the first symptom, occurring in up to 95% of patients, and 75% complain of abnormal vaginal bleeding (such as 'spotting')
- The patient may present in a state of collapse secondary to hypovolaemic shock.

Management

- Manage shock aggressively with oxygen, two large-bore IV cannulae and fluid resuscitation
- Transfer rapidly to hospital as the definitive management is surgery.

Table 50.1 Differential diagnosis of miscarriage and ectopic pregnancy

	Miscarriage	**Ectopic pregnancy**
Timing	5–12 weeks	5–8 weeks
Abdominal pain	Central and cramping	May be unilateral
Pain in relation to bleeding	Follows	Precedes
Vaginal bleeding	Frank May be heavy	Normally scanty Dark brown
Haemodynamic status	Shock rare	Shock common

Vaginal bleeding and abdominal pain in later pregnancy

Third-trimester vaginal bleeding (antepartum haemorrhage) is bleeding that occurs after 28 weeks of pregnancy. It occurs in approximately 4% of pregnancies. All patients require assessment in hospital.

> Abdominal pain and vaginal bleeding in later pregnancy: think of placental abruption and placenta praevia

Placental abruption

- Placental abruption is the separation of a normally located placenta before delivery of the fetus. Bleeding occurs and the blood is initially confined between the placenta and the uterine wall
- There may be simply abdominal pain, however severe cases can present with painful vaginal bleeding associated with a tender, contracting uterus, shock and fetal compromise
- Give oxygen and manage shock with intravenous fluid resuscitation
- If the patient has deteriorating vital signs in transit, then appropriate warning to the receiving obstetric unit should be given enabling staff to prepare for urgent delivery of the baby.

Placenta praevia

- Placenta praevia occurs when the placenta is implanted in the lower uterine segment and subsequent separation will cause blood loss into the vagina

- Patients present with vaginal bleeding, which may be heavy, but may have little or no abdominal pain. The patient should be transferred urgently to hospital for full assessment
- Give oxygen and consider the need for IV fluids.

Eclampsia

- A degree of hypertension occurs in approximately 8% of pregnancies
- The most severe manifestation is *eclampsia*, in which a combination of hypertension, cerebral oedema, intracerebral haemorrhage and seizures
- Eclampsia results in the death of about 1000 babies and 10 women each year in the UK
- Patients usually have a known history of hypertension earlier in their pregnancy
- On examination, the patient may be fitting, will be hypertensive and will have peripheral oedema.

Box 50.1 **Clinical features of eclampsia**

- Hypertension
- Cerebral oedema and haemorrhage
- Seizures
- Headaches
- Visual disturbance
- Weight gain and peripheral oedema
- Abdominal pain.

Management

- Urgent transfer to hospital is essential, since definitive treatment requires urgent delivery of the baby
- If there is fitting, the first priority is to establish an airway and administer oxygen. In a fitting patient the most practical means of achieving an airway may be the nasopharyngeal route
- Intravenous or rectal diazepam (10–20 mg) should be given in an attempt to terminate the seizures
- Alert the receiving unit that you are arriving with a pregnant patient with seizures.

Common general medical emergencies in pregnancy

Common sense and first principles apply and these are the same whether the patient is pregnant or not.

Asthma

The effect of pregnancy on asthma is variable. The majority of patients experience less frequent attacks, but a few experience more frequent attacks. Asthma has no effect on the course of pregnancy. The management of an acute exacerbation is the same as in a non-pregnant woman, with oxygen, nebulised salbutamol and transfer to hospital for assessment.

Epilepsy

Seizures may occur in pregnancy unrelated to hypertension, simply as a manifestation of pre-existing epilepsy. Treatment regimens may have been modified prior to or early in pregnancy, in order to avoid fetal damage, and control may have been lost. Management of seizures is conventional and consists of prevention of harm to the patient during a seizure, attention to the airway, administration of oxygen, diazepam if the fit is prolonged, and transfer to hospital.

Diabetes mellitus

When a diabetic woman becomes pregnant, close attention is required to maintain good control of the disease throughout the pregnancy. Hypoglycaemic and hyperglycaemic emergencies may occur and will be rapidly identified clinically using a glucose reagent strip. Standard protocols for control of hypoglycaemia should be followed (Hypostop gel, IV glucose, IM glucagon). Patients with hyperglycaemic emergencies should receive oxygen and fluid resuscitation with normal saline, and be transferred immediately to hospital.

For further information, see Ch. 51 in *Emergency Care: A Textbook for Paramedics*.

CHAPTER 51

Trauma in pregnancy

The approach to the pregnant trauma victim is exactly the same as for the non-pregnant trauma victim, except that there are two patients – mother and fetus – to consider.

The mother is treated directly, the fetus is treated indirectly by optimum resuscitation of the mother. The best chance for the fetus is optimum resuscitation of the mother.

Because the mother has reduced oxygen reserves, the spontaneously breathing pregnant trauma victim must *always* receive oxygen at as high a concentration as possible, preferably close to 100%, via a reservoir face mask.

> Always administer high-flow oxygen

The approach to the pregnant trauma victim

The 'SAFE' approach and immediate management of life-threatening injuries is the same for all trauma patients.

Maternal clinical signs of hypovolaemia and haemorrhage present too late to save the fetus in 80% of cases so maintain a high index of suspicion. Treatment precedes formal diagnosis.

> If there is ANY possibility of significant trauma immediate evacuation is essential

- High flow oxygen should be applied immediately or early intubation if unconscious
- Position the patient for relief of vena caval compression
- Do not attempt formal examination of the perineum, however do try and check for bleeding or fluid loss from this area
- An attempt should be made to palpate the abdomen, checking for fetal parts, movements and the fetal heart rate if possible. Undue time must not be wasted on this part of the assessment
- Evacuate rapidly to hospital.

Consequences of trauma in pregnancy

- A pregnant woman sustaining *any* trauma to the abdomen and pelvis, however minor, requires specialist assessment and observation at hospital
- Even small degrees of abdominal trauma can cause the maternal circulation to be contaminated by fetal red blood cells. As a consequence, maternal antibody formation against fetal red cells may result in fetal anaemia and problems with future pregnancies.

Blunt trauma

- Blunt trauma to the abdomen and pelvis is more common than penetrating trauma in UK practice, and in the pregnant woman is most often caused by:
  1. Road traffic collisions
  2. Falls
  3. Assaults
- The three most common pathological mechanisms in blunt abdomino-pelvic trauma in the pregnant mother are:
  1. Placental abruption
  2. Uterine rupture
  3. Pelvic fracture
- In each, both mother and fetus may die from unrecognised, often concealed, hypovolaemic shock resulting from haemorrhage.

Placental abruption

- Placental abruption occurs in as many as 5% of episodes of minor trauma and 50% of major trauma cases, and can present up to 48 hours after trauma
- Direct trauma to the abdominal wall transmitted to the uterus, or deceleration forces applied to the body as a whole causes the placenta to shear off the uterine wall
- Haemorrhage occurs between the placenta and the uterine wall and may be concealed or revealed (per vaginam)
- Premature labour may be precipitated by placental abruption.

Uterine rupture

- Uterine rupture requires considerable direct force and will almost inevitably be associated with other life-threatening injuries
- Signs of uterine rupture include maternal shock, fetal bradycardia (or absence of fetal heart sounds) and obvious palpable fetal parts on abdominal examination. There may or may not be vaginal bleeding or abdominal pain.

Pelvic fracture

- Internal bleeding from pelvic fractures is difficult to control
- The usual causes of pelvic fractures are falls from a height and road traffic accidents
- The signs are those of massive or progressive maternal haemorrhagic shock
- Apply a pelvic splint, taking care not to compress the abdomen
- Copious IV fluids will be indicated in order to prevent or reduce maternal hypotension.

> There must be no delays in getting to hospital

Penetrating trauma

- In the UK, stab wounds are more common than gunshot wounds
- The usual outcome in significant abdominal injuries is fetal death with maternal survival
- The approach is the same as for the non-pregnant woman, with a continuous watch for concealed haemorrhage and the possibility of time-critical but concealed injury to other organs
- Attention to ABC and rapid transport are essential.

Burns

- The management of pregnant patients with burns is exactly the same as for non-pregnant patients, except that they must be taken to a facility where caesarean section can be performed. Once the patient is removed to a safe environment the use of humidified oxygen and early intubation are essential
- Because of the metabolic and fluid requirements of the pregnant and burnt woman, delivery by caesarean section is often the only option
- The mortality rates in pregnant women depend on the body surface area burnt: in those with burns of 33–66% of body surface area, survival will depend crucially on the early management of hypoxia and hypovolaemia.

Summary

- Haemorrhage is frequently concealed in the pregnant victim and hypovolaemic shock is inevitably severe once the signs manifest
- Intravenous fluid therapy should aim to avoid the development of maternal hypotension
- Failure to relieve vena caval-compression can kill both mother and fetus
- The pregnant trauma victim should always be considered to have time-critical injuries and be transported to a surgical facility quickly
- Obstetric and gynaecological diagnoses need not be made in the field.

For further information, see Ch. 52 in *Emergency Care: A Textbook for Paramedics*.

CHAPTER 52

Neonatal resuscitation and transport

Cardiac arrest in a neonate (a baby less than 1 month old) may present from:

- A planned home delivery
- An unplanned birth before arrival in hospital
- An infant who has a normal birth and is discharged home and thereafter becomes ill.

> The general principles remain the same:
> Support of airway (A), breathing (B) and circulation (C).

Neonatal resuscitation

In most instances, the baby born outside hospital will not require any advanced interventions. If the baby is active with a normal respiratory rate and heart rate, then the only treatment required will be to dry and warm the baby, and to use suction as required. A small number of babies will require more active resuscitative measures. Hypothermia is very common and must be avoided, as it leads to poor outcomes.

Meconium

- Fetal distress during labour leads to contamination of the amniotic fluid with meconium from the baby's gastrointestinal tract
- Wait for the baby to be fully born before applying suction

- The baby will require careful suction after the body is delivered to ensure that no further meconium is aspirated into the trachea and lower airways: the morbidity and mortality rates from meconium aspiration syndrome remain high.

Apgar scores

Table 52.1 Apgar scoring			
Sign	**0**	**1**	**2**
Heart rate (bpm)	Absent	Slow (<100)	>100
Respirations	Absent	Slow, irregular	Good, crying
Muscle tone	Limp	Some flexion	Active motion
Reflex irritability (catheter in nares)	No response	Grimace	Cough or sneeze
Colour	Blue or pale	Pink body with blue extremities	Completely pink

This system assesses the baby's overall condition at 1 minute and 5 minutes after birth and later if required. Resuscitative measures should be started immediately, however, and not delayed for evaluation of the Apgar score.

Neonatal basic life support

- The first measure is to stimulate the child. This occurs during drying and warming, and by suctioning of the nasopharyngeal and oropharyngeal passages
- This is often enough to increase the child's respiratory rate which, as a result of better oxygenation, increases the cardiac rate
- If, after a short period of stimulation, the clinical situation remains grave, the next measure is to maintain the airway by placing the baby in a supine position with the neck in a neutral position, thus avoiding hyperextension (a folded towel under the shoulder can facilitate this)
- Supplemental oxygen via a face mask can be applied, with further suction if copious secretions are present. Again, the hoped-for result is improved respiratory effort and consequently increased cardiac output
- If the neonate fails to respond to these measures it will be necessary to ventilate the baby using a self-inflating bag and mask
- For the neonate, the smallest self-inflating bag is used (usually 240 mL capacity). Care needs to be taken not to overinflate the lungs

- The paramedic should ventilate at a rate of 60 breaths/min for approximately 15–30 seconds. In a newborn, the first few breaths are 'inflation' breaths
- The pulse is then checked and if the brachial or femoral pulse rate remains at less than 60/min then chest compressions are started
- The most efficient method of delivering chest compressions is to grip the chest in such a way that the two thumbs can press on the lower third of the sternum, just below an imaginary line joining the nipples, with the fingers over the spine at the back. Compress the chest quickly and firmly reducing the diameter of the chest by one-third
- The sternum should be compressed 100–120 times per minute. The cycle for chest compressions to ventilation is 3 to 1 for a neonate.

> Neonatal CPR: 3 compressions to 1 ventilation

Neonatal advanced life support

- If the neonate fails to respond or indeed goes into full cardiopulmonary arrest, more advanced life support techniques are needed
- The paramedic may elect to intubate the child to improve ventilation and to secure the airway against inhalation
- The usual size of an ET tube for a full-term baby is 3–3.5 mm.

> ET tube size for a full-term baby: 3 or 3.5 mm (uncuffed)

- The next step is to achieve vascular access either through a peripheral vein or by insertion of an intraosseous needle into the tibia
- Adrenaline is given in asystole or profound bradycardia at a dose of 0.01 mg/kg (0.1 mL/kg) of adrenaline 1 in 10 000 solution intravenously or by the intraosseous route.

> Adrenaline dose in neonates is 0.1 mL/kg of 1 in 10 000 solution IV or IO

- In addition to drugs, it is sometimes necessary to give the neonate a fluid challenge of 10–20 mL/kg of normal saline. This treatment is usually carried out during urgent evacuation to hospital
- Care should be taken to maintain the child's temperature, e.g. by using warm blankets. Always remember to cover the head as well as the body. The back of the ambulance should be kept very warm (uncomfortably hot for the adults).

Newborn Life Support

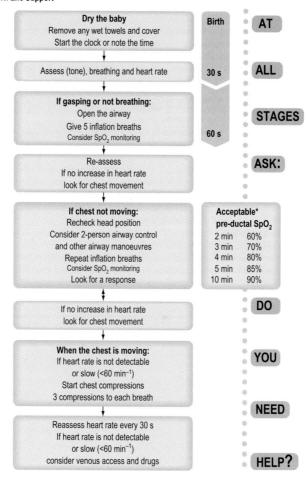

Figure 52.1 Newborn Life Support algorithm (Resuscitation Council UK). The authors are aware of impending changes in resuscitation guidelines (late 2010). Refer to www.resus.org .uk for further up-to-date information.

Neonatal transport

- Neonatal transfers are common between district general hospitals and specialist neonatal or paediatric units
- Nursing staff and doctors from the peripheral hospital will usually travel with the neonate however some regions send out specialist retrieval teams
- The most important point is that the neonate should be stable prior to transfer
- The whole transfer should be well planned by the sending and the receiving hospitals, so that it is known in advance to which part of the receiving hospital the child is to be taken
- Incubators are used to maintain the child's temperature during the transfer and possibly to provide ventilation of the neonate
- The incubator operates on a battery supply and requires the use of cylinders of oxygen and air for ventilation. When preparing for such a transfer, it is mandatory to check that sufficient oxygen and battery life are available for the intended journey, allowing some leeway for unforeseen delays or detours
- Most modern incubators can be plugged into the ambulance electrical system, although it is necessary to check that this is the case
- The transport team must have the necessary equipment and drugs available in case the child deteriorates *en route*
- Facilities for procedures such as reintubation and any other resuscitation techniques such as the reinsertion of intravenous access must be available
- There must be at least one person who can carry out cardiopulmonary resuscitation of the neonate before embarking on the journey.

For further information, see Ch.53 in *Emergency Care: A Textbook for Paramedics*.

CHAPTER 53

Substance abuse

Alcohol dependence

Of the UK population, 2% suffer from alcohol dependence syndrome at any time.

Dependence is most common in:

- Those aged 40–54 years
- The divorced and separated
- Those who have never been married
- Publicans, doctors, journalists and senior businessmen are most vulnerable.

Factors increasing risk of dependence include:

- Cheap or easily available alcohol
- Unsupervised work routine
- Unsociable working hours
- Work involving separation from family or other stabilising social constraints.

Effects of alcohol

Psychological effects of alcohol

- Hallucinations of voices (alcoholic hallucinosis), which are usually derogatory in content, may occur in clear consciousness
- Depressive symptoms occur in 90% of people with alcoholism and there is a 10–15% risk of completed suicide associated with alcoholism
- Pathological jealousy manifests as a morbid delusional belief that a partner is being unfaithful and may put the partner at risk of serious violence.

Box 53.1 **Effects of alcohol on the gastrointestinal tract**

- Liver damage
- Alcoholic hepatitis
- Fatty liver
- Cirrhosis
- Liver failure and hepatic encephalopathy
- Oesophagitis and gastritis causing vomiting and retching
- Mallory–Weiss tear in lower oesophagus causing haematemesis
- Portal hypertension causing oesophageal varices and possible massive haematemesis
- Peptic ulceration
- Acute and chronic pancreatitis (acute has a mortality of 10–40%)
- Carcinoma of upper gastrointestinal tract.

Box 53.2 **Effects of alcohol on the cardiovascular system**

- Cardiac arrhythmias
- Cardiomyopathy
- Coronary artery disease
- Hypertension
- Cerebrovascular accident.

Box 53.3 **Metabolic and haematological effects of alcohol**

Metabolic

- Hypoglycaemia
- Ketoacidosis.

Haematological

- Anaemia
- Thrombocytopenia.

Box 53.4 **The effects of alcohol on the nervous system**

- Diffuse brain damage from cortical shrinkage and ventricular dilation
- Alcoholic dementia
- Wernicke–Korsakoff syndrome
- Seizures from alcohol withdrawal.

Wernicke–Korsakoff syndrome is caused by deficiency of thiamine (vitamin B1).

In acute Wernicke's encephalopathy, symptoms include alteration in level of consciousness, nystagmus, external ophthalmoplegia, ataxia and peripheral neuropathy.

Alcoholics are frequently prescribed oral thiamine and given IV thiamine preparations in hospital.

Medical emergencies specifically related to alcohol

Acute intoxication

Acute intoxication may lead to physical injury from trauma or head injury and predisposes to hypoglycaemia.

> Alcohol alone should never be accepted as a cause of reduced or lost consciousness

Acute alcohol withdrawal

Acute alcohol withdrawal occurs in the dependent state and is characterised by:

- Nausea
- Vomiting
- Tremors
- Excessive sweating
- Tachycardia.

It may begin within 6 hours of cessation or reduction of alcohol and peaks by 48 hours, subsiding over the next 7 days. It can be associated with withdrawal grand mal epileptic seizures 12–24 hours after drinking.

Delirium tremens

Delirium tremens ('the DTs') occurs on days 3–5 following cessation or significant reduction of drinking in an alcohol-dependent person. It is characterised by:

- Confusion
- Disorientation
- Delusions
- Hallucinations
- Vivid imagery (often insects but not the pink elephants of popular belief)
- Intense tremulousness.

There is often a marked lability of emotions and autonomic dysfunction. There is no craving for alcohol. Admission to a medical ward for rehydration, sedation and nutrition is essential. In 50% of cases DTs are precipitated by an intercurrent infection. The mortality rate is up to 10%.

Abuse of other substances

- Unusual behaviour of any sort could be due to substance misuse
- Check patient's arms and legs for evidence of injection sites
- Misusers of volatile solvents often smell of glue or aerosol propellant and may have a rash around their mouth and nose where there has been contact with an inhalation bag
- Street names vary in different geographical areas and also change over time. If in doubt, it is best to ask for, or suggest, the generic name of the substance and seek confirmation from the patient.

Opiates

Overdose or ingestion of opiates is characterised by:

- Altered level of consciousness
- Respiratory depression
- Pinpoint pupils
- Euphoric or stuporous mental state
- Convulsions (rare)
- Hypotension (rare)
- Hypothermia. (rare)

The initial management of an opiate overdose or respiratory depression due to opiate ingestion is:

- Maintenance of the airway and oxygenation followed by
- Administration of naloxone.

Naloxone will wear off faster than the opiate

Table 53.1 Opiates and their potentially fatal doses

Opiate	Potentially fatal doses
Opium	Preparations are variable
Heroin	As little as 0.2 g, fatalities can occur when an unusually pure batch of heroin is sold
Morphine	20 mg
Methadone	As low as 5 mg for children and 25 mg for intolerant adults
Dipipanone (Diconal)	Not known
Pethidine	About 1 g
Fentanyl	Not known
Dextromoramide (Palfium)	About 500 mg
Codeine	>1 g
Co-proxamol (codeine and dextropropoxyphene)	1–1.5 g

Hallucinogens

Lysergic acid diethylamide (LSD)

- LSD is a synthetic psychedelic drug of low toxicity. Symptoms include confusion, agitation, hallucinations, dilated pupils, and (rarely) coma and respiratory arrest. Supportive measures only are required.

Psilocybin (magic mushrooms)

- Ingestion of magic mushrooms is a seasonal problem, usually well known in particular localities where the mushrooms can be picked. Cases may occur in small epidemics. The fatal dose is unknown
- Euphoria, anxiety, depression, illusions and psychosis are all common manifestations. Hyperthermia, tachycardia, tremors and dilated pupils are characteristic. There is no specific treatment in the prehospital setting but efforts should be made to calm the victim by giving reassurance that the effects are self-limiting.

Phencyclidine

- Phencyclidine is a psychedelic drug, fatal dose unknown. Symptoms include anxiety and psychosis, ataxia, paraesthesia, catatonic movements, fits, coma, hypotension, respiratory impairment, Cheyne–Stokes breathing and respiratory arrest. Treatment is supportive.

Cannabis

- There is evidence to support the use of cannabis and the development of mental problems, including psychosis
- Of relatively low toxicity (unless ingested by children when coma may ensue), it may be smoked or eaten
- The symptoms of toxicity include excitement, euphoria, drowsiness, panic attacks, toxic psychosis and, rarely, coma and dilated pupils. No specific treatment is required in the prehospital setting apart from supportive measures.

Amyl nitrate

- Amyl nitrate is toxic by ingestion and inhalation. Its principal mode of toxicity is by the formation of methaemoglobin. The fatal dose is unknown, but even small amounts can cause symptoms
- Symptoms occur within a few seconds of inhalation, but may be delayed by ingestion. Headache, nausea and vomiting occur along with sweating and flushing. Tightness of the chest is common, as is confusion and occasionally fits
- Cyanosis due to methaemoglobinaemia may occur. There is no specific prehospital treatment apart from maintenance of the airway and administration of oxygen to treat cyanosis.

> Remember that the presence of methaemoglobinaemia will make pulse oximetry unreliable

Stimulants

Amphetamines

- Dexamphetamine (Dexedrine, 'dexies') and amphetamine-like drugs such as methylphenidate (Ritalin) and diethylpropion (Tenuate) may be abused
- The acute effects of amphetamines include euphoria, anxiety, increased energy, miosis and tachycardia
- Amphetamine psychosis mimics acute symptoms of schizophrenia and manifests with paranoid delusions, auditory, visual and tactile hallucinations and increased arousal and irritability. Consciousness is impaired
- Withdrawal effects include dysphoria, fatigue, lassitude and depression.

Cocaine

- The fatal dose is approximately 1 g when taken orally and 10 mg when injected
- Symptoms include tachycardia, sweating, hallucinations, increased respiratory rate, increased temperature, fits, arrhythmias and rarely cardiac arrest

- There is no specific treatment; fits should be controlled with diazepam and general supportive measures instituted
- Crack is a processed form of cocaine which produces a much quicker 'high' which is of short duration. It is much more addictive than cocaine.

Ecstasy (MDMA)

- A semisynthetic amphetamine (3,4-methylenedioxymethamphetamine)
- Two causes of death are commonly recognised: early deaths are due to arrhythmias and late deaths are due to an effect on muscles associated with a fatal rise in body temperature
- Deaths can occur after exposure to doses previously tolerated and are thought to be due to an idiosyncratic reaction
- Symptoms range from mild to life-threatening and include muscle spasms, dilated pupils, anxiety, tachycardia, increased temperature, abdominal pain, hypotension, fits, coma and stroke
- The fatal dose is unknown
- There are no specific treatments other than supportive measures in the prehospital setting
- Gamma-hydroxybutyrate (GHB) or 'liquid ecstasy' has similar effects and is dangerous when mixed with alcohol or other recreational drugs.

Ephedrine

- Ephedrine is a sympathomimetic drug with a fatal dose of 200 mg in children and over 2 g in adults. It causes restlessness, tachycardia, dilated pupils, arrhythmias and hallucinations
- Apart from treating fits with diazepam, there is no specific prehospital treatment but supportive measures should be instituted.

Sedatives

Barbiturates

- The barbiturates are a group of drugs that include amylobarbitone (Amytal), barbitone, pentobarbitone (Nembutal), phenobarbitone and sodium amylobarbitone (sodium Amytal)
- Symptoms of overdose include ataxia, dysarthria, decreased conscious level, coma, respiratory depression, hypothermia and hypotension
- There are no specific treatments apart from general supportive measures. Withdrawal seizures may occur and should be controlled with diazepam.

Volatile solvents

Glue

- Toluene is the most common solvent in glues available over the counter. Effects include excitement, chest tightness, fits, coma, arrhythmias and death

• Supportive measures should be instituted with particular emphasis on oxygenation to reduce the likelihood of arrhythmias.

Butane

• Butane is a colourless, odourless gas, commonly used as the propellant in 'ozone-friendly' sprays but also available in cigarette lighters. It is generally inhaled from a bag. Symptoms include respiratory depression, coma, hypotension and arrhythmias. Treatment is supportive only.

Butyl nitrate

• An industrial solvent, butyl nitrate is also used as a room deodoriser. It can be fatal when ingested in even small quantities, but the fatal dose is unknown. Symptoms include flushing, tachycardia, hypotension, confusion, shortness of breath and cyanosis (from the formation of methaemoglobin), coma and fits. Treatment is supportive. Remember that pulse oximetry readings are likely to be inaccurate.

For further information, see Ch. 54 in *Emergency Care: A Textbook for Paramedics*.

CHAPTER 54

The uncooperative or violent patient

Ambulance crews are frequently exposed to violent situations and threatening behaviour from patients and bystanders. Ambulance control should communicate to crews any factors that may increase their risk when attending a scene. Factors suggesting the possibility of violence include:

- Location – such as night-club, party, rave, etc
- Historical – are violent incidents known to have happened at this location in the past?
- Type of call – fighting, stabbing, domestic violence
- Illness related – head injury, pain, delusions.

Police support should be requested early.

Prior to arrival

It is important to think about equipment that may be used against personnel, e.g.:

- Equipment bags
- Scissors, pens, pencils
- Stethoscopes.

All communication equipment, including hand-held devices, must be checked to avoid communications breakdown when help is needed in a violent or potentially violent situation.

On arrival

On arrival, initial considerations must include:

- Protective clothing – is there a need for a helmet and eye protection? Should high-visibility clothing be worn?
- Vehicle positioning – position safely with an easily accessible exit

- Survey the scene
- Establish if there are other services present. Who is in charge?
- Determine whether support (ambulance officer, police, fire brigade) will be needed
- Clear bystanders.

Systematic approach to the uncooperative or violent patient

- Maintain safety
- Introduce yourself
- Establish a rapport
- Set the ground rules
- Seek a history
- Seek clarification.

Principles of assessment

As mentioned above, it is essential to complete a brief survey of the scene.

- Is it safe to enter?
- Where is the person? Is he standing, sitting or lying?
- Is the person calm, upset or angry?
- Are there objects nearby he could use to inflict harm? (If there are, they should be discreetly removed to a safe distance.)

Attempt to treat the person in the same manner in which one would like to be treated oneself, with respect and maintenance of dignity.

Attempt to establish a rapport with the patient by engaging them calmly, clearly and in a non-threatening manner.

Try and identify if a specific issue is making the patient angry.

Assessment and identification of the problem are vital to:

- Provide a clear history
- Prevent frustration
- Prevent violence and non-cooperation with ambulance personnel and others.

Transportation of the uncooperative or violent person

- Consider whether it will be necessary for a police officer to accompany the patient to hospital and to ensure that ambulance control is fully aware of the situation
- Before entering the ambulance with the patient, any potentially dangerous objects should be stowed securely away

---

Box 54.1 **Dealing with a potentially violent patient**

- Remain calm
- Ensure that there is an exit
- Maintain a 2-metre distance from the person and stand side-on
- Maintain non-threatening eye contact
- Seek extra help (in the background, e.g. in another room)
- Be careful what one says
- Try to negotiate and so defuse the situation
- Do not lie, or promise outcomes one cannot guarantee
- Recognise the need for rapid intervention if the situation deteriorates further.

Box 54.2 **Dealing with a violent patient**

- Immediately call for police assistance
- Use only the minimum of physical restraint to control the situation
- Never restrain a person in a way that could impair breathing, e.g. pushing the person's face down or sitting on his chest
- Never restrain the person around the neck
- When restraining, use only the legs and arms
- Check pulses in these limbs to ensure circulation
- Reassure the person at all times
- Keeps calm and avoid threats
- Negotiate with the person
- When the person is calm, slowly release the physical restraint
- Liaise with the police to decide appropriate management – hospital care or police custody.

- Attention should be paid to the seating arrangements, bearing in mind the patient's potential for violence or escape and crew safety
- Only when it is clear that one has enough information should a decision be made to transport the patient
- Reference should be made to service guidelines and policies on transporting violent or uncooperative patients
- If the person is to be admitted under the Mental Health Act 1983, then an Approved Social Worker or Community Psychiatric Nurse may accompany the patient
- If male ambulance personnel are transporting a disturbed woman, then a female chaperone is essential to protect the crew from allegations of misconduct.

What to do after an incident

- After an incident involving violence has occurred, ambulance control must be informed
- Medical attention should be sought for any injuries and the police will need to be informed
- An incident form should be completed. Completing the incident form is the responsibility of the staff member involved in the incident. Other personnel may be at risk in the future if the form is not completed.

For further information, see Ch. 55 in *Emergency Care: A Textbook for Paramedics*.

CHAPTER 55

Psychiatric emergencies

Mentally ill patients may be admitted to hospital involuntarily under the Mental Health Act if they are deemed to be a risk to themselves or to others, however most do not need this level of intervention.

Box 55.1 **Important components of the history**

- Nature and onset of presenting symptoms
- Past psychiatric history
- Past medical history
- Current medication
- History of substance misuse
- Social support.

Physical examination

- A brief physical examination should be carried out in every case, as far as possible, even if there appears to be no apparent physical disorder
- Common organic causes of psychiatric emergencies include hypoglycaemia, infection, cardiac failure, delirium tremens and subdural haematoma
- Recreational drug use and alcohol misuse are commonly implicated.

Mental state examination

This includes:

- Appearance and behaviour
- Speech form (i.e. coherence) and content
- Beliefs and thoughts
- Overall mood state and whether it is congruent with the thought content
- Observable abnormal perceptions or experiences (e.g. hallucinations)
- Assessment of level of consciousness, orientation to time, place and person, concentration and short-term memory
- Presence of insight (the acknowledgement by the patient that there are psychological problems that need to be resolved)
- Suicidal ideation.

Psychosis: recognition and treatment

Psychosis refers to disturbances in thinking and behaviour, usually involving delusions, hallucinations and thought disorder. They may be attributable to a diagnosis such as schizophrenia, mania or psychotic depression.

Delusions

- A delusion is a firmly held but false belief that is out of context with the person's social and cultural background
- Paranoid delusions may be that they are being persecuted or hounded by others or that others are watching or listening to them through bugging devices.

Hallucinations

- Hallucinations refer to the experience of perceptions (e.g. hearing voices or noises, seeing vivid images or tasting particular flavours) in the absence of a stimulus causing the perception. They appear real to the patient.

Dangerous behaviour

- Occasionally, psychiatric patients have a tendency to be violent, usually as a direct consequence of their illness
- Clearly it is inadvisable to enter a situation that puts the paramedic in physical danger and if there is a likelihood that this will occur, the police should be involved
- It is inadvisable to assess an acutely psychotic patient alone because of the risk of unpredictable behaviour that may lead to injury.

> Always have an escape route

Management of psychosis

Controlling a patient's behaviour can often be achieved by use of good interpersonal skills of empathy, reassurance, a non-threatening posture and an air of calmness and confidence.

Antipsychotic drugs

Antipsychotic drugs have an initial sedative action that precedes any antipsychotic effect. They need to be prescribed and administered by a doctor.

Parasuicide: recognition and treatment

- The first consideration must be safeguarding the physical welfare of the patient and this will usually entail transportation to the Emergency Department
- Do not be deceived by any apparent evidence that only a small quantity of tablets have been ingested or the patient's protestations that the overdose was not life-threatening
- Patients are often unaware of the lack of toxicity of the medication that they have taken and believe that the quantity ingested was sufficient to cause death
- More violent methods of attempted self-harm (e.g. hanging, shooting or deep lacerations) should always be assessed by a psychiatrist
- Attempted suicide should be considered as a possibility at any single-occupant road traffic collision where the conditions of the accident are unclear
- Self-harm is not in itself a mental illness and the majority of people who harm themselves have no psychiatric illness
- If the person agrees to admission to hospital and this is appropriate, then it should be expedited. If the person does not agree, but is detainable under the Mental Health Act, then the appropriate procedures should be followed with the patient being closely supervised until admission takes place
- The paramedic has no powers under the Mental Health Act but the police may take an individual to a place of safety (e.g. psychiatric unit or police station) under Section 136
- Persons who appear to be actively attempting to end their own life, or seem to be about to do so, can be restrained from doing so (under common law), pending a psychiatric assessment.

Depression and mania

- Clinical depression refers to a persistent and debilitating disorder of mood characterised by sadness, an inability to derive pleasure from any activity, low self-worth and lethargy
- Patients may neglect themselves and become physically at risk through not eating or drinking
- Often depressed mood is associated with poor social circumstances and deprivation

- Manic depression is characterised by elation and overactivity with increased speed of thought and pressure of speech. They may have grandiose delusions and see themselves as being rich, famous or wealthy
- A patient suffering from manic depression may dress inappropriately or be sexually disinhibited.

Features of depression:

- Sadness
- Inability to derive pleasure from any activity
- Low self-worth
- Lethargy
- Lack of motivation
- Sleep disturbance
- Appetite disturbance
- Lack of libido
- Thoughts of guilt and self-blame.

Anxiety disorders

- Anxiety disorders include anxiety states, phobias and obsessive compulsive disorder
- Hyperventilation is the result of excessive breathing from the upper chest (ribcage) and results in hypocapnia, which causes tinnitus, tetany, tingling, weakness and chest pains
- The experience of these physical symptoms may exacerbate the feeling of anxiety, causing more hyperventilation
- An explanation of the symptoms and reassurance that the patient will not come to any harm as a result of them is the first step, and may need frequent and authoritative repetition.

Box 55.2 **Symptoms of anxiety states**

- Fearfulness
- Irritability
- Difficulty in concentration
- Sensitivity to noise
- Feelings of restlessness
- Hyperventilation
- Sweating
- Increased heart rate
- Dry mouth.

Management of hyperventilation

- Make sure the patient is sitting or lying in a supported posture
- Stress the need to regulate the breathing by breathing more slowly and taking shallower breaths (not deeper ones), ideally until the patient can breathe through the nose
- Demonstrate how the patient can breathe using the diaphragm by placing one hand on the chest and one on the abdomen. The hand on the abdomen should move more than the one on the chest
- Provide ongoing explanation for the symptoms and plenty of reassurance
- Always rule out other possible causes of the symptoms (such as an acute coronary syndrome) before treating any patient for hyperventilation.

Delirium

- Acute toxic confusional state (delirium) is easily confused with psychiatric presentations. An elderly person suffering from dementia may develop a toxic confusional state as a complication
- Delirium tends to be variable in its nature, whereas dementia is altogether a more gradual and constant deterioration in functioning and behaviour
- Causes include infections such as urinary or respiratory infections or conditions such as acute urinary retention.

Box 55.3 **Features of acute toxic confusional states**

- Clouding and fluctuation of consciousness
- Periods of drowsiness
- Poor concentration
- Lack of lucidity
- Increased arousal
- Acute anxiety
- Fearfulness
- Disturbances in perception
- Illusions or hallucinations
- Disorientation to time, place and person.

Alcohol and illicit drugs

- It may not be easy to decide whether an intoxicated individual requires hospital assessment or (if causing a disturbance) whether police custody is more appropriate.

Beware of the drunk, head-injured patient – if in doubt, take them to hospital

- Alcoholism is often associated with conditions such as head injuries and alcohol withdrawal is a common cause of seizures
- Delirium tremens, which occurs after reduction in drinking, is characterised by tremulousness, disorientation and vivid hallucinations, is associated with a mortality of 10% and should always be managed in a general hospital
- Certain hallucinogens (such as LSD or magic mushrooms) can trigger a psychotic reaction in a previously undiagnosed or vulnerable person.

Personality disorder

- These patients are often frequent users of the emergency services
- They often harm themselves or express suicidal ideation and are frequently admitted to hospital. They may be hostile and impatient and lack the ability to form a rapport
- They appear to induce feelings of irritability and antagonism in staff and it is easy to lose an objective approach to their problems.

The Mental Health Act 1983

- If, after assessment, it is felt that a patient needs to be in a psychiatric hospital, a patient who refuses admission can be admitted compulsorily under the provisions of the Mental Health Act 1983
- The sections that are most likely to be used in an emergency are Sections 2, 3, 4, 135 and 136. The section papers must be filled in before the patient is taken to hospital
- The Mental Health Act does not apply to persons who are intoxicated by alcohol or drugs.

Section 2: Admission for assessment

- Section 2 is for assessment in hospital, or for assessment followed by treatment, and it is usually applied when a patient has no past history of mental disorder or is not known to the local psychiatric service
- The section is valid for 28 days
- The procedure requires an application by an approved social worker or nearest relative and medical recommendations by two doctors, one of whom is usually a psychiatrist.

Section 3: Admission for treatment

- Section 3 allows the compulsory admission of a patient and treatment for up to 6 months. It is usually applied when there is a known diagnosis
- The application is made by the patient's nearest relative or an approved social worker.

Section 4: Admission in an emergency

- This Section allows for a patient to be detained for not more than 72 hours in order to obtain the second medical opinion. It is expected that it will be converted to a Section 2 as soon as possible.

Section 135

- A social worker who believes that someone is suffering from a mental disorder and is unable to care for himself, or is being ill treated or neglected, may apply to a magistrate for a warrant for that person's removal to a place of safety.

Section 136

- It is possible that some emergency situations (such as road traffic collisions) will necessitate the removal of apparently mentally ill people to a place of safety without the possibility of obtaining applications from social workers or psychiatrists
- With Section 136, police constables have the power to remove to a place of safety a person whom they find in a public place who appears to be suffering from a mental disorder and to be in need of care and control for his own interests or for the protection of others
- The person should be taken to the nearest convenient place of safety (usually a hospital or police station) to be detained for a period not exceeding 72 hours for the purpose of examination by a doctor and interview by an approved social worker.

For further information, see Ch. 56 in *Emergency Care: A Textbook for Paramedics.*

CHAPTER 56

The major incident: An overview

Classification

- A *simple* major incident is one in which the infrastructure of the community in which it occurs remains intact, e.g. a train or air crash
- A *compound* major incident destroys or damages the infrastructure of the surrounding community
- A *compensated* major incident is one in which there are sufficient local resources to deal with the consequences
- An *uncompensated* major incident is one where the medical and other responding emergency services are destroyed or totally inadequate.

CSCATTT

CSCATT describes the priorities involved in managing a major incident.

Box 56.1 **CSCATTT**
C – **C**OMMAND
S – **S**AFETY
C – **C**OMMUNICATION
A – **A**SSESSMENT
T – **T**RIAGE
T – **T**REATMENT
T – **T**RANSPORT

Responsibilities of the first crew on scene

Attendant

- The attendant assumes the role of *Ambulance commander* until relieved by a senior ambulance officer
- He/she should undertake a rapid reconnaissance of the scene and feed back a situation report to the driver, who can then pass this to control using the METHANE mnemonic (see below)
- Suitable sites for ambulance parking point, control point and the casualty clearing station should be identified
- The *Fire commander* and *Police commander* should be identified and contacted at an early opportunity
- As ambulance commander, he/she must not become involved with the treatment of casualties.

Driver

- The driver is to stay with the vehicle at all times. He will form the communication link between the scene and ambulance control
- Park the vehicle as close to the scene as safety allows and leave the beacon switched on. The driver should then provide control with a brief report, stating the location and type of incident
- The driver must remain in contact with the attendant at all times and should not leave the vehicle until directed to do so by a senior ambulance officer.

Box 56.2 **METHANE report to ambulance control**

Major incident standby/major incident declared
Exact location
Type of incident
Hazards
Access
Number of casualties
Emergency services present and required

Table 56.1 Identifying commanders at the scene

Commander	Tabard
Fire	Red/white
Police	Blue/white
Ambulance	Green/white

Emergency services

- Overall control of the scene is the responsibility of the police who will control the outer cordon
- There will be a police manned *incident control point* through which all staff should enter and leave; all movements will be logged
- If hazards are present, the Fire service will have responsibility inside the inner cordon (the hot zone) until the danger is controlled
- Personnel entering and leaving the inner cordon must also be recorded for safety purposes
- The *bronze* (*operational*) area lies within the inner cordon and is the area where the rescue operation is in place. There will be bronze commanders (*forward commanders*) from each emergency service
- *Silver* (*tactical*) command consists of the area within the outer cordon. The commanders from each service will be within this area, although they may move in and out of the bronze zones
- *Gold* (*strategic*) command is removed from the scene – usually in the police HQ or local authority buildings – and is the location where the chief officers from each emergency service meet.

Silver (tactical) command

Silver command is usually handed over to more senior officers as they arrive. Commanders must not become involved in the rescue or treatment of casualties. There must be frequent documented meetings between the silver commanders from each service. The first priority is to share intelligence and establish what has happened:

- What are the main priorities for the next hour?
- What difficulties need to be resolved?
- Are other resources required?
- Which are the casualty receiving hospitals?
- Where is the survivor reception centre and who is resourcing it?
- Do any of the services present have particular problems or difficulties that another may be able to help with?

The health service response is controlled by the Ambulance commander (AC) at silver level.

There are several areas that should be allocated by the Ambulance commander:

- **Ambulance Control Point** – this is marked with a steady green roof-light. All health service staff are to report here on arrival
- **Forward Control Point** – this is where the forward incident officers meet to direct the rescue operation. The forward commanders report to their respective silver commanders
- **Casualty Clearing Station** – an appropriate site for secondary triage and treatment of patients, ideally sheltered, safe and accessible

---

Box 56.3 **Responsibilities of the Ambulance commander**

- Liaise with other commanders
- Delegate tasks to other ambulance personnel
- Ensure adequate communications for all health service staff
- Determine (with the Medical commander) the receiving hospitals
- Determine (with the Medical commander) where mobile medical teams are drawn from
- Establish triage and treatment
- Determine appropriate transport routes
- Organise replenishment of equipment
- Liaise with police regarding the media.

- **Ambulance Parking Point** – where ambulances wait until called forward to the rear of the casualty clearing station (CCS)
- **Ambulance Loading Point** – where patients are loaded, preferably at the rear of the CCS.

There are several key roles that must be delegated by the Ambulance commander:

- Communications officer
- Forward ambulance commander
- Casualty clearing station officer
- Ambulance parking officer
- Ambulance loading officer
- Primary triage officer
- Ambulance safety officer
- Equipment officer.

The Medical commander

- The AC may be joined by an appropriately trained doctor who will act as *Medical commander*; this may be a doctor from the Ambulance service itself, a practitioner from the local immediate care scheme or a consultant from an Emergency Department and should be known to the Ambulance service
- In the future, this role may be provided by Department of Health MERITs (Medical Emergency Response and Intervention Teams)
- The primary role of the Medical commander is to work in close conjunction with the Ambulance commander and to this end, they should usually be found in close proximity to each other
- The Medical commander should establish and maintain direct contact with the receiving hospitals and decide if specialist medical teams should be called
- Communication with hospitals should go through the Medical commander
- To aid communication between hospitals and the scene, the Ambulance service should despatch a liaison team to each receiving hospital

- One officer should ensure smooth turnaround and re-equipping of ambulances and document the number of casualties. The other should join the hospital coordination team to advise and update the hospital staff on progress at the scene.

Triage

Primary triage occurs in the bronze area and aims to rapidly identify those in need of immediate life-saving treatments. The *triage sieve* is used for primary triage. *Secondary triage* occurs at the entrance to the CCS, where a more detailed system involving the triage revised trauma score (TRTS) is used.
The triage categories are:

- Delayed (green)
- Urgent (yellow)
- Immediate (red)
- Dead (white).

In extreme circumstances, an *expectant* category (*blue*) may be used on patients who have a very high likelihood of dying anyway, in order to conserve resources for patients who can be saved. The expectant category will only be implemented on the joint agreement of the Ambulance and Medical commanders.

Once triaged, casualties must be marked, preferably with triage labels. Triage is a dynamic process and should be repeated at different stages and triage categories amended as required.

Ambulances

- Ambulances are parked at the ambulance parking point under the direction of the Parking officer
- Always leave the keys in the ignition so that vehicles can be moved
- Ambulance traffic should be directed in a circuit to prevent traffic jams. Ambulances are usually the only vehicles which will need to come and go from the scene
- All patients must be adequately packaged for transport, including securing of all lines and tubes, supply of sufficient oxygen and drugs for the journey and provision of relevant paperwork
- Casualties requiring specialist centre treatment (e.g. burns or neurosurgery) should be transported directly to a centre providing that speciality, to avoid delays later in secondary transportation
- Vehicles other than land ambulances may be used for transport: helicopters have advantages of speed, but can only transport one patient
- Patients with minor injuries may be sent to hospital by recruited buses or vans.

The dead

In England and Wales, the dead are the responsibility of the Coroner and in Scotland of the Procurator Fiscal. The police act as the Coroner's agents and will control all further management of the deceased. Those casualties triaged as dead should be labelled as such and covered with a blanket where they are found unless they are blocking access to the living. An attached label should indicate the date and time, location found and the name of the doctor and police officer. Subsequently, when the pressure of the incident is reduced, a doctor accompanied by a nominated police officer should formally confirm death. Photographs of the body *in situ* should be taken, before it is removed to a body-holding point or temporary mortuary.

Terrorist incidents

- Bomb explosions result in devastation over a wide area
- Secondary devices are a common hazard and all attending emergency service personnel need to remember the basic rule – *protect yourself*
- The location of the rendezvous point for attending vehicles should be chosen with great care. A search of this area to confirm safety is of paramount importance
- Use of radios and mobile phones may be restricted, as these devices can trigger secondary devices
- A minimal number of personnel should be deployed in the explosion site, at least until safety has been established
- Considerable importance is attached to the preservation of forensic evidence after a bomb explosion
- The dressings, clothing and other belongings of the casualties may need to be preserved. Pieces of shrapnel must also be preserved and the scene disturbed as little as possible.

Civil disorder

The key to a successful operation in a civil disorder situation is neutrality. The paramedic must not take sides with the police or with demonstrators, with left-wing or right-wing political protestors or with racial groups
Three distinct patterns of civil disorder can occur:

1. Prearranged demonstrations along a prescribed route with preplanning and preparation by the emergency services
2. Static confrontation, usually with an area of conflict which is clearly defined

3. Uncontrolled rioting with no set pattern or direction, sometimes with changing focus of casualties.

Rival groups should be taken to separate hospitals. If the police form a third group then they too should ideally have a dedicated emergency department. Full riot protective clothing and in some situations flak jackets may be required by crews and ambulances should have a crew of three whenever possible.

Treatment facilities at a static point may avoid the need for a large number of people with minor injuries being moved to hospital. Police should recover their own personnel, evacuating them to *paramedic forward aid points*. An ambulance liaison officer in the police control room is vital in informing paramedic teams of police tactics to ensure their safety when working among demonstrators or rioters.

Underground incidents

Major incidents underground may present special problems since communications can be particularly difficult.

For caves and coal mines specialist rescue teams are usually available.

In the underground railway system, ambulance paramedics will be required to work in conditions of very high temperatures. In the London Underground railway system, temperatures regularly rise to 40°C.

Evacuation of trains with over 1000 passengers is often necessary. On occasion, the scene may have to be approached from two different stations either side of the incident.

Chemical and radiation incidents

The Fire service will of necessity take a lead role in ascertaining safety.

Only fire officers and HART (Hazardous Area Response Team) trained paramedics should enter the 'hot zone'.

The National Arrangements for Incidents Involving Radiation (NAIR) scheme will direct the planning for incidents involving nuclear power stations, medical or military sources of radiation.

Debriefing

When paramedical staff have finished their duties at the scene of a major incident, it is most important that a senior officer takes the trouble to thank them personally and check that they are safe to travel home. This *hot debrief* can either occur at the scene or back at a suitable station. It should not last for very long and should be directed towards welfare issues.

Within a few days, it is necessary to arrange a more *formal debrief* for those involved. This should be directed towards fact finding. A final, full written report can then be prepared for all interested parties. The inevitable public enquiry will follow, so documentation and recording of all times and decisions are essential.

For further information, see Ch. 58 in *Emergency Care: A Textbook for Paramedics*.

CHAPTER 57

Triage

Triage is the sorting of casualties according to clinical priorities and is a dynamic process which can be used to assess priorities for treatment *and* for evacuation. Triage should be undertaken whenever the number of casualties exceeds the number of skilled helpers available. Different triage methods are available depending on the circumstances: generally triage 'sieve' is applied then refined, using triage 'sort'.

Priorities

The systems of priorities in common use are referred to as the treatment (T) system and the priority (P) system:

Table 57.1 Triage priority systems

Description	Colour	T system	P system
Immediate	Red	1	1
Urgent	Yellow	2	2
Delayed	Green	3	3
Expectant	Blue	4	
Dead	White		

Definitions

Table 57.2 Triage category definitions	
Category	**Definition**
Immediate	Casualties who require immediate life-saving treatment
Urgent	Casualties who require treatment within 6 hours
Delayed	Less serious cases who require treatment but not within a set time
Expectant	Casualties whose injuries are so severe that either: they cannot survive despite treatment; or the degree of intervention required is such that, in the circumstances, their treatment would seriously compromise the provision of treatment for others

Use of the fourth category

Whether or not the *expectant* category is used is a decision for the senior personnel involved (the ambulance and medical incident officers at the scene and the chief triage officer at the hospital). Patients in the expectant category will be treated and transported *after* those in the T1 category but *before* those in the T2 and T3 categories.

Triage at major incidents

There may be a large number of casualties at a major incident and thus an enormous number of decisions need to be made as quickly and efficiently as possible.

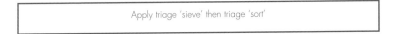

Apply triage 'sieve' then triage 'sort'

Triage sieve

- Anybody that can walk is a Category 3 for the time being
- Any patient who is not breathing has their airway opened. If they still do not breathe then they are dead
- The rest can be divided into Category 1 and Category 2, depending on their breathing and pulse.

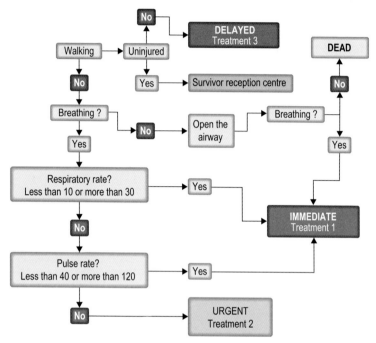

Figure 57.1 The triage sieve – summary.

Triage sort

Following the triage sieve, on arrival in the casualty clearing centre, patients are triaged using a more detailed method. This is the *triage sort* which is based on three parameters:

    Respiratory rate
    Systolic blood pressure
    Glasgow Coma Scale.

A score for each of these is assigned to the patient.

The sum of these three scores is the *triage revised trauma score* (TRTS). This method can be used to assign triage priorities.

Although more time consuming than the triage sieve, the triage sort is more accurate and can be used to prioritise further treatment and evacuation.

Table 57.3 The triage sort 1–1 scoring

Physiological parameter	Measured value	Score
Respiratory rate (breaths/min)	10–29	4
	>29	3
	6–9	2
	1–5	1
	0	0
Systolic blood pressure (mmHg)	90	4
	76–89	3
	50–75	2
	1–49	1
	0	0
Glasgow Coma Scale score	13–15	4
	9–12	3
	6–8	2
	4–5	1
	3	0

Table 57.4 Triage priorities using the TRTS

Category	Priority	TRTS
Immediate	T1	1–9
Urgent	T2	10–11
Delayed	T3	12
Dead	T4	0

CRAMS

An alternative triage system used by some UK ambulance services is the CRAMS system:

C – **C**irculation
R – **R**espiration
A – **A**bdomen and thorax
M – **M**otor response
S – **S**peech

The CRAMS score is calculated by adding the five values together. The triage category is then assigned as shown in Table 57.1.

Table 57.5 Triage categories using the CRAMS score

Priority	CRAMS score	Mortality (%)
Immediate (red)	<6	15–100
Urgent (yellow)	7	3
Delayed (green)	8–10	0–0.5

Box 57.1 **The CRAMS score**

Circulation
2 Normal capillary refill or systolic BP >100 mmHg
1 Delayed capillary refill or systolic BP 85–99 mmHg
0 No capillary refill or systolic BP <85 mmHg

Respiration
2 Normal respiration
1 Laboured, shallow or rate above 20/min
0 Respiration absent

Abdomen thorax
2 Abdomen not tender
1 Abdomen tender
0 Abdomen rigid, flail chest or penetrating injury

Motor response
2 Normal (obeys commands)
1 Responds only to pain
0 Postures or no response

Speech
2 Normal speech (oriented)
1 Confused or inappropriate
0 Nil or unintelligible sounds

Triage labelling

The patients must be labelled to allow orderly evacuation and to prevent duplication of effort. Cruciform triage cards allow category/colour allocation and allow for the allocation to be changed as required.

For further information, see Ch. 59 in *Emergency Care: A Textbook for Paramedics.*

CHAPTER 58

The Ambulance service at mass gatherings

Casualty figures reported at mass gatherings range from 0.11 per thousand to 9.0 per thousand. Weather conditions and other factors cause wide daily variations at similar events.

> A mass gathering is defined as a collection of 1000 people or more

Casualty types

- About 20–25% of the work is caused by pre-existing disease (such as diabetes mellitus, bronchitis, epilepsy and ischaemic heart disease)
- 20–30% is due to trauma such as sprains, strains and abrasions, burns and scalds, foreign bodies in the eye and blisters
- Environment-related illnesses such as heatstroke are common
- Their will be occasional collapse due to cardiac arrest, stroke or a drug-related incident
- Minor complaints such as sore throats and non-specific maladies make up the rest.

Planning

Familiarity with the local geography, evacuation routes and specific amendments to baseline plans for a specific event is mandatory. Contingency planning for such events should always include a review of the major incident plan.

The Guide for Safety at Sports Grounds (the green guide) is published by the Department for Culture, Media and Sport. Section 18 covers the provision of medical support to events. This should be read in association with The Event Safety Guide (the purple guide, published by the Health and Safety Executive).

Table 58.1 Ambulance provision according to anticipated attendance

Anticipated attendance	Minimum paramedic ambulance provision	Statutory ambulance officer	Statutory ambulance authority vehicles
5000–25 000	1	1	
25 000–45 000	1	1	1 major incident equipment vehicle; 1 control unit
45 000 or more	2	1	1 major incident equipment vehicle; 1 control unit

For further information, see Ch. 60 in *Emergency Care: A Textbook for Paramedics*.

CHAPTER 59

Legal issues

Record-keeping

A *Patient Report Form* (PRF) should be completed for each patient treated and a copy handed over to the receiving hospital. Written records are the only defence when faced with complaints and legal action.

- Good notes – good defence
- Poor notes – poor defence
- No notes – no defence.

The names of all professionals who have been involved in the care of a patient should be clearly recorded in full. If a patient (or his relatives or friends) is aggressive or uncooperative, this should also be recorded. The form must be viewed as a legal document and stored safely for future recall.

If it was not written down, it was not done

Consent

Patient consent is required before providing any form of treatment

Consent may take one of three forms according to the circumstances of the incident:

1. *Express* consent is where a patient grants specific permission for a treatment to be carried out
2. *Implied* consent is where patients, by their actions, present themselves for treatment but without specific verbal or written authorisation

3. *Presumed* consent can be used, e.g. in the unconscious patient, where the patient is not able to give consent but it could be presumed that if they were able to give consent, they would do so in the given circumstances.

Informed consent implies that the patient has been informed of the foreseeable benefits and possible side-effects of the treatment concerned and understands their right to refuse treatment and the consequences of doing so. Failure to obtain consent is, in legal terms, an assault and such an action brings with it the risk of prosecution.

Capacity

In order to provide consent a patient must have capacity. This means that a patient must be able to make their own decisions by:

- Understanding the information and choices presented
- Weighing up the information to determine what the decision will mean for them
- Then communicating that decision.

Failures of any of these areas mean that the patient may lack capacity. Difficult situations arise with patients who refuse treatment but lack capacity. Clearly, the hypoglycaemic diabetic who is violently resisting treatment needs to be treated anyway.

Refusal of treatment

- Every patient with capacity has the right to refuse treatment
- In this situation, the patient should ideally sign the medical documentation to show that they have had the possible consequences of their actions explained to them
- If they refuse to sign, then the documentation should be signed by another witness, such as another ambulance crew member
- Ambulance control should be informed of the incident and any further information carefully documented
- Any patient who wishes to be taken to hospital should be transported, as there is, as yet, no clearly defined policy which allows an ambulance service to refuse to convey a patient
- If a patient is properly examined and there appear to be no grounds for attending hospital, the patient must be fully in agreement with the decision to stay at home.

Children

- A minor (under 16 years of age) may consent to or refuse treatment without reference to an adult where they are of sufficient maturity to understand the full implications of what is happening to them
- A child may consent to treatment against the wishes of their parents, but may not refuse treatment of a serious or life-threatening illness if the parents consent.

Living wills

Living wills (also known as 'advance directives') are a method of withholding consent to treatment in the event that any future illness incapacitates them to the extent that they cannot express their wishes. The circumstances in which an advance directive will have the greatest impact for paramedics are where an individual with a 'living will' suffers a cardiac arrest out of hospital.

Ethically, it is obvious that the wishes of the patient should be honoured, however there may not be incontrovertible evidence that the document is genuine or does indeed represent the patient's current wishes.

If ambulance staff are *not* satisfied that the patient had made a prior and specific request to refuse treatment, then all clinical care should be provided in the normal way. Local ambulance trusts may have specific guidance to follow if presented with an advance directive, e.g. to discuss the situation with the medical director.

'Do not resuscitate' (DNR) orders

DNR orders take the form of written and signed instructions from the physician responsible for the care of the patient concerned. They must always be in writing. Ideally, the DNR order should be confirmed face-to-face with the responsible doctor.

The wishes of the patient, the family and the responsible doctor should be followed if possible. If the situation is different from that predicted, then the DNR may not be valid. For example, a patient who has a simple blocked airway after choking on food should not be left untreated simply because of a DNR order relating to an ongoing terminal condition.

> Any decision to withhold treatment of a patient must be documented thoroughly

Confidentiality

The ethical obligation to maintain confidentiality is also a legal duty and applies to all professions where a practitioner has a privileged relationship with a client. The HPC, responsible for the state registration of paramedics, includes breach of confidentiality as an example of infamous conduct.

Maintaining confidentiality includes not talking about specific patients while off-duty and correct handling of patient records. Confidentiality continues to apply *after the patient's death*.

Restraint or assault

Ambulance personnel have no legal right to restrain a patient over and above that of the ordinary citizen. Should restraint or forced transportation be necessary for any reason, the assistance of the police should be requested. In the event of an assault, one has a legal right to defend oneself but it is only permissible to use 'reasonable force' to prevent harm being inflicted.

Breaking and entering

Ambulance personnel have no legal rights to force entry into private property, even if they suspect that an individual's life is at risk. The assistance of the police should be requested and their arrival awaited before forcing an entry. In practice, if the police were not immediately available, it seems unlikely that anyone would press charges for breaking and entering in the event of a paramedic having strong suspicion that a patient was at risk.

Pronouncing death

In law, the ability to certify death is confined to registered medical practitioners. This should not be confused with the pronouncement that death has occurred, specifically that the patient has a non-salvageable condition.

There will be some circumstances where it is not appropriate for the paramedic to attempt resuscitation.

Some ambulance services widen the definition to allow paramedics to identify 'irreversible death' and thus not commence resuscitation.

Any pronouncement of death by a paramedic must be unquestionable. If in doubt, resuscitate and let a doctor at the receiving hospital make the decision to stop.

Stopping resuscitation

The outcomes of patients receiving full advanced cardiac life support in the field who do not develop a perfusing rhythm prior to transportation are universally poor and transporting a patient with CPR in progress is potentially hazardous for unrestrained staff in the back of the ambulance.

Some services are now introducing appropriate policies which have medical approval, authorising paramedics to abandon resuscitation attempts in specific circumstances.

If resuscitation is stopped in the field, it will be necessary to inform the patient's general practitioner and the police, who will act for the coroner's officer.

Box 59.1 **Example of irreversible death**

History

- Patient in a lifeless condition for at least 10 minutes with no bystander CPR.

Vital signs

- No carotid or femoral pulses
- No spontaneous respirations
- Fixed and dilated pupils
- 30-second trace of continuous asystole.

Drug security

Controlled drugs such as morphine sulphate must, by law, be kept in a locked container within a locked cabinet fixed to an immovable surface.

An ambulance suffices for legal purposes, however, there have been many instances of the theft of these substances from ambulances.

Unaccounted for controlled drugs must be declared at the first opportunity to allow an immediate investigation. Controlled drugs that are 'out-of-date' must be returned to the supplying pharmacy for witnessed disposal with the correct documentation.

For further information, see Chs 61 and 64 in *Emergency Care: A Textbook for Paramedics.*

INDEX

Note: Page numbers followed by *b* indicate boxes, *f* indicate figures and *t* indicate tables